THE CIRCULATION:
*An Integrative
Physiologic Study*

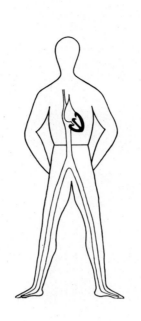
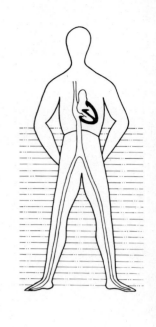

An Integrative Physiologic Study

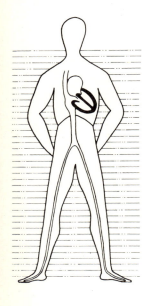

The CIRCULATION

JAMES P. HENRY, M.D.
Professor, Department of Physiology

JOHN P. MEEHAN, M.D.
Professor and Chairman, Department of Physiology
University of Southern California School of Medicine

YEAR BOOK MEDICAL PUBLISHERS, INC.
35 EAST WACKER DRIVE • CHICAGO

Copyright © 1971 by Year Book Medical Publishers, Inc. All rights reserved. No part of this publication may be reproduced, stored in a retrieval system, or transmitted, in any form or by any means, electronic, mechanical, photocopying, recording, or otherwise, without prior written permission from the publisher. Printed in the United States of America.

Library of Congress Catalog Card Number: 70-125801

International Standard Book Number: 0-8151-4279-X

Preface

THE TITLE OF THIS BOOK betrays its bias. This is an attempt at an integrative physiology of the cardiovascular system. As such, it must necessarily be eclectic, and our indebtedness stands out in the names scattered throughout its pages, in the acknowledgments accompanying the legends, and in the references.

It owes its inception to our friend and collaborator, Dr. Otto H. Gauer, Physiology Institute, Berlin-Dahlem. Ten years ago, he recognized the didactic merits of a separate consideration of the high- and low-pressure systems, and his presentation in the Landois-Rosemann *Lehrbuch der Physiologies des Menschen* adopted this format.

In addition, we are particularly grateful to the late Dr. Chester Hyman, Department of Physiology, University of Southern California, for his advice and contributions on the microcirculation; to Dr. Bernard C. Abbott, Department of Biology, University of Southern California, for his great help in the section on the intrinsic and extrinsic determinants of cardiac function; to Dr. Travis Winsor, Department of Medicine, University of Southern California, for permitting us to draw on his expertise in the section on the electrocardiogram; to Dr. Michael O'Rourke, Department of Physiology, University of New South Wales, for writing a resumé of the new viewpoints that are emerging from the British schools' fresh approach to arterial hemodynamics; and to Dr. John C. Cassel, Department of Epidemiology, University of North Carolina, for his contribution to the section on hypertension.

Finally, we wish to express our appreciation of how much we owe to Mrs. Beverly Rhue and to Miss Jo Kolsum for the many tedious hours spent in preparing this manuscript for the press, and to Mrs. Patricia Stephens for her skill and equal patience in the preparation of the art work.

JAMES P. HENRY
JOHN P. MEEHAN

Table of Contents

1. General Properties of the Circulation. **15**
    Introduction 15
    The High- and Low-Pressure Systems 15
    Pressure Flow Relationships in the Vascular Bed. 17
        Hydrostatic Columns 17
        Flow of Blood. 17
        Velocity and Lateral Pressure at a Constriction 18
        Intramural Tension and Radius 19
        Viscosity 19
        Elasticity of the Vascular Bed 20
        Distribution of Blood Volume in Different Regions 20
    Control and Integration 21
        Strategic Stretch Receptors in the High- and Low-Pressure Systems 21
        Central Integration of Exteroceptive and Interoceptive Information 22
        Efferent Nervous and Hormonal Control 22

2. The Heart as a Reservoir and Pump **24**
    Introduction 24
    Cardiac Chambers as Muscular Pumps 24
        Muscular Arrangement 24
        Pericardial Assistance to Heart Filling 25
        Function of Valves 25
    Sequence of Events in the Cardiac Cycle 26
        Ventricular Systole 26
        Influence of Frequency on the Ratio of Systole to Diastole. 28
    Some Factors Determining Cardiac Output. 28
        Heart Chambers as a Reservoir of the Low-Pressure System 28
        Control of Heart Rate 29

TABLE OF CONTENTS

    Elastic Forces, Viscosity, and Laplace's Equation. 30
    Cardiac Output 30
    Cardiac Efficiency 30
    Work of the Heart 30
Heart Sounds 31
    Introduction 31
    Causes and Timing of Heart Sounds 32
    Areas for Auscultation of Normal Heart Sounds 33
    Murmurs 33
    Aortic Stenosis 34
    Mitral Regurgitation. 34
    Aortic Regurgitation. 34
    Mitral Stenosis 34
    Patent Ductus Arteriosus 34

3. The Heart as a Specialized Muscle **35**
    Introduction 35
    Intrinsic and Extrinsic Determinants of Cardiac Function 35
        The Mechanism of Muscular Contraction 35
        Activation of the Contractile Mechanism. 37
        The Frank-Starling Law of the Heart 38
        Exceptions to the Law of the Heart 39
        Studies of the Contractility of Isolated Cardiac Muscle 41
        Variations in Contractility Versus Effects of Preloading. 44
        Diagrams of the Force-Velocity-Length Relationship. 45
        Work Versus Power. 46
        Clinical Aspects of Contractility Studies 46
    The Special Conducting System and the Electrocardiogram 47
        Differences Between Skeletal and Cardiac Muscle. 47
        The Excitatory and Conductive System of the Heart. 47
        The Electrocardiogram 50
        Determination of the Electrical Axis of the Heart 52
        Vectorcardiography 53
        Exploring Electrodes 53
        Abnormalities of Rhythm 54
        Conduction Disturbances 55
        Effects of Ions on the Heart 56
        Influence of Innervation of the Heart 57

4. The High-Pressure System **59**
    Pulse and Blood Pressure. 59

TABLE OF CONTENTS 9

    Introduction 59
        Branching of the Arterial Tree 60
        Applicability of Poiseuille's Law to the Circulation 61
    Elements in the Vascular Wall 61
    Practical Aspects of the Laplace Relation 63
    Pressure Volume Diagram of the Vessels 64
        Methods. 64
        Volume Elasticity Coefficient. 65
        Elastic Reservoir Function of the Aorta 66
    The Arterial Pulse 68
        Pulse Wave Velocity 68
        Pulse Contour. 68
        Wave Reflection and Vascular Impedance 70
    Causes of Variations in the Blood Pressure. 72
    Estimation of Mean Blood Pressure 73

5.. Exchange of Substances Through the Capillary Wall and the Role of the Lymphatics . . . **75**
    Capillary Function 75
        General Considerations. 75
        Filtration and Absorption 76
        Hydrostatic Pressure in the Capillary 76
        Morphology of the Fluid Exchange Network 77
        Functional Changes of Capillary Blood Pressure 80
    Osmotic Pressure of the Plasma Proteins 82
    Interstitial Fluid 84
        Pressure in the Interstitial Fluid Compartment 84
        Osmotic Pressure of Proteins in Interstitial Fluid Outside Capillary Walls and the
            Function of the Lymphatics 84
        Circulation of Interstitial Fluid 86
    Capillary Permeability to Lipid Soluble Molecules., i.e., Respiratory Gases 90

6. The Low-Pressure System, Orthostasis, and the Return of Blood to the
        Central Reservoir **92**
    Introduction 92
    Blood Volume and its Divisions 93
        General Considerations 93
        The Central Blood Volume 95
        Position of the Left Ventricle in the Low-Pressure System 97
        Blood Volume of the Extrathoracic Circulation. 97
    Relation Between Blood Volume and Interstitial Fluid Space. 98
    Venous Pressure Gradient 98

　　　　Influence of Respiration on Venous Circulation 99
　　　　Influence of Orthostasis on Distribution of Blood Volume. 99
　　　　　　The Hydrostatic Indifference Point. 99
　　　　　　Acute Changes and Redistribution of Blood Volume in Orthostasis 102
　　　　　　Influence of Posture on Cardiac Performance 103
　　　　Venous Tone. 103
　　　　Effects of Weightlessness and Bed Rest Upon Blood Volume. 104
　　　　The Muscle Pump and Orthostasis 105
　　　　　　Factors Regulating Venous Pressure in the Foot 105
　　　　　　Action of the Calf and Thigh Pumps 106
　　　　Venous Pressure Measurements 107

7. **Local Regulation and Central Integration of Cardiovascular Function** **110**
　　　　Introduction 110
　　　　Local Regulation 110
　　　　Stretch Receptors in the Low- and High-Pressure Systems 111
　　　　　　Stretch Receptors in the Low-Pressure System. 112
　　　　　　Stretch Receptors in the High-Pressure System 114
　　　　　　Afferent Pathways and Central Representation 115
　　　　Efferent Pathways and Hormones Controlling the Cardiovascular System 116
　　　　　　Introduction 116
　　　　　　Volume Regulatory Responses 116
　　　　　　Pressure Regulatory Responses 118
　　　　Reflex Central Nervous Regulation of Pressure and Volume 121
　　　　Carotid Sinus Perfusion Experiments 121
　　　　Changes in Atrial Pressure by Use of a Balloon 122
　　　　Responses of Atrial and Aortic Baroreceptors to Progressive Blood Loss 124

8. **Characteristics of Responses of Local Circulations** **129**
　　　　Coronary 129
　　　　　　Characteristics of the Coronary Vessels 129
　　　　　　Phasic Flow 131
　　　　　　Coronary Innervation 132
　　　　Cerebral Circulation 133
　　　　　　Methods of Measuring Flow 133
　　　　　　The Effects of the Rigidity of the Cranium 134
　　　　Circulation in the Skin. 135
　　　　　　Environmental Factors. 135
　　　　　　Nervous Control 136
　　　　　　Vasodilator Effects of Bradykinin 136

Color of the Skin. 136

White Reaction of the Skin 137

Triple Response 137

Splanchnic Circulation. 138

Hepatic Blood Supply and Its Measurement. 138

Stomach. 139

Intestine. 139

Spleen 140

Kidney 141

Regulation of the Pulmonary Circulation. 142

Vasomotor Nerves 142

Effects of Hypoxia on the Pulmonary Circulation 143

The Reproductive System 143

Erectile Tissue 143

Menstruation 143

Placental and Fetal Circulation 144

Changes at Birth 145

9. Special Responses of the Cardiovascular System **146**

Straining and Coughing and the Valsalva Maneuver 146

Straining and the Elevation of Intrathoracic Pressure. 146

Coughing 147

Paradoxic Lack of Effect of Straining During Heart Failure 147

Exercise 148

Introduction 148

Respiration. 148

Peripheral Vascular Bed 150

Heart. 150

Effects of the Supine and Erect Postures. 150

Changes Occurring During Exercise: Integrative Aspects 151

Circulatory Changes During Underwater Exposure 152

Altitude Hypoxia 153

Circulatory Changes During Digestion 154

Circulatory Changes During Heat Exposure 154

Circulatory Changes During Exposure to Cold 155

Circulatory Changes in Emotion 157

Defense-Alarm Response 157

Vasodepressor Syncope 158

10. Circulatory Failure: Shock and Syncope and Chronic Congestive Failure **160**

Introduction 160
Syncope 160
   Introduction 160
   Orthostatic Hypotension 160
   Cardiac Syncope 161
Acute Circulatory Failure 161
   Factors Inducing Failure 161
   Mechanism for Compensatory Responses During
      Nonhypotensive Hemorrhage 162
   Acute Circulatory Failure: Irreversible Shock 163
   Treatment of Acute Circulatory Failure 164
Congestive Heart Failure: A Disorder of Regulation of the Low-Pressure System. . 164
   Symptoms 164
   Exercise, Adrenergic Activity and Heart Failure 165
   A Suggested Role for Receptors in Heart Failure 168
   Treatment of Chronic (Congestive) Heart Failure 170
   Postmitral Commissurotomy Dilutional Syndrome. 171
   Paroxysmal Atrial Tachycardia 173

11. High Blood Pressure 174
   Introduction 174
   High Blood Pressure and Mechanisms Distal to the Hypothalamus. 174
   Experimental Observations Demonstrating the Role of Subhypothalamic
      Mechanisms in the Development of High Blood Pressure. 175
   High Blood Pressure and Mechanisms from the Hypothalamus Upward
      Involving Higher Centers in Inducing High Blood Pressure 177
   Role of Various Environmental Factors in the Development of
      High Blood Pressure 182
      Introduction 182
      Exercise. 182
      Salt 183
      Fat and Protein 184
      Malnutrition 184
      Disease 184
      Obesity 185
      Heredity. 186
      Smoking. 186
   Role of Psychosocial Stimuli and the Increase of Blood Pressure of
      Human Populations 186
     Pressure Changes with Age in Different Communities 186

Analysis of Groups with Unexpected Blood Pressure Changes with Age 190

12. Cardiovascular Changes in Certain Adaptive States: A Summary **194**

    Reflex Mechanisms and Their Integration 194

        Description of Diagrams 194

        Exercise. 195

        Reduced Central Blood Volume. 197

        Congestive Heart Failure 198

        Essential Hypertension. 199

    Conclusions: Levels of Integration of Cardiovascular Function 199

Index **203**

1

General Properties of the Circulation

Introduction

THE CIRCULATION has a huge variety of demands placed on it by the varying conditions of life. Consider, for example, the sequence of getting up in the morning and going to work. Dreaming sleep is accompanied by the adjustments appropriate for the emotions being experienced by the dreamer. Suddenly, he is aroused, perhaps angered and alarmed by being late; then food is ingested and the stomach must receive a blood supply appropriate for its secretory functions. A hurried trip to the bathroom may be accompanied by huge rises in intrathoracic pressure, obstructing venous return and precipitating near syncope. A few tender moments as he bids the family goodbye are followed by a violent burst of muscular activity as he sprints to catch the bus.

Clearly, there is need for an effective regulatory mechanism that will determine the force as well as the rate of cardiac contraction, in order to assure that there is always a head of pressure in the arterial system and that the resistances in the network always provide sufficient flow for the particular organ system in use in response to the particular environmental demand, be it the digestion of food or the running in pursuit of it.

In what follows, the emphasis will be on the way in which the various components of the circulation mesh to meet demands such as those sketched above. The initial description is of certain basic physical and operating characteristics that are held in common by vertebrate circulatory systems. The rest of the chapter is concerned with a brief résumé in general terms of the regulatory mechanisms that will be the principal concern of this book.

The High- and Low-Pressure Systems

The vertebrate cardiovascular system is composed of the heart and blood vessels that form a closed circulatory loop. The arrangement consists of a single, powerful, regularly contractile muscle pump, the heart, which forces blood under pressure into the arteries, the delivery system. These break up into the fine and universal microcirculatory vessels, whence the circulating fluid returns via low-pressure ducts, the veins, to reservoirs at the portals of the pump. Muscle also surrounds the walls of the arteries where it controls the regional distribution of blood flow in accordance with the changing needs of the various tissues. The walls of veins contain much less muscle tissue, and their function here appears to be one of adjusting the capacity of the system.

Finally, the nervous and humoral control mechanisms necessary for the integration of cardiovascular function with the requirements of the body form a very necessary component of any cardiovascular system. Figure 1-1 summarizes some of the main features. Notice the division into two main parts, namely, the high-pressure and the low-pressure systems. The former includes the left ventricle in systole, as well as those vessels that distribute blood to the systemic capillary beds. Systole is the term used to denote the active or contracting state of the heart muscle. The low-pressure system includes the capillary beds and all vascular elements returning the blood to the left ventricle, which is a part of the

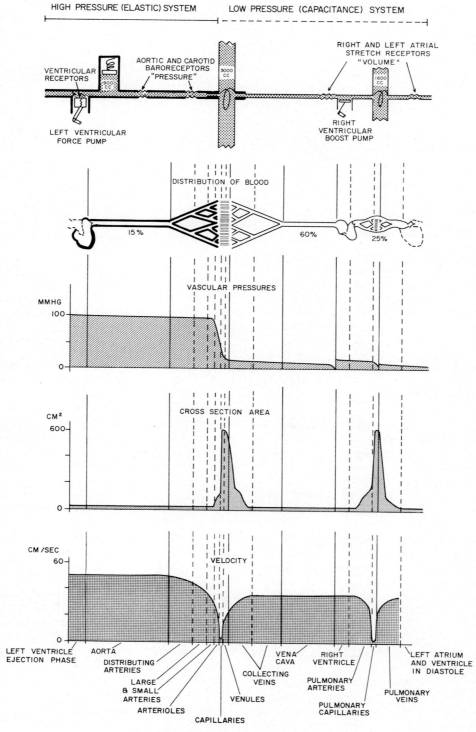

See legend on facing page.

low-pressure system when relaxed, i.e., in diastole. The pulmonary circulation with its massive blood content is a vital part of the low-pressure system.

Pressure Flow Relationships in the Vascular Bed

HYDROSTATIC COLUMNS

The data diagrammed in Figure 1-1 applies to man in the horizontal position, that is, when the cardiovascular axis is essentially horizontal to the ground. In man, as well as in a few other homeothermic animals, special problems resulting from hydrostatic loading develop with assumption of the upright posture for a large portion of the soft tissues will then be located well below the level of the heart.

Contrast, for example, the cardiovascular system of a dachshund with that of a giraffe. The cardiovascular axis of the dachshund is essentially parallel to the ground. The giraffe, on the other hand, can move his head up and down through a maximum vertical distance of 17 feet. The heart not only has to supply enough energy to overcome ordinary vascular resistances, but also must be capable of pumping blood to the giraffe's brain through a hydrostatic distance that can attain 7 feet, corresponding to a pressure of approximately 160 mm Hg above the level of the heart.

In an erect man, the hydrostatic pressure difference between the brain and the heart is 25 mm Hg or one quarter of the mean arterial pressure. In addition, as a result of the posture, the vessels of the lower extremities are subjected to a considerable distending pressure that is of special significance to the compliant venous system.

FLOW OF BLOOD

The dynamics of blood movement through the vascular system depend on the relationships that exist between driving pressure, rate of flow, and resistance to flow. The simplest relationship is analogous to Ohm's law concerning the flow of electric current. The following equation is essentially Ohm's law (i.e., $E = IR$ where E is voltage, R electrical resistance, and I current flow) adapted to the movement of fluid in the vascular system.

(a) $\qquad (P_a - P_b) = RF$

i.e.,
P_a = point of high pressure
P_b = point of low pressure
R = vascular resistance
F = blood flow per unit time

The movement of fluid through the vascular system involves a number of additional subtle considerations that must be taken into account. In the early nineteenth century, a French physician, Jean Poiseuille; a Swiss physicist, Jacques Bernoulli; and an English physicist, Osborne Reynolds, each provided important insights into the physics of blood flow through vascular structures.

Poiseuille was the first to study the flow of fluids through tubes. He used a model constructed of rigid tubes; water and a large reservoir provided the driving pressure. He was able to show that the resistance to movement of fluid was directly related to the length of the tube and the viscosity of the fluid and inversely related to the fourth power of the radius:

(b) $\qquad R = \frac{\eta L}{r^4}$

η = viscosity of the fluid
L = length of the tube
r = radius of the tube

Substituting (b) for R in (a) and using the constant $\pi/8$ yields the classical expression describing the movement of fluid in a system of rigid tubes, i.e., the Poiseuille-Hagen formula for flow:

$$F = \frac{\pi}{8} \times \frac{(P_a - P_b) r^4}{L\eta}$$

Implicit in the equation is the fact that the blood flows from a region of high to a region of rela-

---

Fig. 1-1.—A schematic diagram showing the interrelationships between various parameters of the human cardiovascular system. The left ventricle is depicted twice—for it is a part of the high-pressure system during systole and of the low-pressure system during diastole.

The two top figures delineate the elasticity of the system by the thickness of the lines. The extent of the reservoir functions of the high- and low-pressure systems is indicated with figures to show the percentage distribution and volumes held by each subdivision.

The three bottom figures present the mean pressure, the cross-sectional area of the bed, and the flow velocity in the different divisions.

The cross-section is the greatest and the flow the slowest, i.e., <.1 cm/sec, in the capillary bed. The horizontal spacing of the various vertical bars subdividing the different diagrams indicates the relative lengths of each subdivision of the cardiovascular system. The pulmonary and systemic capillary beds have the highest cross-sectional area, the lowest flow rates, and are the shortest segments.

tively lower pressure. Of particular physiologic significance is the importance of the radius of the vessel in determining the resistance to flow through it. The terminal vessels of the arterial system, the arterioles, are of a small caliber compared with the arteries leading up to them. They are capable of big changes in diameter because of the many muscular cells surrounding them. These are the "resistance" vessels of the circulation, and they actively control the flow of blood to the various body tissues. A 16% increase in the radius of these vessels is enough to double the blood flow if the driving pressure remains constant.

The Poiseuille equation is satisfactory as long as the fluid flow is laminar or streamline in character. The fluid passing along a tube can be considered as a concentric series of very thin cylinders. The one next to the wall of the vessel is almost motionless. Within this is another that moves more rapidly, and so on, so that the cylindrical elements nearest the center of the tube have the highest linear velocity.

Data from Poiseuille's experiments show a sudden break point when the driving pressure is relatively high and flow becomes markedly accelerated. Osborne Reynolds showed that this was due to the intervention of yet another characteristic of liquids in motion. He pointed out that turbulence develops above a critical flow velocity. With this, the flow breaks up into vortices, and resistance is vastly increased (Fig. 1-2).

The critical velocity is a function of the viscosity and density of the fluid and may be calculated from the following expression:

$$U = \frac{K\eta}{\rho R}$$

K = Reynolds' number
η = viscosity
ρ = density
R = radius of the tube

Reynolds' number for whole blood is approximately 1,000 in grams per milliliter where the radius is in centimeters. It represents the ratio of the viscous to the inertial forces acting when a fluid is in motion.

VELOCITY AND LATERAL PRESSURE AT A CONSTRICTION

Jacques Bernoulli pointed out that, when blood flow is rapid, side pressure declines and vice versa. In all normal arteries, this effect is negligible, and the "end" pressure, which is measured by occluding the femoral artery with a cannula, will be within a few millimeters of the lateral pressure recorded from a T cannula inserted in the vessel. Bernoulli's principle states that:

$$W = PV + Mgh + \tfrac{1}{2} Mu^2$$

where W is the total energy of the fluid and equals the sum of the potential energy due to the pressure PV, the potential energy due to gravity Mgh, and the kinetic energy due to the velocity of flow $\tfrac{1}{2} Mu^2$. (This principle extends the concept of fluid movement given by the Poiseuille equation and states that fluid will move from a region of high total energy to one of lower total energy. This partially accounts for occasional discrepancies in the pressure-determined pattern of blood flow found in the vascular system.)

The hydrostatic component due to gravity is, of course, an important factor in determining blood flow when the subject is erect. The inertial factor, $\tfrac{1}{2} Mu^2$, becomes important where large masses of blood are moving at low pressure differences as, for example, through the pulmonary artery. Under these circumstances, end pressures will differ significantly from side pressures. Finally, the effects of Bernoulli's principle show up clearly when considering the closure of the valves of the heart. The rapid flow of blood past the aortic orifice helps to keep the valve leaflets mobilized from the vessel wall, thus facilitating punctual closure at the onset of diastole.

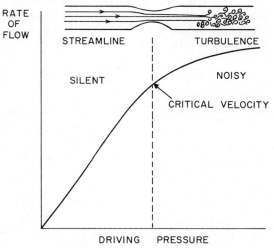

Fig. 1-2.—Change in type of flow from streamline to turbulent at the critical velocity. (From Burton, A. C.: in Ruch, T. C., and Patton, H. D. (eds.): *Physiology and Biophysics* [Philadelphia: W. B. Saunders Co., 1965].)

Intramural Tension and Radius

In 1820, another Frenchman, Laplace, formulated a mathematical principle that applies to cardiovascular physiology in general and to the arterial tree in particular. It concerns the relationship between the pressure in a hollow organ and the tension in the wall. If the membrane is curved, as in the case of a blood vessel, then the tension can be expressed as dynes/cm across an imaginary slit in the membrane (Fig. 1-3). The difference in tension between the inside and outside of the membrane, P, or the "transmural pressure," is given by the equation:

$$P = T \left(\frac{1}{R_1} + \frac{1}{R_2} \right)$$

For a blood vessel, one term vanishes since the radius of a cylinder is infinite. Thus, for blood vessels, Laplace's law may be written: $P = T/R$. This explains why an aorta with a diameter of 2 cm has a tension of 200 dynes/cm at 100 mm Hg; yet, the thin-walled capillaries in the foot can withstand a similar transmural pressure. The reason is that the radius of curvature is so small that the capillary will have a wall tension of no more than 14 dynes/cm. From this it follows that the larger the heart, the greater the wall tension will have to be in order to eject blood at the same pressure (Fig. 1-3). Thus the grossly distended atria of the chronically failing heart require greatly increased wall tension if they are to contract and empty. Furthermore, if the aorta begins to stretch—as it may—when arteriosclerotic changes cause deterioration of the media, then a vicious circle ensues. The larger the vessel is at a given blood pressure, the more likely it is to rupture. To some degree, this effect is countered by the presence of collagenous as well as elastic fibers in the artery wall. These fibers do not stretch as easily and serve as reinforcing bands countering a dangerous degree of stretch of the vessel.

Viscosity

The characteristics of blood as a fluid are complicated by the suspension of red cells in a homogenous liquid—the plasma. For this reason, the apparent viscosity of whole blood varies as the hematocrit ratio, i.e., the ratio of the volume of red cells to the volume of whole blood. Thus plasma has a viscosity only 1.2 to 1.3 times that of water. Whole blood, however, has an apparent viscosity 2.4 times that of plasma.

The blood of animals using a high-pressure delivery system contains considerable amounts of albumin and some low-molecular-weight globulins. These are primarily responsible for the high colloid osmotic pressure in spite of a minor increase in plasma viscosity over that of water. The albumin has a molecular weight of about 70,000 and, were it not for this compact molecular shape, the viscosity of the plasma would be far greater.

The apparent viscosity of whole blood depends critically on the size of the vessel through which it flows. When blood is flowing through vessels narrower than 1.5 to 2 mm in internal diameter, the apparent viscosity falls until it is close to that of plasma (Fig. 1-4). This is known as the Fahraeus-Lindquist effect. Fahraeus and Lindquist attributed the influence of vessel diameter upon apparent viscosity to changes in the actual composition of blood as it flows through small vessels. The red cells tend to move in the faster axial stream, while the plasma flows in the slower marginal layers, with the result that the ratio of red cells to plasma is reduced in the smaller vessels. The red cells "slow up" when blood reaches larger vessels, and the apparent viscosity of blood increases. The axial separation of red cells and plasma in the smaller vessels becomes less distinct, and plasma does not move along as readily in the larger vessels. The net

Fig. 1-3.—Diagram of forces operating in equilibrium of wall of cylindrical vessel. Tension, *T*, is in dynes per cm of length of vessel. Pressure, *P*, is in dynes per sq cm. Radius, *R*, is in cm. (From Burton, A. C.: in Ruch, T. C., and Patton, H. D. (eds.): *Physiology and Biophysics* [Philadelphia: W. B. Saunders Co., 1965].)

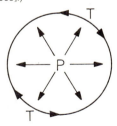

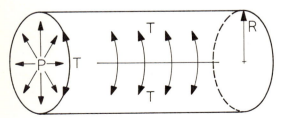

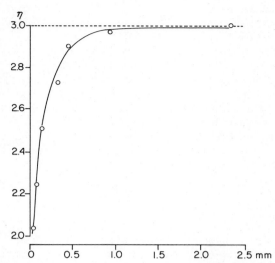

Fig. 1-4.—The decrease in relative viscosity of blood (η) when viscometers having very small-bore tubes are used. For tubes of more than 1 mm radius, there is no further change in relative viscosity. (From Burton, A. C.: *Physiology and Biophysics of the Circulation* [Chicago: Year Book Medical Publishers, Inc., 1965].)

effect is that the hematocrit is reduced only in the very small vessels. The actual volume of red cells and plasma flowing through the small vessels is, of course, the same as that pumped by the heart.

These features of the circulating fluid solve the complex problems of supplying the tissues with enough osmotic pressure to control fluid loss and of providing a great oxygen-carrying capacity. Undue viscosity is avoided, and the blood behaves hydrodynamically approximately like water.

Elasticity of the Vascular Bed

The extent to which the vascular bed will stretch as the amount and, consequently, the pressure of the fluid within it increases varies from one part to another. There is a sharp difference between the high-pressure (elastic) system and the more compliant low-pressure capacitance (reservoir) system.

The elasticity E of a reservoir is the inverse of its compliance or distensibility D and is measured by determining the pressure-volume diagram, i.e., $E = \frac{1}{D} = \frac{P}{V}$ dynes/cm^{-5}. Where compartments of different distensibility are interconnected, as in the cardiovascular system, E total = $E_1 + E_2 + \cdots + E_n$; i.e., E total = E high-pressure system + E low-pressure system.

In man, the aorta and the peripheral arteries together take up about 50 cc as a stroke volume is ejected; this raises the pressure by about 40 mm Hg. Very approximately, then:

$$\text{E high pressure} = \frac{40 \text{ mm Hg}}{50 \text{ ml}} = \frac{54 \text{ cm H}_2\text{O}}{50 \text{ ml}}$$

or approximately 1,100 dynes cm^{-5}.

On the other hand, the low-pressure system is vastly more distensible. A total volume change of 1,000 cc induces a change of pressure of only 7 cm H$_2$O; i.e., $\text{E low pressure} = \frac{7 \text{ cm H}_2\text{O}}{1,000 \text{ ml}} = 7$ dynes cm^{-5}.

Hence, when the various distensibilities are summed, the low-pressure system will store or give up 990 ml for every liter that is infused or withdrawn. Thus the roles of the two portions of the cardiovascular system are determined by their respective elasticities or distensibilities. The vessels of the high-pressure system serve primarily as conduits, and the low-pressure system serves as a reservoir. The high-pressure distributing system working at a pressure of 80–120 mm Hg (i.e., 110 to 160 cm H$_2$O) depends upon the balance between flow resistance and the dynamics of cardiac output for its pressure relationship. The primary effect of an infusion or withdrawal of blood is to raise or lower the pressure in the low-pressure system by a small but very significant increment or decrement of a few centimeters of water.

Distribution of Blood Volume in Different Regions

The arterial tree contains approximately 15% of the blood volume. In a 70-kg man whose blood volume is about 8% of the body weight, there would be 840 cc of arterial blood (Fig. 1-1). This amount stays constant, despite considerable changes in the total blood volume, because it is contained between the left ventricle and the arteriolar network at the relatively steady, elevated pressure needed to permit control of its distribution by the arteriolar sluice gates (Fig. 1-1). The central blood volume in the thorax is of the order of 1,600 cm. The exact amount varies as the lungs are filled and emptied of air. The intrathoracic vessels are not surrounded by tissue, but are suspended in the elastic network of the lungs. This, combined with the large radius of the heart chambers, makes the intrathoracic circulation an elastic reservoir into which relatively large volumes of blood can readily be moved from the periphery, either as a result of mechanical compression (as by water immersion), vasoconstriction (as in cold), or change in posture from standing to lying. Although it contains only 25–30% of the total blood volume, this region will provide one half of any blood taken from the person.

The blood volume of the extrathoracic circulation is approximately 70% of the total. The visceral circulation contains about 20–25% of the total volume. With active muscular work, the content of this region drops sharply, whereas the muscle blood content increases fivefold when the full potential of its massive capillary bed is being used.

Finally, one comes full circle back to the left ventricle—the force pump of the circulation (Fig. 1-1). The left ventricle stands alternately between the low-pressure reservoir and the high-pressure arterial delivery system. During diastole, it is part of the reservoir. During systole, it is the pump chamber. The heart's portion of the intrathoracic reservoir is of the order of 12% of the total blood volume. It forms the primary reserve to meet moment-to-moment changes in the demands for stroke output. Thus it participates passively in the reservoir function, and blood can be instantly taken from the store in its chambers in order to maintain constant filling of the high-pressure delivery tubes, despite sudden acute alterations in the rates of inflow of blood into the reservoir region. The need for this constancy is pointed up by the fact that, if the necessary 50–60 mm Hg perfusion pressure across the brain fails for only 7 seconds, unconsciousness supervenes.

Control and Integration

Strategic Stretch Receptors in the High- and Low-Pressure Systems

Well-defined neural receptor areas are found in the cardiovascular system at strategic locations. From an engineering viewpoint, it is to be expected that the system would monitor at least the volume of fluid held in reserve, the force of the beat of the pump, and the pressure in the arterial delivering channels (Fig. 1-1). Information as to which channels in the distributing diffusion networks are open would be valuable, together with some measure of the over-all work demanded of the system.

Knowledge as to how this integrated regulation is accomplished is still very incomplete. Nevertheless, there is information about the receptors in the reservoir and delivery systems, and their effectiveness is readily demonstrable. Two locations in the high-pressure system are equipped with stretch receptors (Fig. 1-1). These are the carotid sinus, located at the bifurcation of the carotid artery in the neck, and the general region of the arch of the aorta. Extensively branched, coiled, and intertwined, myelinated fibers resembling Golgi tendon stretch receptors are found in the adventitia of these arteries. Supplied by the glossopharyngeal and vagus nerves, they discharge primarily during systole. When pressure in the arterial tree rises, the discharge rate rises and vice versa. They respond less well to sustained pressure than they do to change in pressure and constitute an effective reflex feedback mechanism that operates to stabilize blood pressure. Any fall in arterial pressure decreases the inhibitory discharge in these so-called buffer nerves, activates the brain stem reticular formation, and induces a compensatory rise in blood pressure. A rise in arterial pressure produces the opposite effect, starting with a dilatation of the arterioles and going on to a whole complex of related and supporting changes. The corresponding sensors on the low-pressure side of the circulation are the atrial stretch receptors (Fig. 1-1). One type, the complex unencapsulated endings of Nonidez (CUE), consists of a freely interwoven network of repeatedly branching endings located in the subendocardium of the pulmonary veins, the intrapericardial portion of the vena cava, and in the atria themselves. Their position in the most distensible portion of the venous system is ideal for recording the filling of this representative part of the low-pressure system. Another type, the end nets, consists of a meshwork of delicate dendrites whose role is not yet defined. Bursts of impulses from the CUE atrial stretch receptors occur during the V wave of atrial diastole at the time that the atrium is most distended during the cardiac cycle. Very small changes in reservoir capacity (for example, as little as a 10% reduction in blood volume) will lead to a sharp fall in CUE atrial receptor discharge rate, and vice versa. The end networks may also be affected. These various changes in impulse rates set in motion compensatory adaptations. The fall in atrial pressure is accompanied by a rise in pulse rate. Probably thirst is experienced. There is a rise in antidiuretic hormone output, helping conserve fluid volume. Renin is released, and there may be a relative increase of blood flow in the renal medulla—both of which promote sodium retention. In the later stages, there may be splenic contraction that discharges extra red cells into the circulation. In addition, changes in the ratio of arteriolar and venous resistances in skeletal muscle favor transfer of fluids from muscle tissue into the capillaries.

Central Integration of Exteroceptive and Interoceptive Information

The impulses arising from the above two main monitoring regions in the cardiovascular system eventually arrive at the tractus solitarius nucleus of the vagus nerve. They converge at locations as close to each other as might be expected in view of the interdependence between the low- and high-pressure portions of the system. In a continuous pumping circuit, it is as critical to ensure filling of the pump chamber as it is to maintain pressure in the distributing network. Although basic integration of cardiovascular function is accomplished at the rhombencephalic level, the diencephalon including the hypothalamus is also involved, especially in the adaptation to the demands of the environment such as emotion, exercise, and temperature change.

Efferent Nervous and Hormonal Control

In direct response to an acute loss of blood volume, there is an increase in sympathetic discharge to the heart, which greatly increases both its contractility, i.e., maximum velocity of contraction, as well as the force with which it contracts. A simultaneous discharge to peripheral vessels sustains or even raises arterial pressure. Antidiuretic hormone, sustaining fluid volume, is released via the supraopticohypophyseal pathway as the result of changes in the afferent impulses from the low-pressure system. The response to activation of the high-pressure system receptors by a reduction of systemic arterial pressure is very similar. If, however, pressure is reduced in the carotid sinus region, without at the same time reducing central blood volume, the control effects are far less marked. It is probable that the system is programmed for simultaneous change in both high- and low-pressure systems in the same direction and that any changes in opposite directions in the two systems —changes that would not occur in nature—are less effective. The control of the resistance in the peripheral vascular bed of the various organs differs in its central connections. Thus, for instance, skeletal muscle is equipped with special sympathetic cholinergic vasodilator nerves that may work under emotion to provide quick starts in hunt and flight. In general, sympathetic stimulation occurs when blood volume or blood pressure, or both, are reduced. Sweating and vasodilation in the heat-dissipating arteriovenous complexes of the hands appears to be under control of noncardiovascular inputs, namely, the sensation of heat or cold on the skin. With strong stimulation, the onus shifts from direct sympathetic nervous control to the overriding effects of the catecholamines that are released from the adrenal glands.

Summary

In keeping with our central theme of the integrative physiology of the cardiovascular system, this book discusses the continual interplay between the flow of impulses from the mechanoreceptors in the heart and great vessels, on the one hand, and the data coming from higher centers and the environment, on the other. The points of interaction between these two information flows are in the brain stem extending downward from the hypothalamus to the medulla. From these regions go nervous impulses and hormonal messages carried by the circulation that appropriately modify blood volume, blood pressure, and, most importantly, local blood flow. It is probable that incorporated into the picture in some way as yet unknown are schematics or preprogrammed nervous patterns determining the normal responses of the organism. Their location may not be confined to the central nervous system.

REFERENCES

Burton, A. C.: *Physiology and Biophysics of the Circulation* (Chicago: Year Book Medical Publishers, Inc., 1965).

Gauer, O. H., and Henry, J. P.: Circulatory Basis of Fluid Volume Control, Physiol. Rev. 43:423, 1963.

Gauer, O. H., Henry, J. P., and Behn, C.: The Regulation of Extracellular Fluid Volume, Ann. Rev. Physiol. 32:547, 1970.

Ruch, T. C., and Patton, H. D.: *Physiology and Biophysics* (Philadelphia: W. B. Saunders Co., 1965).

Rushmer, R. F.: *Cardiovascular Dynamics,* 2d ed. (Philadelphia: W. B. Saunders Co., 1961).

Weale, F. E.: *An Introduction to Surgical Haemodynamics* (Chicago: Year Book Medical Publishers, Inc., 1967).

Winsor, T., and Hyman, C.: *A Primer of Peripheral Vascular Diseases* (Philadelphia: Lea & Febiger, 1965), chap. 1–7.

2

The Heart as a Reservoir and Pump

Introduction

THIS CHAPTER is concerned with the heart as the pump that, with the arterioles, effectively divides the circulation into its two principal parts, the high-pressure or arterial system and the low-pressure system. Since it holds a significant proportion of the blood volume, it is further described as a reservoir.

Cardiac Chambers as Muscular Pumps

MUSCULAR ARRANGEMENT

In the adult, the left ventricle consists of over 400 grams of spirally wound muscles lying in two sheets. One surrounds both ventricles; the other, the left ventricle only. The muscle of the left ventricle spirals so gradually that it is, in effect, circular. Considerable information on changes in the shape of the heart during contraction has been obtained from special transducers sewn into the heart chambers and from x-ray motion pictures. The first change occurs while the heart is tightening up on the mass of blood prior to ejection. There is no absolute decrease in volume, but the ventricle becomes more spherical. This occurs because the apex of the heart moves towards the fibrous atrioventricular plane in which the four cardiac valves are located. As the force of contraction raises the pressure above that of the aorta, ejection starts and there is a further shortening of the distance between the apex and the atrioventricular septum. At the same time, the powerful constrictor band curving around the interventricular septum contracts and the transverse diameter decreases. Because the spiral muscles are wound in opposite directions, there is very little rolling or rotation of the apex during contraction.

The atria themselves are primarily reservoirs for blood flowing toward the heart during ventricular contraction, and their contraction provides only a slight boost to the refilling of the ventricle. Active contraction of the right ventricle provides only a part of the energy propelling blood to the lungs; for the rest, its action is

Fig. 2-1.—Changes in the cross-section of the ventricles during myocardial contraction. In **A**, the left ventricle contains a normal 150 cc at diastole; and in **B**, the volume is reduced to 75 cc at systole. In **C**, there is no residual volume. In moving from **A** to **B**, there is no serious change in fiber length, but in passing from **B** to **C**, there is a serious distortion and marked tangential pull between the adjacent muscle bundles. The diagram also demonstrates the fact that even a flaccid right ventricle will be partially emptied by the systole of the left ventricle to which it is attached like a pouch. (From Rushmer, R. F.: *Cardiovascular Dynamics,* 2d. ed. [Philadelphia: W. B. Saunders Co., 1961].)

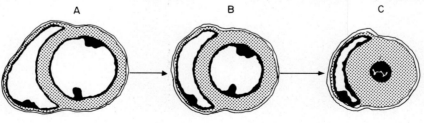

passive. In fact, to a large degree, it serves as a valved pouch fastened to the wall of the left ventricle. As the latter becomes more spherical during its ejection phase, the interventricular septum encroaches upon the cavity of the right ventricle, which is, in effect, progressively stretched over the spherical left ventricle, and its capacity is thereby reduced. The result is that, as long as the left ventricle is contracting effectively, even a completely inoperative right ventricle can maintain flow through the pulmonary circuit (Fig. 2-1).

For these reasons, the right ventricle and atria can be regarded at best as auxiliary "booster" pumps that maintain flow through the valve orifices and the pulmonary circuit and serve to fill the primary pump—the left ventricle—during its period of relaxation.

Pericardial Assistance to Heart Filling

As the distance between the apex and the base of the ventricle decreases during its contraction, the atria and large vessels are stretched since they are enclosed within a cavity formed by the pericardial sac. The consequent reduction of pressure accelerates flow into the atria so that, in a passive sense, the intact pericardium aids the inflow of blood into the atria during left ventricular systole. The evidence for this is that, in early ventricular contraction, the difference between right atrial pressure and intrapericardial pressure increases sharply; i.e., the pressure gradient from thoracic veins to right atrium is increased and blood is drawn into the right atrium. In this way, the better part of a stroke volume is readied for the return of the atrioventricular ring during ventricular diastole (Fig. 2-2). Pericardectomized animals survive perfectly well, but they perform poorly when exercising, probably because this mechanism is more important when the heart rate is high. Another function of the pericardium is to splint the heart, equalizing pressure as the organism changes posture from recumbent to vertical and preventing overdistension when the volume of blood in the thorax is greatly increased.

Function of Valves

Unidirectional flow of blood through the circulatory system depends on the function of four cardiac valves. They are embedded in approximately the same plane in the fibrous base of the ventricles. The semilunar valves separate the ventricles from their associated arteries. The atrioventricular valves separate the atria from their respective ventricles.

The structure of the aortic semilunar valve is particularly critical. The three outpouchings of the sinuses of Valsalva just above the cusps are precisely designed to fulfill a role. During systolic ejection, the high-velocity blood stream develops turbulent flow as it encounters these expansions (Fig. 1-2). The resultant eddy currents keep the valve flaps located in the stream. This not only maintains them in the proper position for instant closure, but, if the flaps were to be forced right back to the aortic wall, the coronary orifices would be blocked (Fig. 2-3).

The atrioventricular valves, tricuspid on the right and mitral on the left, prevent the ventricles from ejecting blood back into the atria. Their

Fig. 2-2.—Movements of the valve ring: **left,** ventricular diastole and atrial systole; **right,** atrial diastole and ventricular systole. The blood is sucked into the heart by the downward movement of the valve ring during ventricular systole. (From Landois-Rosemann: *Lehrbuch der Physiologie des Menschen,* 28th ed. [Munich: Urban & Schwarzenberg, 1960].)

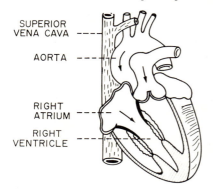
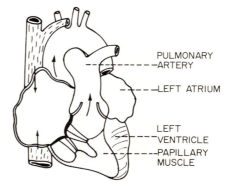

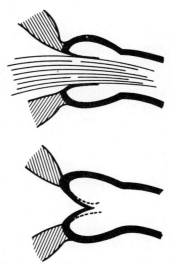

Fig. 2-3.—Flow patterns during systole **(above)** and diastole **(below)**. Because of the rapid flow, side pressure declines and the valve leaflet stays mobilized, ready for rapid closure when the flow reverses. (From Rushmer, R. F.: *Cardiovascular Dynamics*, 2d. ed. [Philadelphia: W. B. Saunders Co., 1961].)

cusps are large because the valves change size, shape, and position during different phases of the heart cycle. They must, therefore, be larger than the area to be covered at rest. The chordae tendinae leading to the papillary muscles prevent eversion of the flexible cusps as intraventricular pressure rises. Further, because the Purkinje fibers enter the myocardium over the endocardial surface at the roots of the papillary muscles, these are the first parts of the ventricles to contract; because they are located on the inner wall of the ventricle, these "guywires" tighten at the beginning of systole, thus helping to hold the cusps together during the rise of intraventricular pressure (Fig. 2-2). This active prevention of valvular eversion makes the ejection phase more efficient since a bulging valve would have the effect of a leak of the same volume. The mechanism of closure is not simply a matter of snapping shut with the rise of systolic pressure. There is evidence that a wave of slightly negative pressure at the end of atrial systole brings the cusps somewhat forward into the stream in a position ready for closing (Fig. 2-3). The sequence occurs so rapidly that it forms a single movement that is completed by ventricular systole. This approximation of the valve cusps induced by atrial systole prevents any significant reflux and is a contribution of the atrium to the effectiveness of the cardiac pump.

Sequence of Events in the Cardiac Cycle

The action of the heart valves with each beat is associated with a series of events whose sequence is described by referring to the action of the left ventricle. Figure 2-4 outlines these events for a heart beating at 75 cycles per minute. Two cycles are presented, and the various phases and events are presented in their temporal relationships.

VENTRICULAR SYSTOLE

Systole at this heart rate is briefer than diastole. During isometric ventricular contraction, the ventricle is tightening up on the "bolus" of blood. The atrioventricular valves have snapped shut, but the semilunar valves are not yet open. The ventricular muscle is contracting, and tension in the cardiac wall is increasing, but no shortening has occurred, hence the term isometric. As can be seen from the curve, tension rapidly develops in the muscle and the pressure rises very fast, i.e., in less than a tenth of a second. The mitral and tricuspid valves bulge slightly into the atrium, causing small peaks in the corresponding atrial pressure waves. The moment the pressure in the left ventricle exceeds that in the aorta, the aortic and pulmonary valves open and ventricular ejection commences as the muscle fibers shorten on their load. Flow into the aortic reservoir is rapid at first. As the ventricular volume curve also shows, about 70 cc are ejected with each stroke of the cycle, leaving about 50 cc as a reserve. Diastole begins when isometric ventricular relaxation ends; filling commences as ventricular pressure falls below atrial pressure. The valves open, and the atrioventricular rings move back toward their original position at the beginning of systole. Because of the inertia of the mass of the blood in the atria, much of it stays in place while the valve rings actually move over the "bolus" of blood (Fig. 2-2). The filling of the ventricles is by no means a passive process depending only on a pressure gradient between the atria and ventricles. Indeed, atrial systole is a final event in the process; it is far too feeble to make it more than an auxiliary mode. At high heart rates and outputs, this action of "swallowing" the waiting "bolus" of blood is a major contribution to cardiac filling.

Intraventricular pressure soon starts to decline in the course of systole and, due to the momentum

THE HEART AS A RESERVOIR AND PUMP 27

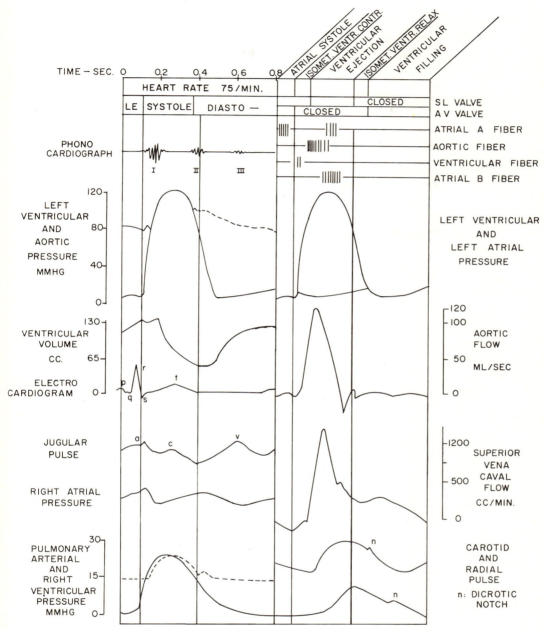

Fig. 2-4.—Composite diagram showing the relative timing of various pressure, volume, and flow events during the resting human cardiac cycle. The principal components of the phonocardiograph, the electrocardiogram, and the firing times of important receptors are also included.

of the blood, is actually exceeded in the later phases by the aortic pressure. Then this, too, rapidly falls as the elastic force of the aorta exceeds the fading intraventricular pressure and the semilunar valves snap shut. At this point, the tension decreases without further change in fiber length in so-called isometric ventricular relaxation.

Flow in the aorta is now zero near the semilunar valves. However, the blood ejected from the heart goes on flowing into the peripheral vascular bed, driven forward by its momentum and urged on by the elastic recoil of the aorta and large arteries. Thus the peak of pressure in the carotid artery occurs significantly later than the peak aortic pressure. The peak of pressure in the radial artery actually occurs at the time when the ventricle is relaxing after closure of the semilunar valves. A pulse wave passes down the elastic arterial tree with a velocity determined by the rigidity of the vessels—a velocity that greatly exceeds the actual flow of blood down the vessels.

The decrease of ventricular volume during systole is associated with a considerable change in ventricular shape as the AV valves are pulled downward. The pull on the atria drops the pressure in them. The ventricles, by a combination of pulling on the atrial rings and pulling away from the pericardial sac, induce a rapid influx of blood into the atria. Indeed, recordings of the superior vena caval flow rate show an increase during the powerful systolic contraction of the ventricular muscle. As the ventricular volume curve shows, at normal heart rates, there is a considerable end-systolic ventricular blood volume. In late diastole, especially with bradycardia, the rate of filling declines, and the cusps of the AV valves drift toward each other, propelled by the eddies behind them. It is important to realize that, at slow rates, atrial systole provides no more than 20% of the blood that is in the ventricle at the start of the ejection phase. The rest is made up from the previously described movement of the valve ring plus what remains in the ventricle from the preceding beat. However, although the heart can continue to work effectively despite inactivity of the atria, at high heart rates (i.e., when diastolic time is short) a vigorous atrial contraction is a true asset and can account for as much as 40% of the stroke volume.

Pulmonary arterial and right-ventricular pressure curves follow the left-ventricular pattern except that the pressures are far lower.

INFLUENCE OF FREQUENCY ON THE RATIO OF SYSTOLE TO DIASTOLE

When the frequency of the heart cycle increases, it does so at the expense of diastole (Fig. 2-5). At 75/minute as shown in the figure, the duration of diastole significantly exceeds systole. But at 90–100/minute, the two phases are equal. And at 150/minute, the duration of diastole of an athlete whose resting pulse had

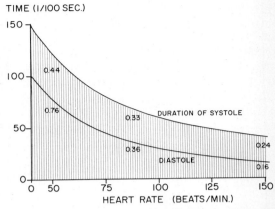

Fig. 2-5.—Duration of systole and diastole in relation to heart rate. At low frequencies, the duration of diastole is about ⅔ of the duration of the cycle. With increasing rate, the filling phase loses out to the work phase. (From Gauer, O. H. in Landois-Rosemann: *Lehrbuch der Physiologie des Menschen*, 28th ed. [Munich: Urban & Schwarzenberg, 1960].)

been 50/minute will have decreased from 0.76 to 0.16 sec., i.e., by 80%; whereas, the duration of his systole falls from 0.44 to 0.24 or only 55%. Since coronary blood flow proceeds principally during diastole, the progressive loss of this rest period as the rate increases is unfavorable for the heart. Indeed, in excess of 200/minute, the heart of the exercising man begins to fail and the output drops. Rates in excess of 150/minute, which are commonly found during exertion, demand the above-mentioned mechanism of movement of the valve ring over the waiting blood during systole (Fig. 2-2) so that inflow during diastole is merely a "topping-up" process. It is only at slow rates that the process of diastolic inflow from the veins predominates.

Some Factors Determining Cardiac Output

HEART CHAMBERS AS A RESERVOIR OF THE LOW-PRESSURE SYSTEM

Although the stroke volume at rest is small in keeping with the modest cardiac output, the heart nearly fills the pericardial sac. Hence, its content of blood is large, i.e., some 12% of the total blood volume or some 600 cc in a normal man. The larger heart of the athlete holds an even larger proportion of the total blood volume. In the event of the high loads of violent exertion, such a heart can increase stroke volume at the expense of the systolic reserve left at diastole.

Thus the heart of the healthy relaxed man is a reservoir that can provide a significant fraction of several stroke volumes. In sudden exertion, this helps to make an acutely accelerated cardiac output feasible until the accessory pumps, i.e., the muscles and respiratory action, have delivered sufficient blood to make up the deficiency and establish a new balance between inflow and outflow.

Control of Heart Rate

Cardiac output, the quantity of blood pumped by the heart in unit time, is the product of the stroke volume and the heart rate as determined by the sinoauricular node. The frequency of this pacemaker depends on the balance between vagal slowing and sympathetic accelerating influences. In the normal adult, it averages about 70 beats/minute with a range from 50 for the athlete up to 200. In the fetus, it is about 135; in the mouse, 400; and in the elephant, 25/minute.

This variability is crucial because, in the healthy animal, stroke volume is held contant, and the heart rate is the major factor determining cardiac output. The ventricle is emptied so rapidly in the early phases of increased demand that the rate can be greatly increased without seriously affecting the filling. The to-and-fro piston-like action of the AV ring is sufficient for all but the highest heart frequencies as long as the venous reservoirs are kept full. Thus, unlike a pump in which inflow is constant, the athlete's heart rate can increase to well over 180/minute and still develop a proportionate increase in cardiac output.

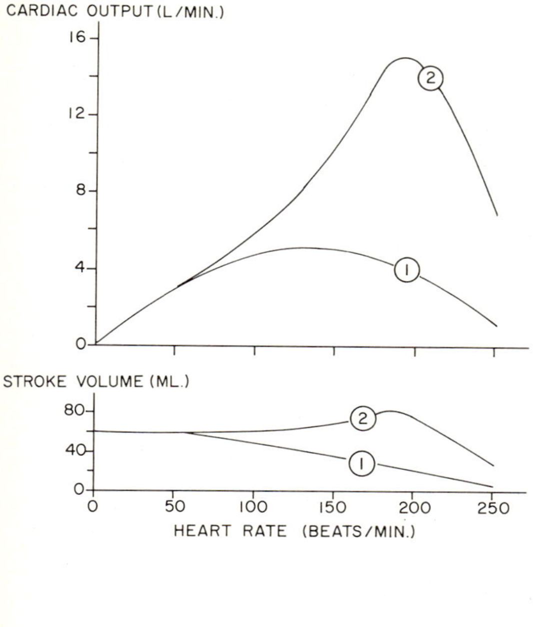

When at rest, the limit of effective heart rate in man is about 180/minute. The maximum attainable during exertion falls progressively with age and, in the 60-year-old, is no more than 150–160/minute.

Tachycardias or heart rates in the resting individual in excess of 150/minute are associated with a decrease in cardiac output as ventricular filling becomes deficient. The mechanism of this deficiency in output at the higher rates is illustrated in Figure 2-6. Since cardiac output is the product of stroke volume and heart rate, if stroke volume remains constant, the cardiac output will increase linearly with an increase of heart rate. This is shown in curves 1 and 2 up to rates of 100. If the individual is exercising and thus assisting in the maintenance of central filling by vigorous action of the accessory muscular and respiratory pumps, there is no significant fall in diastolic filling despite the tachycardia. If the filling is less adequate, as when the subject is at rest, then stroke volume will decline as pulse rate increases, and cardiac output will eventually decrease (Fig. 2-6, curve 1). This can occur in paroxysmal atrial tachycardia when the pulse rate exceeds 150/minute. Curve 2 represents the contrasting state of affairs when filling is maintained despite the tachycardia, as in the exercising athlete. Here the pulse rate may rise to 200/minute and still be accompanied by a corresponding increase in cardiac output.

In contradistinction to the above, at very low ventricular rates, filling time may be completely adequate, but the output is limited by the low rate. Atrioventricular block with pulse rates of less than 50/minute is an example of this situation.

One important factor determining heart rate is body temperature. For every 1° F rise, there is a 7–11 beat/minute increase in rate. The major control of rate is by the vagus and the sympathetic nerves, as will be discussed in the section on nervous control.

Fig. 2-6.—The effect of heart rate on cardiac output. Since cardiac output is the product of stroke volume and heart rate, as long as the stroke remains constant, the output increases linearly with an increase in heart rate. If filling diminishes at the higher rates, as in a tachycardia at rest, then output decreases, *curve 1*. In violent athletics, assistance from the respiratory and muscular pumps and other compensatory mechanisms sustains the stroke volume and cardiac output increases, despite rates approaching 200/minute, *curve 2*. (From Selkurt, E. E.: *Physiology*, 2d. ed. [Boston: Little, Brown & Co., 1966].)

Elastic Forces, Viscosity, and Laplace's Equation

The heart of the recumbent, resting athlete is large and fills the pericardium. Stroke volume is increased by encroaching on the large end-systolic volume. The healthy, well-nourished heart gains from this because less work is done against viscous resistance. Further, when the end-systolic volume is grossly reduced, energy must be used to compress the myocardial chamber around this small residuum (Fig. 2-1). A larger heart can expel the same stroke volume without the added work expenditure needed for tissue compression. Only when the muscle loses contractile force does it become advantageous to have a small heart. Then, as Laplace's law indicates, with the smaller heart, less muscle tension will be needed to produce the same intraventricular pressure.

TABLE 2-1

	Rest	Work	Rest Work Ratio
O_2 consumption cc/min	260	3,120	12:1
Cardiac output cc/min	5,800	22,300	3.8:1
Arteriovenous O_2 difference cc/liter blood	45	140	3.1:1
Stroke volume cc	91	128	1.4:1
Pulse rate/min	64	174	2.7:1

Cardiac Output

As a pump, it is the heart's task to put out fluid; the critical question is the minute volume that it can achieve. In the average man at rest, on applying the formula: Minute volume = stroke volume × frequency, we get the figure: 70–80 cc × 70/min = 5–6 liters/min. In order to reduce this to terms applicable to people of different size, the body surface area is used to calculate the cardiac index, i.e., the cardiac output expressed as liters per minute per square meter. In most people, this is about 3.5 liters. Resting values less than 2 liters and above 5 liters are definitely abnormal. Even in moderately severe heart failure, it is often scarcely reduced. In pregnancy, thyrotoxicosis, and fever, it is increased. In hypothermia, as is used in heart surgery, it may be down to a small fraction of normal.

The end-systolic volume of the trained athlete at rest may be as much as twice his normal stroke volume. This makes it possible for him to increase stroke output without danger of emptying the heart during severe exertion.

However, the normal and the most important way in which the heart increases output is by acceleration. Studies with intact animals have shown that changes in stroke volume are relatively unimportant. As stated, in athletes 180/minute can be sustained for hours with transient peak frequencies up to 240/minute.

If failure forces a reduction of cardiac output, it is first met by an increase in the arteriovenous oxygen differences. As can be seen from Table 2-1, there is plenty of room for an increase in the volume of oxygen taken out of the blood. In fact, a reduction in the saturation of mixed venous blood, causing the AV O_2 differences to exceed the normal 5–6 volumes per cent, is an even more reliable symptom of a deficiency of cardiac function than is the measurement of cardiac output itself.

Cardiac Efficiency

The oxygen consumption of the heart is closely related to the product of arterial pressure and the duration of systole. The heat production of the muscle is measured by the tension maintained times the duration of this tension. Thus an increase in blood pressure increases the demands on the heart. Since the capillary bed is perfused at the same low pressure in a man with high blood pressure, hypertension is wasteful. The efficient heart works at a low blood pressure, dissipating less energy in the arteriolar control channels. The combination of hypertension with the impairment of oxygen delivery to the laboring heart muscle by coronary sclerosis is disastrous. Aortic stenosis is critical because it demands prolonged tension in the laboring ventricular muscle to induce the sustained high-intraventricular pressure needed to expel the stroke volume through the narrowed orifice. The increase of stroke volume demanded by insufficient leaking valves is not as taxing as might be expected, since the heart does not have to work for a prolonged time at a high pressure.

Work of the Heart

The heart must not only accelerate a certain mass of blood down the aorta, it must also eject this volume against the arterial pressure. The total work done is the sum of this volume work plus the kinetic energy provided to the "bolus" of blood. In the resting man, the total comes to

THE HEART AS A RESERVOIR AND PUMP

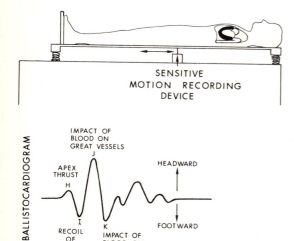

Fig. 2-7.—Ballistocardiography uses a low-frequency spring-mounted table that is critically damped. However, the tissues in contact with the table determine the transmission characteristics from heart to table affecting the consistency of the relationship between the deflection and the stroke volume. (From Rushmer, R. F.: *Cardiovascular Dynamics*, 2d ed. [Philadelphia: W. B. Saunders Co., 1961].)

some 8 kilogram meters per minute, and, in the performing athlete, it can rise as high as 80 kilogram meters per minute. At these peak loads, as much as 27% of the work is going into acceleration of the blood.

In the intact organism, the ballistocardiograph gives a crude measure of this parameter (Fig. 2-7). The subject is placed on a table that can move freely in the horizontal plane. The inertial changes as the heart ejects its quota of blood can be recorded with an appropriate device for registering small movements, i.e., a strain gauge. A related phenomenon is the rhythmic movement of the bathroom scale when a man with a vigorously beating heart stands on it.

In valvular insufficiency, much work is also spent in accelerating blood. The more resistant and stiffer the aorta becomes, as in the aged with arteriosclerotic change, the more work the heart must do to accelerate the blood down the delivery system. The increase can be up to double the values in a normally elastic arterial tree.

Heart Sounds

INTRODUCTION

By listening to the heart, it is often possible to recognize signs of organic disease long before there are any clues elsewhere in the system. Characteristic murmurs and changes in the normal sounds will occur in a heart that can fully compensate and as yet shows no disturbance of power output. Auscultation is, however, very much of an art, for the sounds are faint and not easy to recognize. One reason for the difficulty is that they are in the low-frequency range where the sensitivity of the human ear is least. As Figure 2-8 shows, only a fraction of the total sounds produced are audible. The stethoscope, which is used to detect them, does not amplify but damps and distorts the sounds whose greatest intensity is at 24 cycles/sec. The lowest frequencies that we can perceive are in the range of 30–50 cycles/sec; there are few heart sound

Fig. 2-8.—Showing how small a proportion of the total range of vibrations produced by the heart are audible. This is because the more intense vibrations are in the low frequencies where auditory acuity falls off sharply. (Modified from Butterworth, J. S., Chassin, M. R., and McGrath, R.: *Cardiac Auscultation* [New York: Grune & Stratton, Inc., 1955].)

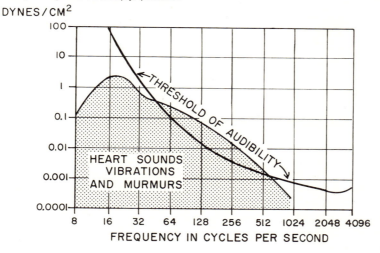

components above 500 cycles/sec where we have our highest auditory acuity. The picture changes if electrical recording is employed. With a microphone sensitive to low frequencies, heart sound records can be made that not only give information imperceptible to the ear, but also record it in its exact relationship to other events in the cardiac cycle. These phonocardiograms can be of value in detecting fleeting sounds at or below the limit of auditory acuity and in comparing sounds at one time with those developing a few months later.

CAUSES AND TIMING OF HEART SOUNDS

Since the heart cycle is arbitrarily defined as beginning with the systole, the first heart sound is that heard as the ventricle contracts. Reference to Figure 2-9 shows the timing of this sound corresponds with the beginning of ventricular systole coincident with the rise in ventricular pressure. The second sound is associated with the dicrotic notch on the aortic pressure curve that is caused by the closure of the semilunar valves. The mechanisms responsible for these complex sounds is still controversial. Nevertheless, it is illuminating to break the first sound into the four components described by Rushmer (Fig. 2-9). All originate from the development of vibrations in the heart and its blood content that are transmitted through the lungs and other tissues to the chest wall. The first component of the first sound is regarded as due to the surge of blood toward the AV valves, initiating closure as the ventricle starts to contract. The second phase develops as the now-tense AV valves suddenly decelerate the blood and the whole chamber is set into vibration. The third component may be due to oscillation of the blood between the root of the aorta and ventricular walls, and the fourth to turbulence of the stream as it is ejected into the pulmonary artery and aorta.

The diagram (Fig. 2-9) also indicates the origins of the second heart sound. It is primarily due to vibrations induced by the closure and tensing of the semilunar valves. These start in the aorta and pulmonary artery but are transmitted to the ventricles and atria by the vibrations of the tightly shut valves locked into their fibrous rings in the heart structure.

Phonocardiography frequently reveals a very low-frequency third sound, which is rarely heard because of the low sensitivity of the ear. It occurs at the sudden termination of the rapid-filling phase of diastole and appears to be due to vibra-

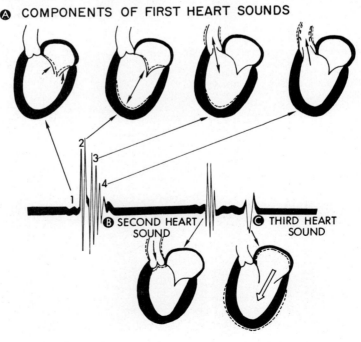

Fig. 2-9.—Schematic drawings of the causes of various components of heart sounds based on the concept that vibrations are induced by acceleration or deceleration of blood within the elastic chambers. For details see text. (From Rushmer, R. F.: *Cardiovascular Dynamics*, 2d. ed. [Philadelphia: W. B. Saunders Co., 1961].)

THE HEART AS A RESERVOIR AND PUMP

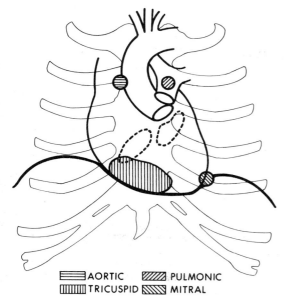

Fig. 2-10.—Locations on body surface at which sounds from particular valve regions are best perceived. (From Scher, A. M.: in Ruch, T. C., and Patton, H. D. (eds.): *Physiology and Biophysics*, 19th ed. [Philadelphia: W. B. Saunders Co., 1965].)

one to determine which of two valves closing simultaneously has a defect. The anatomy of the heart determines that sounds from the pulmonary and tricuspid valves, which are closest to the chest wall, are heard the best near the underlying valves (Fig. 2-10). For the mitral and aortic valves, which are farther from the chest wall, the best hearing conditions are at the apex of the heart for the mitral and to the right of the sternum in the second right intercostal space for the aortic valve.

Murmurs

The heart sounds are induced by the vibration resulting from the sudden acceleration or deceleration of the blood and of the actual structures of the heart chambers containing it. Murmurs are the result of turbulence developing in rapidly flowing blood. In almost the entire arterial tree, the flow is smoothly laminar and noiseless. Systolic murmurs heard in early systole may be regarded as a prolongation of the fourth component of the first heart sound. They occur as the blood leaves the pulmonary and aortic valves, especially in children, and in anemia when turbulence flow rates are high and the viscosity lower. Another place where turbulence creates a murmur is under the compressing cuff of the sphygmomanometer. These Korotkoff sounds are due to turbulent flow as the blood jets out of the half-compressed artery into the open vessel beyond.

Figure 2-11 shows phonocardiograms from a number of common abnormalities of the heart valves.

tions of the chamber walls. These vibrations would be at a low frequency because the walls are relaxed and flaccid.

Areas for Auscultation of Normal Heart Sounds

Knowledge of the locations where the various valves can best be heard is an important part of auscultatory technique. For example, it permits

Fig. 2-11.—Phonocardiograms from normal and abnormal hearts. (Modified from Guyton, A. C.: *Textbook of Medical Physiology*, 3d ed. [Philadelphia: W. B. Saunders Co., 1966].)

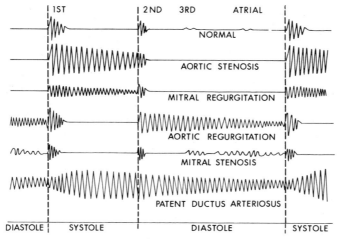

Aortic Stenosis

In aortic stenosis, blood is ejected from the left ventricle through a small opening in the aortic valve. Sometimes as little as 10% of the original aperture is left. Resistance to ejection leads to a very high left-ventricular pressure (450 mm Hg) while the pressure in the aorta remains normal. There is a nozzle effect as the blood jets through the narrow orifice and intense vibrations are set up in the aorta.

Mitral Regurgitation

Mitral regurgitation occurs when the blood flows backward through the mitral valve during systole, creating a high-frequency sound which is actually best heard in the left atrium if an intravascular microphone is used. As stated above, on the chest wall, it is best heard at the apex. The murmur is caused by the "swish" as the blood is driven into the atrium by the force of ventricular systole.

Aortic Regurgitation

Aortic regurgitation is caused by the return of blood from the elastic aorta through the defective valve during diastole. Because the pressures are not as high as in aortic stenosis, the sound is not as loud. However, size of orifice is no measure of intensity of sound; the worst inadequacies of the valves will lead to little resistance to backflow and so to a less impressive sound than a smaller orifice.

Mitral Stenosis

In the common condition of mitral stenosis, there is an obstruction to flow through the orifice so that blood must be forced from the atrium in diastole. The rate of ventricular filling is thus delayed until in the latter part of diastole. The ventricle is stretched enough to permit the system to resonate. The murmur is of such low frequency that often it is more readily felt as a vibration over the apex than it can be heard. In severe cases, there is a prolonged murmur due to the forcing of a jet of blood through the valve aperture in what is—in effect—an intensified third heart sound.

Patent Ductus Arteriosus

If the ductus arteriosus fails to close in infancy, blood ejected by the left ventricle surges through this shunt into the pulmonary artery. The high velocity of flow through the restricted channel into the big pulmonary artery produces continuous turbulence. Unlike the valvular lesions, the murmur is continuous because the pressure differential between aorta and the low-pressure system is a sustained one. Similar continuous murmurs are heard where, as occasionally happens due to injury, an arteriovenous shunt develops between an artery and a vein. These lesions may be quite small and yet produce a lot of noise—examples of the fact that the largest lesions are not necessarily responsible for the loudest murmurs.

Summary

The amount of blood pumped by the heart in unit time depends upon heart rate and stroke volume. Heart rate is determined by the play of sympathetic and vagal influences on the pacemaker cells of the sinoauricular node. The stroke volume is the difference between the diastolic- and systolic-end volumes.

The residual volume of blood retained in the heart by the normal person remains large, and the heart maintains much the same stroke volume despite fluctuations in cardiac output. This is done by varying rate, rather than stroke volume.

Auscultation of the sounds made by the heart in action gives good indications, not only of the major events in the cycle, but of disturbances that often cannot be detected by other means. Phonocardiography also gives valuable physiological information and has the advantage of giving a permanent registration of events that are fleeting, hard to perceive, and difficult to time.

REFERENCES

Gauer, O. H.: Volume Changes of the Left Ventricle during Blood Pooling and Exercise in the Intact Animal, Physiol. Rev. 35:143-155, 1955.

Guyton, A. C.: *Textbook of Medical Physiology*, 3d ed. (Philadelphia: W. B. Saunders Co., 1966).

Keele, C. A., and Neil, E., in Wright, S.: *Applied Physiology*, 11th ed. (New York: Oxford University Press, 1965).

Riecher, G. A., and Galletti, P. M.: Functional Anatomy of Cardiac Pumping, in *Handbook of Physiology: Circulation* (Washington: American Physiological Society, 1962), Chap. 23.

Ruch, T. C., and Patton, H. D.: *Physiology and Biophysics*, 19th ed. (Philadelphia: W. B. Saunders Co., 1965).

Selkurt, E. E.: *Physiology*, 2d ed. (Boston: Little, Brown & Co., 1966).

3

The Heart as a Specialized Muscle

Introduction

THE PRECEDING CHAPTER discussed the mechanical characteristics of the heart as a pump. It outlined the sequence of events in the cycle and pointed to the importance of heart rate in determining cardiac output. This section will consider the heart as a muscle and attempt to interpret its responses in terms of the physiology of muscle in general and of the specializations that have evolved to provide a cyclic operation that can be sustained for many years without pause and yet still remain adaptable to the grossly varying demands of the moment.

Intrinsic and Extrinsic Determinants of Cardiac Function

THE MECHANISM OF MUSCULAR CONTRACTION

Remarkable discoveries in molecular biology during the past few years have confirmed the basic features of H. E. Huxley's brilliant sliding filament concept of the mechanism of contraction of striated muscle. The contractile material consists of a long series of partially overlapping arrays of "thick" (160 Å) myosin and "thin" (50 Å) actin filaments. The cross striations of the muscle, so readily observable with the light microscope, are an expression of their regular arrangement. There are dense A bands, so called because they are strongly anisotropic in polarized light. They contain the myosin filaments, which can be seen in longitudinal electron microscopic sections to be stacked in parallel register. In transverse sections they show up as a tightly packed hexagonal arrangement. The less opaque I bands contain actin filaments extending from a dense, thin z line, through a clear zone, and partly into the A band. Here the actin and myosin filaments overlap. The general arrangement is shown in Fig. 3-1-A.

Because the length of the A band remains constant despite changes in muscle length, it appears that the A filaments do not change length. Since the distance between the Z line and the H-zone edge also stays constant, it was concluded that the same holds for the thin filaments. However, the width of the H zone changes as the muscle contracts and relaxes. Therefore, the hypothesis was put forward and eventually substantiated that changes in muscle length are due to a sliding process in which the adjustment is in the extent of the overlap of the filaments.

Figure 3-1-B shows the situation when the muscle is relaxed and sarcomere length is at a minimum. The first effect of pulling on a muscle in such a state will be to eliminate the overriding of the thin filaments. This will bring the muscle to the optimum point at which there is a maximally effective side-by-side placement of the actin and myosin filaments. Figure 3-1-C shows the filament bundles in a partially extended state, i.e., somewhat past this optimum point. As extension continues still further, shorter and shorter lengths of actin will be exposed to interaction with the myosin until, finally, at extremes of tension, there will be no overlap at all.

Electron microscopy shows that cross-bridges occur at regular intervals between the thick and thin filaments (Fig. 3-1-A). These are the only mechanical linkages between the filaments, and it was concluded that these cross-bridges must generate the tension developed by the muscle.

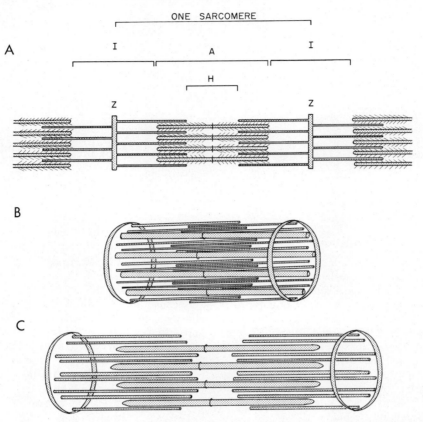

Fig. 3-1.—**A,** Diagram showing the limits of one sarcomere and how the A band composed of thick myosin filaments interdigitates with the I band composed of thinner actin filaments. Limits of the sarcomere are set by the cell membranes, i.e., the Z lines. The fine hairs on the myosin indicate meromyosin cross-bridges (see Fig. 3-2). **B,** Schematic illustration of a muscle fibril in extreme shortening. The actin filaments overlap each other and are therefore doubled in number relative to the myosin for a significant part of their length. **C,** In the prestretched muscle fiber, there is a lower ratio of actin to myosin, and yet individual actin-myosin filaments overlap extensively, presenting near-optimal opportunity for cross-bridge attachment. (Modified from Huxley, H. E.: The Mechanism of Muscular Contraction, Scient. Am. 213:18-24, 1965, and Science 164:1356-1366, 1969. Copyright 1969 by the American Association for the Advancement of Science, Washington, D.C.)

Because in the course of contraction the filaments move great distances, up to 10,000 Å or more, a mechanism was sought by which the relatively short cross-bridges could operate in a cyclic fashion, first attaching to one site on the filament and then detaching and reattaching themselves to a new site farther along.

Figure 3-2 shows a concept recently put forward by H. E. Huxley that suggests one possible form this remarkable mechanochemical conversion apparatus might take. It has been found that the myosin filaments can be split into light and heavy meromyosin halves. The light half has an affinity for other molecules of the same type, and it is bound into myosin filament bundles. The other half, the heavy meromyosin, consists of a 400 Å molecular chain with a 50 Å globular head that has an affinity for actin. One of Huxley's suggestions is that this globular head might be so arranged—perhaps in two subunits—that, during the energy releasing of adenosin triphosphate (ATP), the relative positions of the subunits change. Thus, in moving from contraction phase I to contraction phase II (Fig. 3-2), the release of the ATP's phosphate bond energy may lead to a significant tilt of the globular head, which, however, remains attached to the actin. As a result of the tilt, tension would be exerted on the filamentous linear portion. This would create a shearing force between the actin and myosin filaments. In this way, the chemical energy of the ATP could be converted into a small but significant mechanical movement. The movement could be magnified by repeated formation and breaking of bonds between the actin and myosin at a regular progression of sites, passing up the helical actin molecule. The cycling rate of this "rachet" mechanism would then determine the velocity of shortening of the muscles. On the other hand, the force of contraction would be determined by the total number of cross-bridges acting together at any one moment, i.e., on the extent of filament overlap. This latter is determined by the length of the fiber, i.e., by the initial stretch put on the muscle.

ACTIVATION OF THE CONTRACTILE MECHANISM

The brilliant concepts and related experiments that have led to the proposal of this mechano-chemical device have given clues at the molecular level as to how muscles contract. A further puzzle was how the effects of the nerve impulse could be transmitted to the huge number of filaments that make up the individual sarcomere sufficiently rapidly to account for the speed of a muscle twitch. Recently, electron microscopy has established the existence of a transverse system of impulse-conducting tubules. These are most highly developed in fast-acting muscles, such as those responsible for the bat's ultrasonic squeak. They are extensions of the sarcolemma or cell membrane surrounding the muscle fiber. Their conductive role is suggested by experiments that have shown that ferritin granules will

Fig. 3-2.—Illustrating one of several possible mechanisms for producing relative sliding movement by the tilting of cross-bridges. ATP, derived from the nearby mitochondria and triggered by fibrillar ATPase, provides energy for work by the subdivided tilting globular meromyosin head *(solid arrows).* During relaxation, the head is detached and the connecting heavy meromyosin filament is under no tension. With cycling activity *(contraction I and II),* the heads of the cross-bridges repeatedly attach and tilt, progressing in rachet fashion up the fiber and exerting a shearing force between the myosin and actin.

Initiation and frequency of cycling are determined by Ca^{++} ions whose level in the myoplasm depends on the amount passing through the membrane from the longitudinal elements of sarcoplasmic reticulum. This system is controlled by the cell membrane and its extensions, the transverse tubules, which pass into the fiber depths and transmit effects of the wave of depolarization to the longitudinal elements of the sarcoplasmic reticulum. (Since the distance from the cell membrane to an individual filament can be many thousands of angstroms, this portion is drawn out of scale.) (Modified from Huxley, H. E.: The Mechanism of Muscular Contraction, Science 164:1356-1366, 1969. Copyright 1969 by the American Association for the Advancement of Science, Washington, D.C.)

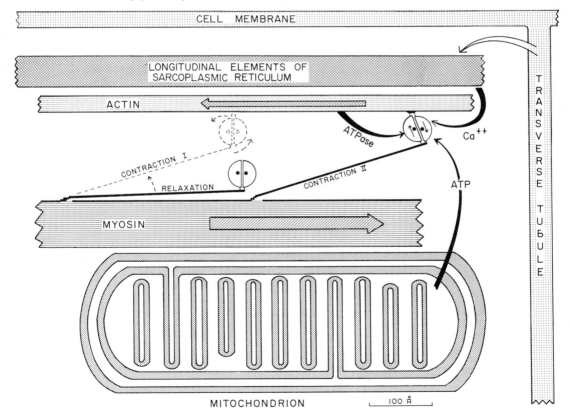

pass rapidly along the special invaginations of this membrane that penetrate into the depths of the fiber in the form of tiny 30 Å transverse tubules. The transverse system serves a supporting longitudinal network that stores calcium and is a powerful Ca^{++} pump. The entire complex facilitates transmission of the effects of the wave of depolarization from the nerve ending on the sarcolemma to all parts of the fiber. As the wave is transmitted by the tubular system, membrane permeability alters in the longitudinal tubules, and free calcium ions appear in the myoplasm or muscle cytoplasm adjacent to the contractile proteins. Contraction is activated when this cation exceeds a critical level in the presence of energy-rich, mitochondrial-produced adenosine triphosphate (ATP) and of the enzyme ATPase, which is intrinsic to the myofibrils (Fig. 3-2).

THE FRANK-STARLING LAW OF THE HEART

The preceding section on the mechanism of muscular contraction points out that the force with which such a system of sliding filaments will contract is determined by the amount of initial overlap. If the overlap is extensive, the redundant actin filaments will interfere with each other, and the force will be less than maximal. If the fiber is stretched far enough, the cross-bridging between myosin and actin will eventually diminish, and less force will be generated. Hence, the force generated will at first rise, then reach a maximum, and, finally, as the stretch becomes excessive, the strength of contraction will fall off. The sliding-filament model of the mechanism of muscle contraction explains this curve, confirming and explaining in molecular terms the conclusions reached in studies with skeletal muscles and with isolated hearts nearly a century ago.

Figure 3-3 shows on the left the effects of the progressive stretching of an isolated strip of human muscle and illustrates the fundamental relationship between the tension developed during maximum voluntary effort and the initial length. At first, the maximum active tension increases dramatically with slight increases in resting length; later, the increase is more gradual until a peak is attained, after which there is actually a falling off as the tension develops. At the turn of the century, the German investigator Otto Frank and the English physiologist Ernest Starling showed, in their respective ingenious experiments with cold-blooded animals and with dogs, that the same principles apply to the heart and that the contractile tension developed during systole depends on the preceding ventricular diastolic volume. The right-hand diagram of Figure 3-3 shows that this response is so sensitive that minute changes in filling pressure are responsible for great increases in stroke work.

Starling studied this relationship between length of fiber and strength of contraction of the heart with his "heart-lung" preparation. Using artificial respiration, the thorax was opened widely and the dog's major vessels were canulated so that the blood flowed from the aorta through tubing and reservoirs to the right atrium and thence through the heart and back to the aorta. By changing the caliber of the outflow tubing, the "peripheral resistance" and hence

Fig. 3-3.—This diagram illustrates that the responses of both skeletal and ventricular muscles to a stimulus are similarly determined by the initial stretch of the fibers.

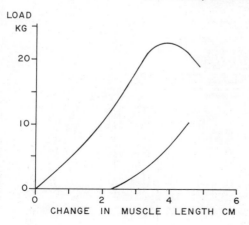
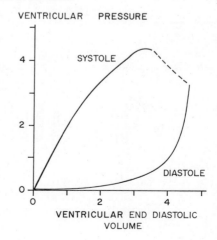

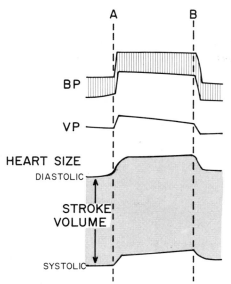

Fig. 3-4.—*A*, Effect of increasing arterial resistance on pressures in a heart-lung preparation. At *B*, the resistance was reduced to its previous level. (From Ganong, W. F.: *Review of Medical Physiology*, 3d ed. [Los Altos, Calif.: Lange Medical Publishers, 1967].)

the blood pressure could be varied. By raising or lowering the reservoir emptying into the right atrium, the venous filling could be changed. Finally, by enclosing the ventricles in a cardiometer cup, the volume changes of the combined ventricles could be measured throughout the cardiac cycle.

As early as 1914, Starling formulated the following generalization that carries his name: "The law of the heart is the same as the law of initial length for skeletal muscle. The strength of contraction is a function of muscle fiber length, i.e., stroke volume is directly proportional to diastolic filling." Using the heart-lung preparation, he showed that, at higher end-diastolic volumes, the peak isovolumetric pressure increases (Fig. 3-3). Just as the tension developed by skeletal muscle increases when its initial length is increased, so the increase of heart filling causes the pressure upon the heart's contents to rise. If peripheral resistance also increased, then the end-systolic and end-diastolic volumes both increased. The heart beat more vigorously, and a new level of blood pressure was established (Fig. 3-4).

The work done by the ventricle is determined by the force against which it is pumping and the volume of the blood pumped. In the Starling preparation, this can be approximated by the product of stroke volume times pressure; in Figure 3-3, the two curves for skeletal and heart muscle are seen to be similar. If this measure of work output of the ventricle is plotted against the left-ventricular end-diastolic pressure or, in fact, filling pressure anywhere in the low-pressure system (for example, in the right atrium), then a curve will be obtained (Fig. 3-5). This basal curve can be determined in the intact organism by appropriately varying the pressures in the low-pressure system by graded transfusion and hemorrhage. By this means, heart rate, blood pressure, and cardiac output data can be obtained, and one can measure the left-ventricular stroke work under basal conditions for the cardiovascular system.

The important Frank-Starling observation that the strength of contraction is determined by the initial fiber length is termed heterometric autoregulation. It is described as autoregulation because it is an intrinsic response of the isolated ventricle, and heterometric because the fiber length must be altered to gain an effect. In normal physiologic processes, it is one of the mechanisms that comes into play to increase heart output during severe exertion, for this is an occasion when the filling pressure of the vigorously contracting heart is usually increased. It probably also has a role in balancing the outputs of the right and left ventricles in the normal animal; for, if the right ventricle pumps more blood than the left, the difference must accumulate in the lung reservoir, and pulmonary venous pressure will rise. The resulting increased diastolic filling of the left ventricle will result in an increase of its output, so correcting the right-left imbalance.

Exceptions to the Law of the Heart

Starling's basic concept points to the dependence of force generation on myofilament overlap —that is, on the length of the contractile element. But there are limitations to a view of the dynamics of cardiac function that places emphasis on this admittedly important intrinsic property of heart muscle. Muscle physiologists have expended much effort on a second critical characteristic of muscle: its contractility or the kinetics of the active process of contraction. In order to dissociate the two, attempts have been made to set up experimental conditions that will permit study of the active state without complication by dimensional changes of the contractile elements.

Starling himself once wrote: "Broadly speaking, there are two main avenues of approach in the attempt to unravel the complicated processes

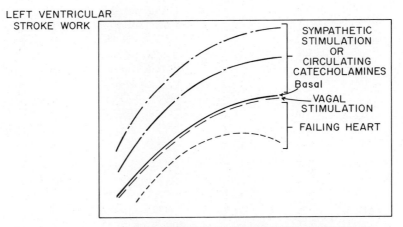

Fig. 3-5.—Ventricular function curve. The inotropic effect of sympathetic agents alters the curves relating stroke work (stroke volume times mean systolic blood pressure) and left-ventricular end-diastolic pressure. Under normal conditions, there is some minor sympathetic activity that sustains the cardiac function curve above basal levels. (From Selkurt, E. E. (ed.): *Physiology*, 2d ed. [Boston: Little, Brown & Co., 1966].)

which determine the function of any individual organ. On the one hand, we may study its reaction in the intact animal to comparatively small environmental changes—a method of inestimable value since it is one which may readily be applied to man; on the other hand, we may remove the organ and study its reaction under grossly artificial conditions." The Starling heart-lung preparation is an example of the latter; Rushmer, whose recent work with the intact animal is already a cardiologic classic, has detailed the objections that apply to it.

To mention only three:

1. The rest of the animal is dead, eliminating all nervous and hormonal control.
2. The cardiometer covers the whole apex and does not distinguish between the two ventricles.
3. The chest is open, disturbing pressure relations significantly.

Rushmer's own work was with active normal animals, and the picture that developed was a different one. In contradistinction to the effect to be anticipated from application of the "law of the heart," the initial length of the fibers seemed to be ignored by the healthy, conscious, active animal, and large changes in atrial filling pressure occurred without alterations of cardiac output. Indeed, heart size including end-diastolic volume was near maximum in the resting state. In fact, the increase in cardiac output with increased venous filling is due to an increased heart rate and is actually accompanied by a decreased end-systolic volume. Rushmer attributed the greater vigor of myocardial contraction to increased sympathetic activity. He noted that, despite huge changes in cardiac output, i.e., in the work of the heart, stroke volume was little affected. Indeed, as the legend to Figure 3-5 indicates, the basal curve can be affected by a number of different factors, the most important being sympathetic stimulation, which significantly increases stroke work, and vagus control, which decreases it somewhat.

It is true that the initial length of the fiber at the beginning of contraction will determine the force of systole; so, the higher the end-diastolic filling pressure, the greater the force of contraction. This gives the classic curve shown in Figure 3-3, which is also the curve described as basal in Figure 3-5. Rising steeply at first, it then flattens out with extremes of diastolic filling. However, as Figure 3-5 indicates, a whole family of left-ventricular stroke-work curves can be obtained as a result of the effects of various agents upon the contractility of the muscle.

For example, the nutrition of the muscle cells by the coronary blood supply must be sufficient in volume and in oxygen content or power will fail, leading to a curve that falls below the basal value. Nutrients such as glucose and the calcium and potassium ions must be in proper balance, and there should be no directly deleterious influence such as bacterial toxins or disease such as rheumatic fever. The curve decreases with vagal stimulation, which has a modest negative inotropic effect. In the failing heart, the curve flattens and the reversal of slope occurs at a lower end-diastolic pressure. On the other hand, stroke work for a given end-diastolic pressure will increase greatly as a result of the inotropic stimulation that occurs with activation of the sympathetic system, with an increase of circulating catecholamines, and with certain drugs such as digitalis.

Thus long ago it became clear that it is not possible to explain the performance of the human heart if one holds too rigidly to the classic framework of the Frank-Starling mechanism. The heart cannot be considered a disconnected muscle in which cardiac output is related primarily to filling pressure. Such a view overemphasizes the role of initial muscle length and does not sufficiently consider another critical dimension of myocardial response—that is, the effects of various nervous and hormonal agents upon its contractility (Fig. 3-5).

Studies of the Contractility of Isolated Cardiac Muscle

Recently, Sonnenblick and Braunwald and their associates at the National Institutes of Health completed a challenging series of investigations that used both of Starling's "avenues of approach." Their work involved isolated papillary muscle, animal hearts, and, finally, the "intact animal," the patient himself. They looked at the dynamics of the heart from the viewpoint of the factors that influence the time course and velocity of contraction as the muscle works against a load. Their studies of the heart as a muscle focus about an approach first outlined by A. V. Hill in his presentation of the force-velocity relationship and by his ensuing studies of the active state or the factors governing force development at constant contractile element length. This pioneer muscle physiologist showed that the velocity of shortening in skeletal muscle is lower when the load is greater, and vice versa. The same facts apply to cardiac muscle. However, there are differences between the velocity responses of the two. For any given length, the activity of individual skeletal muscle fibers remains unchanged, and the muscle force is increased by recruiting more fibers. On the other hand, the active state or contractility of heart muscle is highly variable. It is affected by the length of the contractile elements, by velocity, and by load, and is under constant control of inotropic agents such as nor-epinephrine and of sympathetic nervous activity.

Sonnenblick attempted to disentangle the complex interplay of the influences of initial fiber length or preload and of inotropic agents affecting the active state (contractility) of cardiac muscle. His studies of the isolated papillary muscle from the cat used a modification of an experimental approach made familiar by the muscle physiologists Abbott and Mommaerts (Fig. 3-6).

In the isolated muscle preparation, an adjustable stop determines the initial length of the papillary muscle while it is at rest and sets the preloading tension. With contraction, the afterload is lifted, following an insignificant degree of shortening. Tracings at the bottom of the

Fig. 3-6.—**Left,** Diagram of method of study of the afterloaded isotonic contraction of papillary muscle. The initial length of the muscle is set by adjustment of the preloading stop above the lever and is held constant by it. As the muscle attempts to shorten, it picks up the afterload. **Right,** A typical afterloaded contraction, stimulation at time zero. Tension rises sharply, but no shortening occurs until the afterload has been picked up. The muscle then shortens with constant tension, rapidly at first, then reaching a plateau, i.e., ΔL, and finally falling off. The tangent to the initial stage of the shortening trace denotes dl/dt the initial velocity of shortening. (From Sonnenblick, E. H.: The Mechanics of Myocardial Contraction, in Briller, S. A., and Conn, H. L. [eds.]: *The Myocardial Cell* [Philadelphia: University of Pennsylvania Press, 1966].)

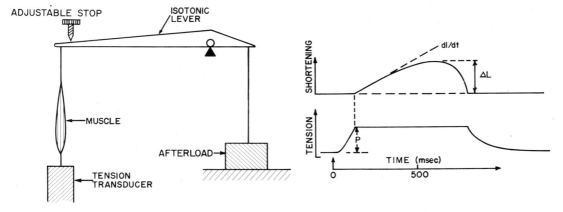

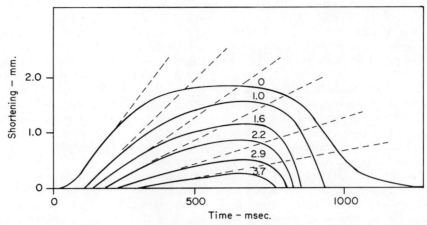

Fig. 3-7.—A sample of heart muscle (papillary), held at constant length in the apparatus shown in Figure 3-6, shows progressively longer isometric phases as the time to the onset of shortening is delayed by the increasing load on the muscle. The initial velocity of shortening is depicted by the dashed tangent to the base of each. The velocity decreases with increasing load. (From Sonnenblick, E. H.: The Mechanics of Myocardial Contraction, in Briller, S. A., and Conn, H. L. [eds.]: *The Myocardial Cell* [Philadelphia: University of Pennsylvania Press, 1966].)

figure show how the tension rises during the isometric phase up to the point at which the afterload is picked up at P. From then on, the tension line remains at a plateau until it tapers off again as the muscle relaxes and the tension sinks to the preload level. The upper curve shows that, while the tension is rising, there is an initial isometric period until the afterload is lifted. Shortening follows, proceeding rapidly at first, and then more slowly. It reaches a plateau and then falls off with the end of the contraction as the afterload is returned and the tension released.

Figure 3-7 is derived from the study of a series of contractions in which the initial length as determined by the preload was kept constant, but the afterload was increased in six stages. The velocity of shortening, i.e., dl/dt (see Fig. 3-6), was high when the afterload was low, but, as the load increased, the initial velocity decreased. This velocity is expressed in Figures 3-6 and 3-7 as the dotted tangent to the initiation of the curve. If the initial velocities of shortening indicated by the six dotted tangents of Figure 3-7 are plotted against the afterloads responsible for their particular curves, then the control force-velocity curve plotted with open circles in Figure 3-8 is obtained. In this curve, the theoretically highest velocity of shortening Vmax is obtained by extrapolating the curve back to zero loading. At the other end of the scale, as force increases to the maximum that the muscle can just lift, the initial velocity of shortening becomes zero and the curve cuts the abscissa at this maximum load.

Thus force and velocity of shortening are inversely related.

If, in an extension of Figure 3-8, control, the

Fig. 3-8.—The effect on the force-velocity relationship of the addition of nor-epinephrine. Initial velocity of shortening is plotted as a function of afterload (see Fig. 3-7). There is an increase in contractility over the control curve; the maximal velocity of shortening increases as well as the force. (From Braunwald, E., Ross, J., Jr., and Sonnenblick, E. H.: *Mechanisms of Contraction of the Normal and Failing Heart*, [Boston: Little, Brown & Co., 1968].)

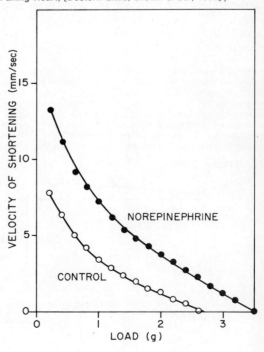

initial velocity of shortening in mm/sec, is plotted against load for a number of different preloading conditions (i.e., for a number of initial fiber lengths), a fresh series of curves will be obtained (Fig. 3-9). Each will range from the maximum velocity Vmax attained at zero load to various maximum tensions that cut the abscissa at points of progressively increasing load. As is indicated by the insert derived from the same data but depicting force, i.e., load versus length, this experiment also demonstrates the Frank-Starling response; i.e., with increasing preload, there is an increase in actively developed force in response to the change of initial fiber length. (Note the similarity between the curves in the insert and those shown in Figure 3-3.)

Sonnenblick reports an important consistency in the curves on the left of Figure 3-9. Under the circumstances of his experiment, despite the progressive increase in the maximum tension generated, the peak velocity of shortening attained by the muscle is not greatly changed, regardless of intial fiber length. As the preloading of the muscle diagrammed in Figure 3-9 was increased, there was a progressive increase in the maximum force of contraction, that is, of the points of intersection of the curves with the abscissa. But, in addition, on extrapolation of the curves back to zero load, they approximated the same point on the ordinate. This led to his suggestion that Vmax could serve as a measure of the inotropic state of cardiac muscle. Supporting this, in Figure 3-8, nor-epinephrine shows the unquestioned change in the relationship between velocity of shortening and load that occurs under the influence of an inotropic agent. Here, not only is the point of intersection of the curve with the abscissa, i.e., the maximum force of contraction, increased, but extrapolation back to zero load shows that Vmax, the peak velocity of shorten-

Fig. 3-9.—Effects of increasing initial muscle length on the force-velocity relationship. Initial velocity of shortening (see Fig. 3-7) is plotted as a function of afterload for each curve; successive curves are obtained with progressively greater preloads. The insert plotting preload against the maximum force developed relates the study to the classic Frank-Starling curve (see Fig. 3-3). Note that under the circumstances of this experiment, although maximum load increases with initial muscle length, approximately the same maximum velocity (Vmax) is obtained on extrapolating the curve back to zero load. (From Sonnenblick, E. H.: The Mechanics of Myocardial Contraction, in Briller, S. A., and Conn, M. L. [eds.]: *The Myocardial Cell* [Philadelphia: University of Pennsylvania Press, 1966].)

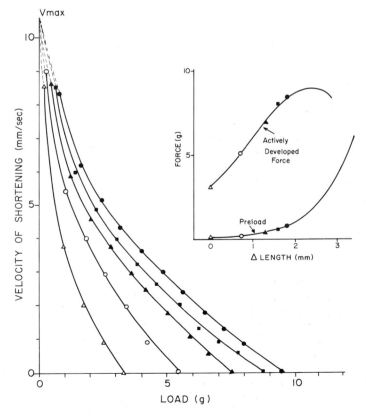

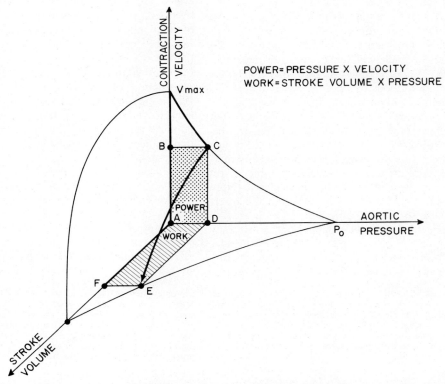

Fig. 3-10.—The force-velocity-volume relationship diagram for a single ventricle. The horizontal axis to the right is afterload or aortic pressure. The vertical axis is velocity of contraction, and the horizontal axis down and to the left is decrease in length or stroke volume. The heavy line represents a single contraction followed through the cycle. After stimulation at initial length (A), Vmax was reached, followed by a decrease in velocity (see Fig. 3-6) as force increased isometrically. At C, the aortic valves open and load remains constant while shortening occurs and velocity falls to zero (E). Pressure then falls to diastolic values (F) and length increases with diastolic filling in the return to A. Power is represented by pressure times velocity (ABDC) and work by stroke volume times pressure (ADEF). (From Sonnenblick, E. H.: The Mechanics of Myocardial Contraction, in Briller, S. A., and Conn, H. L. [eds.]: *The Myocardial Cell* [Philadelphia: University of Pennsylvania Press, 1966].)

ing, i.e., contractility itself, has been very greatly enhanced. Such massive upward shifts of muscle Vmax are accepted by muscle physiologists as a normal sequel to the enhancement of the inotropic level of the contractile elements.

Variations in Contractility Versus Effects of Preloading

A consideration of these results in terms of the mechanics of muscle fiber contraction discussed earlier in this chapter indicates that the mechanisms that underlie the increased force of muscle action associated with increased preloading stretch differ fundamentally from those underlying the increased contractility of inotropic action. It was pointed out that, as muscle fibers are stretched by the increased preloading, there is a decrease in the normal overlapping of the indistensible thin actin and thick myosin filaments that comprise the power source of the muscle (Fig. 3-1). This has the effect of increasing the number of sites at which the molecular rearrangements involved in the contractile process can occur; the more sites, the greater the over-all force with which the muscle fibers contract. Since force × distance is work, this explains the Frank-Starling increase in ventricular stroke work as diastolic filling increases. On the other hand, increased contractility is associated with changes in level of calcium ions at the myofilament. This results from inotropic action playing upon the muscle from the outside. It changes the force-velocity curve itself and greatly affects power or rate of doing work. It has been suggested that the molecular basis of changes in contractility is a change in the cycling rate of the force-generating processes at the sites of energy transfer within the contractile elements. It would appear that these can occur in independence of the extent of filament overlap, i.e., of the muscle length at which shortening begins. This would seem to be the phenomenon underlying Rushmer's observations in freely running dogs whose hearts changed force under the influence of a change in sympathetic drive and failed to adhere to the expectation that force of contraction would be determined by filling pressure during diastole.

Diagrams of the Force-Velocity-Length Relationship

These findings point up the desirability of adding velocity to the two-dimensional Frank-Starling muscle length-force relationship. This can be done by using a three-dimensional diagram in which force-velocity-length relationships are plotted for the intact heart. In Figure 3-10, the horizontal axis to the right represents myocardial force, i.e., aortic pressure. This is the equivalent of the afterload of the isolated papillary muscle experiment. The vertical axis represents initial velocity, i.e., Vmax or contractility, and the horizontal axis down and to the left is decrease of fiber length or stroke volume from the initial (preloaded) or end-diastolic state.

In these diagrams, the lines joining the contraction velocity with the aortic pressure curves are force-velocity curves similar to Figure 3-9 for the isolated papillary muscle. Those joining aortic pressure with stroke volume are the classic length-tension Frank-Starling curves (Fig. 3-3). As the cardiac cycle begins at point A on the heavy line, the maximal shortening velocity Vmax is quickly attained. As tension increases

Fig. 3-11.—A three-dimensional plot of the force-velocity-length relationship of the ventricle, showing the effect of an increase in contractility from $Vmax_1$ to $Vmax_2$ on stroke volume (AH to AI), stroke work (ADGH to ADJI), peak power (ABCD to AFED), and the maximum developed tension (PO_1 to PO_2). (From Sonnenblick, E. H.: The Mechanics of Myocardial Contraction, in Briller, S. A., and Conn, H. L. [eds.]: *The Myocardial Cell* [Philadelphia: University of Pennsylvania Press, 1966].)

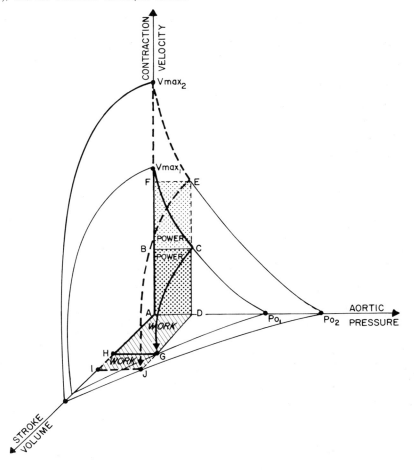

during this isometric phase of contraction, the velocity of shortening of the contractile elements decreases. At C, the aortic valve opens, and a point is reached equivalent to the moment on the papillary muscle contraction curve when the force equals the afterload (see Fig. 3-6, point P). In this case, the afterload is aortic pressure. This remains relatively constant; from C to E, velocity decreases as stroke volume is ejected, and muscle shortening occurs. From E to F, the tension falls off as the aortic valves snap shut; during the diastolic phase, F to A, the muscle lengthens back to its initial value. The area ADEF represents the Frank-Starling stroke work performance, while ABCD represents the peak power generated during contraction, i.e., the maximum rate at which work is done.

The three-dimensional Figure 3-11 shows the effect of increased myocardial contractility induced by cardiac sympathetic nerve stimulation or by the release of the catecholamines, epinephrine or nor-epinephrine. As contractility increased from $Vmax_1$ to $Vmax_2$, the isovolumetric peak force rose from PO_1 to PO_2. (See Fig. 3-8 where the nor-epinephrine curve cuts the abscissa at a greater load than the control.) Peak power increased from ABCD to AFED, and, since stroke volume increased from AH to AI, stroke work grows from ADGH to ADJI. End-diastolic volume, i.e., the initial fiber length, is unchanged because the cardiac muscle is undergoing an increase in contractility. However, similar diagrams can be drawn to show the effects of a change in end-diastolic volume or of aortic pressure. For more detailed presentations, the texts of Braunwald, Sonnenblick, and Berne and Levy should be consulted.

Work Versus Power

Thus the significance of the experimentally based observations made with isolated strips in the laboratory by various muscle physiologists finally becomes apparent. Force-velocity curves provide the data to determine the power or rate of doing work, as well as the work itself—the latter is the integral of the force exerted by the contractile element over distance. In the Starling analysis, the work done was the major consideration. Studies of the active state emphasize power or rate of working as a further important quantity that is tied to the variable contractility characteristics of heart muscle.

As an illustration of the relationship between power and work, consider the crew of a racing shell. At any particular speed of the boat, the rate at which the oar blades impact with and drive through the water is a measure of the power of the crew. The greater their power, the shorter the period of pulling on the oars and the longer the time available to them for relaxed respiration and effective muscle perfusion during their slow forward movement preparatory to the next stroke. As long as the mean velocity of the boat is constant, the work done in propelling it will be the same whether the men take a long or a short time to accomplish the stroke. But the longer the crew takes to drive its blades through the water, the less time, at a given rate of striking, does it have for the recovery period of the forward glide.

Clinical Aspects of Contractility Studies

There are significant clinical applications of the above studies in terms of methods of evaluating the myocardial contractile state. Braunwald points out that the relationship between velocity of shortening of the contractile elements and muscle tension is a sensitive index of cardiac function. Using cineangiograms to determine the mechanical characteristics of ventricular contraction, Gault, Ross, and Braunwald have plotted rate of change of circumference against left-ventricular wall tension at the moment when this is highest during ejection (see Fig. 3-12). Estimates of the contractile state based on these measurements were consistently reduced in a group of patients with left-ventricular deficiency due to coronary artery disease, mitral stenosis, etc. It was concluded that, when the myocardium is failing, there is a reduction of the rate of wall shortening at any given level of tension. Despite this, in some cases the levels of cardiac output were normal. To the authors, this suggested that the tension-velocity relationship is more sensitive than the mere measurement of the resting output. Another valuable measure of the contractile state of the ventricle is the rate of rise of ventricular pressure.

Not surprisingly, myocardial oxygen consumption is closely linked to the contractile state of the myocardium and to its capacity to develop tension. Any enhancement of these parameters is accompanied by an increase in the requirements for oxygen. In keeping with this, when the level of catecholamines or sympathetic discharge increases the contractility of a myocardium suffering from ischemic hypoxia, it is not surprising

THE HEART AS A SPECIALIZED MUSCLE

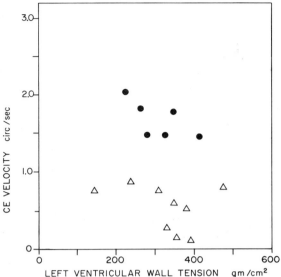

Fig. 3-12.—The contractile state of the left ventricle in patients with normal left ventricular (LV) function *(solid circles)* is contrasted with those with LV disease. *Ordinate:* Maximum velocity of circumferential fiber shortening in circumferences/sec. *Abscissa:* Maximum LV wall tension in G/cm². (From Gault, J. H., Ross, J. Jr., and Braunwald, E.: Contractile State of the Left Ventricle in Man, Circulation Res. 22:459, 1968. By permission of the American Heart Association, New York.)

that anginal symptoms should so frequently develop.

Summary

The energetics of the heart muscle are determined by two basic aspects of contractility. The first is the relationship described by Frank and by Starling showing that the strength of contraction is determined by the initial fiber length. The sliding-filament hypothesis has established the molecular basis for this important intrinsic characteristic. The second factor is Hill's concept of the "active state" or force development at constant contractile element length. The faster the muscle works at any given strength of contraction, the greater is the contractility or power developed. The heart is closely tied through this parameter to the rest of the organism, for one of the variables reflected by the myocardial contractility at any particular instant is the concentration of ionized calcium in the myoplasm, and this, in turn, is determined by nervous and hormonal influences. The sympathetic and vagus nerves, the cardiac glycosides, and the sympathomimetic amines appear to derive their positive or negative effects from the changes they induce in the intracellular concentration of this ion.

The Special Conducting System and the Electrocardiogram

Differences Between Skeletal and Cardiac Muscle

The special features that distinguish cardiac muscle include its submaximal contractile state and capacity to respond to inotropic influences by varying its contractility. Other points of differentiation are that cardiac muscle has a long refractory period and cannot be tetanized, and that 40% by weight consists of noncontractile structures such as mitochondria and nuclei, as compared with 10% for skeletal muscle. Sonnenblick points out that this, together with the fact that cardiac contractility is normally less than maximum, explains why heart muscle appears to be weaker. When taken with the profuse capillary network, these features ensure an adequate supply of metabolites for the molecular processes of contraction and represent adaptations in the interests of endurance and reliability.

Cardiac muscle further differs from skeletal in that the membranes of individual fibers become fixed to their neighbors for some distance. This provides a low-resistance "intercalated disc" that permits excitation to spread laterally from one fiber to another, so that the entire piece of muscle behaves functionally as if it were a syncytium. Ions, on the other hand, can pass with ease down the long axis of the fibers, permitting action potentials to proceed freely.

The Excitatory and Conductive System of the Heart

A further specialization is the excitatory and conductive muscle tissue that times and controls the cycle of contraction. The heart has a built-in system that usurps for this particular organ the impulse-conducting and regulatory function of nervous tissue. It originates the impulse and then organizes its passage through the myocardial mass, so that contraction occurs with a timing and in a sequence best suited for the action of the pump.

As Figure 3-13 indicates, impulses generated in the sinoauricular node (SA node) pass through the atrial muscle to an atrioventricular node (AV node) and thence through the bundle of His and its right and left bundle branches to the

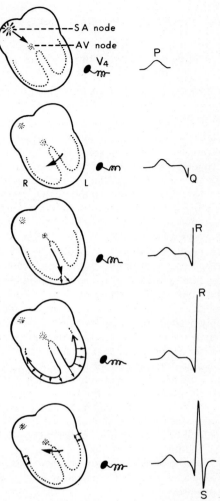

Fig. 3-13.—Normal spread of electrical activity in the heart. From above, downward: *first*, atrial activation; *second*, septal activation from left to right; *third*, activation of anteroseptal region of the ventricular myocardium; *fourth*, activation of major portion of ventricular myocardium from endocardial surfaces; *fifth*, late activation of posterobasal portion of the left ventricle and the pulmonary conus. The stage of the V4 electrocardiogram corresponding to the instant represented by the drawing is presented on the right-hand side of each figure. (From Goldman, M. J.: *Principles of Clinical Electrocardiography*, 6th ed. [Los Altos, Calif.: Lange Medical Publications, 1967].)

Purkinje system. Because muscle acts as a single syncytium, the stimulation of any single atrial fiber induces an action potential that passes over the entire atrial mass. Similarly, stimulation of any ventricular fiber causes the excitation of the whole muscle. If the special conducting tissue is working, an atrial contraction will then be followed by a full ventricular systole. The mechanism is an extension of the all-or-nothing principle that applies to individual skeletal muscle fibers, but the heart muscle contracts as one unit because the interconnections between the fibers permit depolarization to spread. Both skeletal and cardiac muscle have a resting membrane potential of approximately 80 mv with a total action potential of about 105 mv (Fig. 3-14). The transmembrane action potential of an individual cardiac muscle fiber depolarizes with normal speed, but repolarizes far more slowly than skeletal muscle, eliminating the chances of a tetanic contraction. Thus, after each impulse, the membrane potential reverses and repolarization commences. Typical cardiac muscles from different regions of the heart (i.e., the atria, the ventricles, and the conducting tissue) differ significantly in the rate at which depolarization occurs (Fig. 3-14A and B). In all cases, there is a plateau phase before repolarization is rapidly completed. Atrial cells (At) show smaller and ventricular and conducting tissue cells larger plateaus during which the fiber is refractory to stimulus. In the impulse-generating SA and AV nodes, as Figure 3-14-C shows, the entire process of repolarization is gradual, without a plateau and sudden drop. In the atrial fiber (At), the resting potential stays constant until excitation occurs from the outside. But, in the automatic fibers, there is a steady, continuous diastolic repolarization. The result is that the potential builds slowly up to the threshold, and the cell repeats the cycle. This capacity to develop spontaneous depolarization and rhythmic discharge is probably inherent in all heart muscle, but the rapidly declining, unstable membrane potential of the nodal tissue gives it a far more rapid cycling rate than the rest of the heart. It is because of this that changes in the transmembrane potential of the pacemaker cells in the nodes determine the rhythm of the heart. Factors such as autonomic changes not only affect the contractility, excitability, and conduction processes, they also influence the magnitude of the resting potential and the level of the threshold potential (Fig. 3-14-D). By influencing the rate of depolarization, they thus affect the frequency of automatic rhythmic firing.

The anatomical distribution of this rhythmic pacemaker muscle and the special conducting tissues that spread the impulse in its proper sequence, first over the atria and then through the ventricles, is highly appropriate for their

THE HEART AS A SPECIALIZED MUSCLE

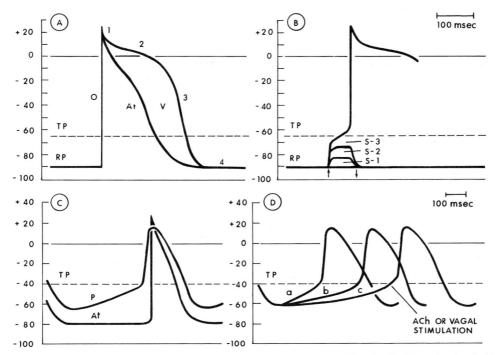

Fig. 3-14.—A: Record of membrane potentials obtained from an atrial fiber *(At)* and a ventricular fiber *(V)*. Note the rapid depolarization *(O)*, the plateauing in the depolarized state *(2)*, repolarization *(3)*, threshold potential *(TP)*, and resting potential *(RP)*.
B: Application of progressively increased cathodal stimuli to cardiac fibers. With a threshold stimulus *(S-3)*, the all-or-none action potential is produced.
C: Progressive self-depolarization occurs in automatic fibers such as the AV node *(P)*. When the threshold level of depolarization is reached, excitation occurs. The atrial fiber *(At)* does not show this progressive change.
D: Epinephrine *(a)* increases the rate by increasing the slope of the diastolic depolarization over that of the control *(b)*. Vagal stimulation *(c)* slows heart rate by decreasing the slope. (From Hoffman, B. F.: in Luisada, A. A. (ed.): *Cardiology: An Encyclopedia of the Cardiovascular System* [New York: McGraw-Hill Book Co., Inc., 1959].)

respective controlling roles. The impulses start with the sinoatrial (SA) node, a crescent-shaped piece of muscle composed of very small caliber fibers that is located at the junction of the superior vena cava with the right atrium. The atrioventricular (AV) node is located in the right posterior part of the interatrial septum, and no special conducting tissue joins the two. However, atrial fibers converge upon and interdigitate with those of the AV node. The latter is continuous with the bundle of His (Fig. 3-15) that divides at the top of the interventricular septum into right and left branches. These run subendocardially down the septum and join the Purkinje system, whose fibers spread to all parts of the ventricular myocardium. Purkinje tissue differs from cardiac muscle in that the fibers are larger, the central cytoplasm has a number of nuclei, and there is more glycogen and peripheral sarcoplasm.

The SA node has the above-mentioned property of permitting decay of the resting membrane potential so that an automatic rhythmic process of firing occurs. During atrial systole, these rhythmic impulses are conducted by the atrial muscle at 0.3 meter/sec toward the AV node. Once the impulse is picked up by the AV node, a complex of events occurs as its passage to the bundle of His is subjected to a timed delay by very small junctional fibers connecting the atrial muscle to the nodal tissue. Thus, whereas the time taken for excitation to pass from the SA to the AV node is only 0.04 sec, another 0.11 sec elapses before the impulse emerges in the AV bundle. Figure 3-15 illustrates this in a diagrammatic form. Potentials were recorded extracellularly at the number of sites about the AV node. The arrows connect the appropriate points in the electrocardiogram with the progression of the impulse. The spike from the atrial muscle

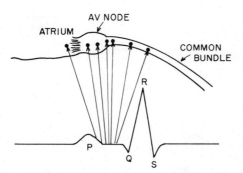

Fig. 3-15.—Diagram correlating the timing of events in the electrocardiogram with the extracellular potentials that develop as the wave of excitation moves from the atrium, through the AV node, into the common bundle. A large part of the time between the end of the P wave and the beginning of the QRS complex is taken up by the passage through the AV node. (From Scher, A. M., et al.: The Mechanism of Atrioventricular Conduction, Circulation Res. 7:54-61, 1959. By permission of the American Heart Association, New York.)

upstream from the AV node occurs during the downstroke of the P wave. A large part of the interval between the end of the P wave and the beginning of the QRS complex is occupied by events in the AV nodal region. Once in the AV bundle, the large fibers of the Purkinje system hurry the impulse at velocities sixfold that of normal cardiac muscle. Their distribution in the ventricular wall, starting at the tip and running back to the base, combined with the high conduction velocity, ensures an almost simultaneous contraction of the whole ventricular muscle mass.

The amphibian heart can be used to demonstrate this remarkable system. By tying a "Stannius" ligature around the sinus venosus (the homologue of the SA node), it can be cut off from the atria. The sinus will continue to beat at the same rate as before, but the atria and ventricles, after a period of arrest, will start at a slower pace initiated by the atrium that is now responding to its own "ectopic" focus. If a second "Stannius" ligature is tied in the groove between atria and ventricle, the ventricle eventually may start on its own still-slower idioventricular rhythm. These famous experiments demonstrate that the nodes set the pace merely because they are contracting faster than the spontaneous rhythm of the undifferentiated cardiac tissue around them. If another part of the heart develops a rhythmic discharge rate faster than that of the SA node, as, for example, if the AV node develops increased excitability, then the pacemaking function will shift to the "ectopic" region. In mammals, these "Stannius" experiments are not possible because the ligature cuts off the coronary circulation on which the muscle depends. However, in the course of disease, conducting tissues can be damaged in various localities, creating the effect of the ligature, and appropriate rate changes with evidence of so-called heart block will then be observed.

The Electrocardiogram

A large proportion of our population suffers from coronary artery disease and will eventually need the diagnostic and therapeutic resources of the cardiologist. The electrocardiogram transmitted by telephone and the telemetered monitoring of the exercising patient are becoming routine practice. The defibrillator, the pacemaker, lidocaine, procaine, and quinidine, and other drugs are extensively employed, together with monitoring in coronary-care units. These developments point to the increasing importance to the physician of a thorough knowledge of the principles of electrocardiography, that is, a knowledge

Fig. 3-16.—Comparing timing of the membrane potential of a single ventricular myocardial fiber with the action potential recorded at the surface of the body, i.e., with the electrocardiogram. Transmembrane alteration of intracellular and extracellular cation concentration is also shown. Depolarization (DE) is accompanied by a shift of Na+ into the cell and a sudden rise in potential (spike action potential). During repolarization (REPOL), K+ leaves the cell. (From Mason, D. T., Spann, J. F., Jr., and Zelis, R.: New Developments in the Understanding of the Actions of the Digitalis Glycosides, Progr. Cardiovasc. Dis. 11:464, 1969. By permission of Grune & Stratton, Inc., New York.)

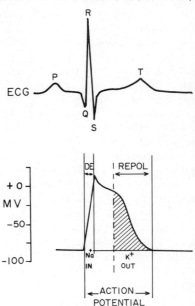

of how to make and interpret a graphic record of the electrical activity of the heart. This record reflects the sum total of electrical events associated with cardiac excitation. It owes its existence to the fortunate circumstance that the body functions as a volume conductor, making it easy to record these internal events by leads applied to the skin. Figure 3-16 compares the events of such an electrocardiogram taken from the surface of the body with the electrical activity of a myocardial fiber as recorded by transmembrane electrodes. The QRS complex signals the moment of depolarization, i.e., of activation, of the myocardial cell, and the T wave is coincident with the process of repolarization.

In 1901, William Einthoven, who had developed the string galvonometer, demonstrated the possibility of applying electrocardiography to clinical medicine. He invented and was responsible for the standardization of the three limb leads and he introduced his triangle concept of the electrical axis of the heart (Fig. 3-17).

Einthoven's hypotheses include the following assumptions:

1. The right arm, left arm, and left leg form the apexes of an equilateral triangle in which the

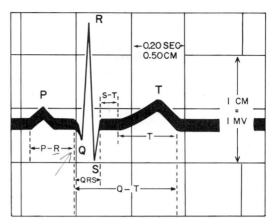

Fig. 3-18.—The normal electrocardiogram showing the time relationships. (From Burch, G. E., and Winsor, T.: *A Primer of Electrocardiography*, 5th ed. [Philadelphia: Lea & Febiger, 1966].)

roots of these extremities are at relatively equal distances from the heart.

2. The body tissues and fluids form a homogeneous volume conductor.

3. The electrical forces resulting from cardiac activation can be represented by a vector at the center of the triangle by appropriate application of the potentials from each of the three leads. The mean polarity of each lead is determined from the sum of the negative and the positive peaks of the QRS complex for that lead.

4. The standard bipolar limb leads provide a time magnitude or scalar record of potential variation in the frontal plane of the body.

The upper tracing on Figure 3-16 is a standard Einthoven lead II electrocardiogram—right arm to left leg—as it appears when recorded by a thin-line penwriter; whereas, for comparison, Figure 3-18 is the same record as made with the Einthoven string galvonometer. The P-R interval represents the time between the onset of atrial and ventricular activation. Its duration ranges from 0.12 to 0.20 seconds. As was seen in Figure 3-15, much of the time between the P wave and the beginning of the QRS complex is taken up by events in the AV node. The duration of the QRS complex ranges from 0.06 to 0.10 seconds. Figure 3-13 indicates the way in which the electrical accession wave passes over the ventricles as this complex is formed. Not only does the duration of the S-T phase show changes of clinical significance with respect to ionic Ca^{++} and K^+ levels and myocardial ischemia, but, because the ventricle is entirely depolarized at

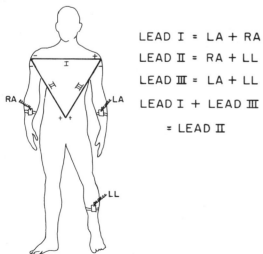

Fig. 3-17.—The location of the standard limb leads and relation to the equilateral triangle of Einthoven. In *lead I*, the deflection is upward when the potential at the L. A. lead exceeds that at the R. A. lead, as shown by the plus and minus signs on the line connecting the left and right shoulders. *Lead II*, left leg and right arm, and *lead III*, left leg and left arm, have deflections that are similarly indicated. (From Berne, R. M., and Levy, M. N.: *Cardiovascular Physiology* [St. Louis: C. V. Mosby Co., 1967].)

this time, the S-T segment should lie on the isoelectric line. Deviations from this isoelectric state are of great clinical interest, for they denote alterations in ventricular excitability. The S-T depression can often be used as a measure of the extent to which the myocardium is suffering from an inadequate oxygen supply, as during the angina of exercise of those with coronary artery disease. The Q-T interval, or electrical systole, varies in duration inversely with the heart rate. It is of interest because it approximates the total period of systole and thus gives the working time of the ventricle. This permits determination of the ratio of work to rest for that particular heart frequency. The T wave represents the repolarization of the ventricle just prior to relaxation of the fibers and the isometric ventricular relaxation phase. It is usually deflected in the same direction as the major components of the QRS complex. This concordance is puzzling since the direction of repolarization normally follows a reverse pattern from that of depolarization. It appears to be connected with the fact that tissue pressure is high in the subendocardial ventricular myocardium during systole. This leads to a delay in repolarization, so that it begins at the epicardium, where the pressure remains low throughout the cycle, and progresses back to the endocardium.

DETERMINATION OF THE ELECTRICAL AXIS OF THE HEART

The nature of the electrocardiogram is determined by the fact that the process of cardiac activation provides a moving potential source located in a volume conductor. The pathway followed by this source is in three dimensions. At any moment, the potential has a magnitude and a direction that is determined by the particular mass of tissue being activated and by the geometric direction being followed by the activation process. Hence, the electrical events of cardiac activation are really vector quantities, and the deflection seen in Einthoven's scalar electrocardiogram is a geometric projection of the vector on a line connecting the two electrodes. The term "scalar" indicates that the electrocardiogram presents the electrical responses in terms of time and magnitude. It may be contrasted with vector cardiography, which is concerned with direction as well as time and magnitude.

The direction of the cardiac vector can, however, be determined from the scalar electro-

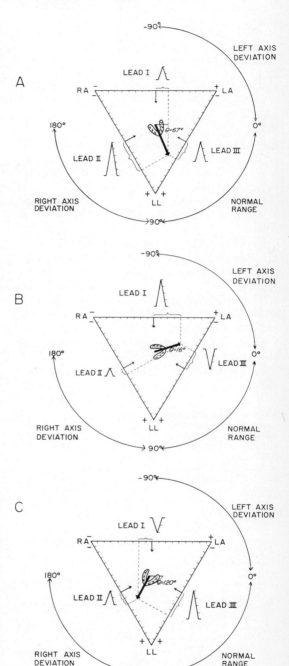

Fig. 3-19.—Relation of electrical axis of the heart to the recorded potentials. In **A**, the arrow indicating the axis or vector of excitation is in the normal range with a θ of 67°. **B**, shows a case of left-axis deviation, i.e., θ is 16°; **C**, indicates deviation to the right, i.e., θ is 120°. The arrow indicates direction, magnitude and orientation of the axis. (From Selkurt, E. E. [ed.]: *Physiology*, 2d ed. [Boston: Little, Brown & Co., 1966].)

cardiogram. The arrows in Figure 3-19, A, B, and C, show various positions of the electrical axis of the heart in the frontal plane as determined by Einthoven's method from electrocardiograms taken on three subjects while using the standard limb leads. The following procedure was followed: the summed potential of the QRS complex on lead I was given an appropriate value along the RA→LA scale of the triangle, i.e., 2 units to the right of center. In this particular subject, the value for lead II was 3 units from the center of the LA→LL side and that for lead III was similarly located, but at 5 units from the center of the RA→LL line. A line drawn between the center of the triangle and the point of intersection of perpendiculars dropped from each of the three above points for the QRS potentials represents the summed vector of the electrical axis of the heart in the frontal plane for this case. Its length is proportional to the magnitude of the summed vectors, and its orientation $\Theta = 67°$ is given by the number of degrees between the horizontal and the direction of the arrow. In this subject, the summed vector is in the normal range.

Figure 3-19-C represents the state of right-axis shift. Because in this case the summed potentials of the QRS complex on the RA→LA arm of the triangle were a negative value, the perpendicular was dropped two units to the left of the midpoint. Leads II and III are 2 and 4 units past the mid-point of RA→LL and LA→LL, respectively. The point of intersection of these perpendiculars gives a Θ of $120°$ in the direction of right-axis deviation. In Figure 3-19-B, lead III has a negative summed potential of 3 units. This time, the point of intersection of the perpendiculars gives an orientation of $-16°$ for the electrical axis of the QRS, showing left-axis deviation.

The determination of axis deviation in the frontal plane has practical implications. First of all, there are physical reasons for a left or right shift. Thus, in short, stocky individuals, one would expect the axis to be shifted to the left; in tall, thin people, it is more often to the right. Variations from these expectations can, therefore, raise the question of cardiovascular malfunction. Furthermore, hypertrophy of one or the other main chambers, the right ventricle (as in pulmonary hypertension) or the left ventricle (as in systemic hypertension), may cause the axis of the heart to deviate to the right or to the left, respectively. The axis may also change abruptly after a myocardial infarction, thus providing information of diagnostic and prognostic value.

Vectorcardiography

Using a cathode-ray oscilloscope, vectorcardiograms can be displayed on a screen and photographed. The technique uses two different lead pairs to drive the horizontal and vertical deflecting plates of an oscilloscope. In this way, the cardiac vector can be projected onto any desired plane, i.e., frontal or sagittal, and its movement throughout the cardiac cycle can be followed as it describes a continuous loop during each heart beat. The advantages to be gained from this method of analysis are important. The sensitive display of phase relationships between the leads gives a highly accurate account of the time sequence of the accession wave of cardiac excitation. By the use of a computer, the patient's mean values can be compared with those of normals, betraying abnormalities in the time course of the wave not perceptible by other means. Previously experimental, it has recently become a proven clinical tool and, in the hands of the experienced cardiologist, this method can be most useful. It is of special value in the determination of aberrant cases of heart block, in the detection of small areas of infarction that would not be recognized with the standard EKG leads, and in the differentiation of chamber size, i.e., in making the distinction between an enlarged atrium and an enlarged ventricle.

Exploring Electrodes

The limb-lead system is useful in studying the time-course of the spread of the process of excitation over the heart. However, when there is a need to detect damage to the heart, as, for example, in coronary occlusion, the electrode needs to be brought closer to the area of injury. The system introduced in 1934 by Frank Wilson is now generally accepted in clinical electrocardiography. He established a "central terminal" or indifferent lead by connecting the three standard extremity leads; 5000–25,000-ohm resistors are placed in each lead. An exploring electrode can then be placed at various points on the chest wall (Fig. 3-20-A). Figure 3-21 shows the location of the commonly used precordial or V leads.

The exploring electrode may also be placed on an extremity. A useful, augmented-level unipolar

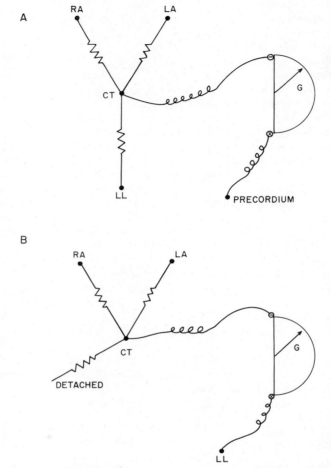

Fig. 3-20.—A, Connections for Wilson's central terminal for precordial leads. *Precordium* indicates the location of the exploring electrode. **B,** With the augmented unipolar lead, the lead to the limb on which the exploring electrode *(LL)* is being placed is detached from the central pole. (From Friedberg, C. K.: *Diseases of the Heart,* 3d ed. [Philadelphia: W. B. Saunders Co., 1966].)

electrocardiogram can be obtained by omitting the wire from the central terminal to the limb under study. These records are approximately 50% greater than those from the standard leads (Fig. 3-20-B). Limb-lead records obtained with such a system are designated according to the placement of the electrodes as: AVR, right arm; AVL, left arm; and AVF, left leg.

Abnormalities of Rhythm

If the control by the SA and AV nodes is disturbed, certain abnormalities of rhythm become apparent. The effects range from a minor, unexpected thump in the chest to fatal cardiac arrest. The normal primacy of the sinoatrial pacemaker (Fig. 3-22-A) may be usurped by a portion of cardiac muscle outside the node that develops increased excitability. Such an atrial premature excitation or ectopic beat produces an unusual P wave, but a normal QRS complex ensues as the AV node picks up the stimulus (Fig. 3-22-B). Because the SA node has responded ahead of time, there will be a compensatory pause while SA excitability recovers prior to the next SA triggering. If the ectopic focus is in the ventricle, contraction will occur early (ventricular premature contraction) and depolarization will be abnormal, resulting in a widened QRS complex. Thereafter, the ventricles will delay the next contraction because they are in a refractory state. Thus there will be a pause

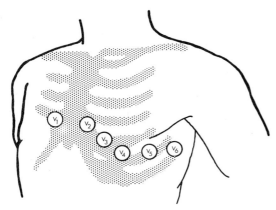

Fig. 3-21.—Location of the customary unipolar precordial leads.

before they recover their excitability and respond to the next sinoatrial impulse as it comes down the normal conducting pathways (Fig. 3-22-C). If the ectopic activity in the atrium is not confined to a single stimulus but becomes intensive and persistent, then the function of the SA node may be overridden as an atrial tachycardia sets in. The frequency of this arrhythmia commonly ranges from 125-plus to 180 beats per minute. Such a tachycardia may last for several hours. It may be so rapid that the cardiac output is inadequate and symptoms of heart failure develop (Fig. 3-22-D). An ectopic focus may be released in the ventricle; by beating faster than the SA node, this region too may take over the pacemaking function. Such a ventricular tachycardia will override the atrial complexes, making the P waves hard to detect. It will have a rate in excess of 100 and reveal distorted QRS waves. Unlike the previous arrhythmias, which are compatible with normal health, this condition is associated with a loss of ventricular efficiency and has a poor prognosis (Fig. 3-22-E).

An ectopic focus in the atrium may fire in rapid sequence from a single point or it may lead to a circus movement. Its activity may be confined to an occasional beat or it may be continuous, persisting for hours or days at frequencies of 260–300/min.

In the latter case, which is termed atrial flutter, the long refractory period of the AV node will usually permit acceptance of only one out of every two or even three pulses (Fig. 3-22-F). The process may progress to persistent, uncoordinated, exceedingly rapid atrial activation, grossly in excess of the rate of flutter. At this point, the atria cease to contract coherently. However, under the control of the AV node, the ventricular contractions proceed normally, and the cardiac output will be sustained with only a moderate deficiency of the order of 20%. Atrial fibrillation, as it is called, can be a late complication of mitral stenosis, and it may persist for very long periods. Its origin in hearts damaged by rheumatic fever or coronary artery disease leads to the current hypothesis that the underlying mechanism is an irregular polarization occurring between islets of atrial tissue having differing refractory periods as a result of varying extents of damage (Fig. 3-22-G).

The ultimate arrhythmic catastrophe is ventricular fibrillation. If this uncoordinated activity of the main muscle mass of the heart is sustained for more than a few seconds, it terminates in cardiac arrest (Fig. 3-22-H).

Conduction Disturbances

If there is a slowing of the normal impulse (Fig. 3-23-A) as it passes through the AV node, the increase in time shows up in the electrocardiogram with a lengthening of the P-R interval beyond an arbitrary "normal" value of 0.21 sec (Fig. 3-23-B). This condition of first-degree AV block is common in infections including diphtheria and rheumatic fever. The lengthening of the P-R interval may extend to a failure of occasional impulses to pass the AV node, i.e., to second-degree AV block. Finally, there is failure of atrioventricular conduction. As the result of this complete or third-degree AV block, the atria contract independently of the ventricles, and the electrocardiogram shows a dissociation of the P waves from the QRS complexes. The condition is associated with exceedingly slow ventricular beats at 20–40/min. The cardiac output may not be sufficient to sustain a normal mean arterial pressure at head level (Fig. 3-23-C). At rates below 20/min, the patient frequently loses consciousness in the so-called Stokes-Adams attack. Impairment of the vascular supply to the AV region is one common cause of this condition. It carries a double threat; not only may the sudden loss of consciousness occur in a life-threatening circumstance, but the lesion itself usually implies a serious cardiac disability. The implantation of a battery-operated pacemaker that gives a constant heart rate of 60–72/min may be a life-saving procedure.

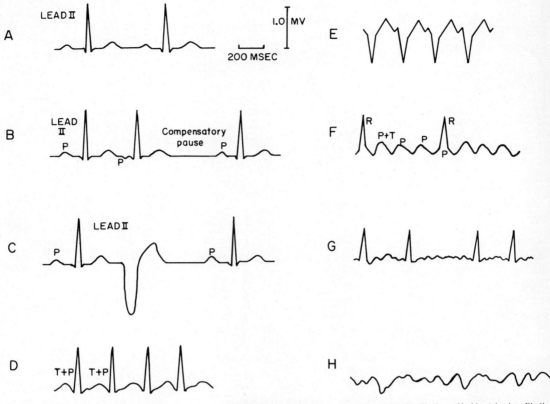

Fig. 3-22.—Cardiac arrhythmias: **A**, Normal rhythms. **B**, Atrial premature excitation. **C**, Ventricular premature excitation. **D**, Atrial tachycardia (T + P indicates superimposition of T and P waves). **E**, Ventricular tachycardia. **F**, Atrial flutter. **G**, Atrial fibrillation. **H**, Ventricular fibrillation. (From Selkurt, E. E. [ed.]: *Physiology,* 2d ed. [Boston: Little, Brown & Co., 1966].)

Local blocks can occur in the conducting system of the ventricles themselves, that is, in the right (Fig. 3-23-D) and in the left (Fig. 3-23-E) branch bundles. The depolarization processes in either the right or left ventricle are disturbed, producing broad, notched QRS complexes, often with a thickened tracing i.e., "slurring," at the apex. The implications of these latter abnormalities of conduction vary and depend on the nature and progress of the coronary artery disease of which they are most commonly an expression.

Effect of Ions on the Heart

Sodium, potassium, and calcium ions all play important and closely interlocked roles in the molecular mechanisms involved in the contraction of heart muscle fibers. This is demonstrated by the simple act of raising the concentration of potassium in the plasma from 4 to 8–15 mg/liter. Cardiac muscle is sharply affected, inducing a cardiac dilation, and a bradycardia develops that can prove fatal. Changes in the plasma concentration of Na^+ or Ca^{++} also significantly affect heart action in vitro. However, the sensitivity of other regions including the brain is even greater, and the plasma sodium or potassium changes needed for a gross effect on heart action are not compatible with life.

There is a close relationship between ion fluxes and myocardial contractility. This contractility is dependent on the relative movements of sodium on the intracellular side of the cell membrane and of potassium on the outside. The biochemical mechanisms yielding the energy for contraction are ultimately controlled by action of the Ca^{++} ions on the enzyme systems of the contractile actin and myosin filaments; the velocity of fiber contraction appears to be determined by the rate of release of Ca^{++} ions. The regulation of the tension developed in the heart muscle fibers thus centers around factors controlling this ion concentration.

As Figure 3-16 indicates, depolarization (DE)

is accompanied by a shift of Na^+ ions into the cell and a sudden rise in spike action potential. The cardiac glycosides appear to potentiate the influx of Ca^{++} into the cell during depolarization. They also increase the rate at which Ca^{++} is released from the sarcoplasmic reticulum. Thus digitalis directly augments myocardial contractility by affecting the level of calcium ions in the myoplasm (Fig. 3-2). This, in turn, controls the rate of the cyclic events responsible for the contraction of the fibrils. On the other hand, the catecholamines appear to increase contractility by a more indirect route. They increase the level of cyclic adenosine 3'5' monophosphate. This, in turn, is associated with an increase in membrane permeability and thereby with an increased uptake of Ca^{++} ions, increased cyclic activity, and, hence, with an increase in cardiac contractility (Fig. 3-2). Caffeine may act by inhibiting an enzyme, phospho-diesterase, that would otherwise decrease the amount of cyclic 3'5' AMP. This maintains an increased membrane permeability and, as is the case with the catecholamines, there is an increase in myoplasmic Ca^{++} and augmented contractions. Thus the cardioactive effects of inotropic drugs appear to be due to their direct or indirect action in increasing the concentration of Ca^{++} in the myoplasm.

INFLUENCE OF INNERVATION OF THE HEART

Both the SA and the AV nodes have many nerve endings and nerve cells serving the vagus. The right vagus supplies the SA node, and the left, the AV node. In addition, these special areas have a rich sympathetic nerve supply, as does the ventricular muscle, which was once thought not to be under the influence of the vagus. Recently, however, it has become recognized that, especially under conditions of high sympathetic drive, vagal stimulation can lead to a significant reduction in contractility (Fig. 3-5). In addition to the negative inotropic effect, stimulation of the vagus or giving acetylcholine will result in a sharp bradycardia that can lead to cardiac arrest. The effect is due to an increase in the time taken for the transmembrane potential to reach threshold (Fig. 3-14-D). This time increases because repolarization is enhanced so that the potential sinks further before recovery and also because the slope of the depolarization rate is decreased. The mechanism of action may be connected with a change in permeability to potassium ions. Strong vagal stimulation will thus either stop rhythmic contraction of the SA node or block conduction through the AV node or both. The result is ventricular arrest until the Purkinje fibers start up on their own at the slow ventricular escape rate of 15–40/min.

Sympathetic stimulation increases the rate of SA nodal discharge up to threefold normal. It also greatly increases the contractility and excitability of all heart muscle, especially the ventricles, which—unlike the vagus—it directly supplies. Thus the sympathetic stimuli induce an increase in myoplasmic Ca^{++} with a significant elevation in the force and rate of contraction. In

Fig. 3-23.—Conduction Disturbances: **A**, Normal. **B**, First-Degree Block. **C**, Complete Block. **D**, Right-Bundle Branch Block. **E**, Left-Bundle Branch Block. (From Selkurt, E. E. [ed.]: *Physiology*, 2d ed. [Boston: Little, Brown & Co., 1966].)

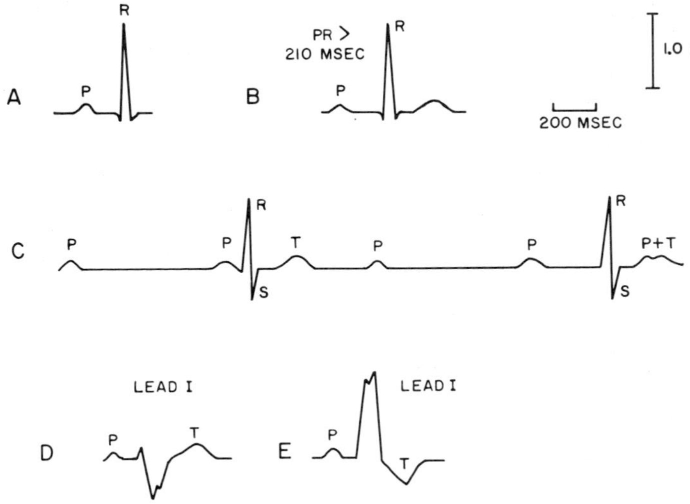

terms of membrane potentials, the mechanism is an increased rate of rise of the spike potential (Fig. 3-14) and an increase in permeability with a more rapid return of the resting membrane potential to the threshold level needed for self-excitation. In the AV node, the sympathetic influence on the minute junctional fibers increases the potentials. They can more easily excite the large nodal fibers, thus decreasing the delay in conduction from atrium to ventricle.

SUMMARY

A complex and highly effective special conduction system ensures the proper coordination of the heart's cyclic operations and increases the efficiency of ventricular contraction. This system gives the organ a needed relative autonomy. At the same time, it permits a degree of nervous and hormonal control over cardiac function that determines its smooth accommodation to the fluctuating demands of the various body states. Disturbances of this intrinsic system can lead to a variety of disorders of rhythm and contractile function.

REFERENCES

Berne, R. M., and Levy, M. N.: *Cardiovascular Physiology* (St. Louis: C. V. Mosby Co., 1967).

Brady, A. J.: Active State in Cardiac Muscle, Physiol. Rev. 48: 570-600, 1968.

Braunwald, E., Ross. J., Jr., and Sonnenblick, E. H.: *Mechanism of Contraction of the Normal and Failing Heart* (Boston: Little, Brown & Co., 1968).

Burch, G. E., and Winsor, T.: *A Primer of Electrocardiography,* 5th ed. (Philadelphia: Lea & Febiger, 1966).

Friedberg, C. K.: *Diseases of the Heart,* 3rd ed. (Philadelphia: W. B. Saunders Co., 1966).

Huxley, H. E.: The Mechanism of Muscular Contraction, Scient. Am. 213:18-24, 1965.

Huxley, H. E.: The Mechanism of Muscular Contraction, Science 164:1356-66, 1969.

Mason, D. T., Spann, J. F., Jr., and Zelis, R.: New Developments in the Understanding of the Actions of the Digitalis Glycosides, Prog. Cardiovasc. Dis. 11:443, 1969.

Nayler, W. G.: Calcium Exchange in Cardiac Muscle: A Basic Mechanism of Drug Action, Am. Heart J. 73:379-93, 1967.

Pollack, G. H.: Maximum Velocity as an Index of Contractility in Cardiac Muscle: A Critical Evaluation, Circulation Res. 26:111-127, 1970.

Rushmer, R. F.: *Cardiovascular Dynamics,* 2d ed.: (Philadelphia: W. B. Saunders Co., 1961).

Sarnoff, S. J.: The Control of the Functions of the Heart, in Hamilton, W. F. (ed.): *Handbook of Physiology: Circulation* (Washington: American Physiological Society, 1962), Vol. I, chap. 15.

Sjostrand, F. S.: Muscle Physiology, in Best, C. H., and Taylor, N. B.: *The Physiological Basis of Medical Practice,* 8th ed. (Baltimore: Williams and Wilkins Co., 1966), chap. 21.

Sonnenblick, E. H.: The Mechanics of Myocardial Contraction, in Briller, S. A., and Conn, H. L. (eds.): *The Myocardial Cell* (Philadelphia: University of Pennsylvania Press, 1966).

4

The High-Pressure System

Pulse and Blood Pressure

INTRODUCTION

THERE ARE two vital pressures in hemodynamics. The first is the driving pressure, which fluctuates between the peak of systole, as the ventricle ejects blood into the arterial tree, and a minimum or diastolic value, as the pressure falls to its lowest ebb just before the next ventricular ejection phase. A normal pulse pressure is the difference between a systolic of some 110 mm Hg and a diastolic of 70 mm Hg and thus approximates 40 mm Hg.

The second critical force is the transmural pressure that stretches the vessel. It is the algebraic sum of the driving pressure and the external restoring forces and is greatest in vessels with muscular walls. If the transmural pressure falls below a certain critical closing value, the vessels will collapse completely and flow will cease, as in the arm vein that goes into spasm after a failure at vein puncture. The effect is also clearly seen in the microcirculation. Here, the counterbalancing tissue pressure represents a significant fraction of the intravascular pressure; in inactive tissues, there are many collapsed capillaries through which flow has ceased because the pressure fell below the critical closing value.

The arterial delivery system operates at a pressure considerably higher than the value needed to hold the capillary open. The way in which this pressure develops—as the left ventricle ejects against the peripheral resistance offered by the end branches of the arterial tree—and the various aspects of the interplay between the force of the beat, the rate of flow, and the resistance offered will be the subject of this chapter.

This interplay can be described as a hydraulic analog of Ohm's law. The heart can be thought of as a pump driving fluid down a tube terminated by a vast number of individual resistances. These can be regarded as collected into one bundle whose total resistance is the sum of all the resistances in the peripheral vascular bed. The energy provided by the pump is used up in overcoming this resistance. Thus the flow rate F in cm^3/sec, the pressure P in $dynes/cm^2$, and the resistance R are related as by Ohm's law:

$$F = \frac{P}{R}, \quad P = FR \text{ and}$$
$$R = \frac{P}{F} = \frac{dynes}{cm^2} \bigg/ \frac{cm^3}{sec} = dynes \ sec \ cm^{-5}$$

The total peripheral resistance that in combination with the cardiac output determines the blood pressure is composed of innumerable tiny resistance vessels $R_1 + R_2 + R_3$ and the conductivity, in turn, is the sum Σ of the reciprocal of these, $\frac{1}{R_1} + \frac{1}{R_2} + \frac{1}{R_3}$. The principal beds into which the human body is divided are presented in Figure 4-1. The table on the right presents the percentage of the total cardiac output taken by each circuit and the flow through it in cc/minute under resting circumstances. The peripheral resistance imposed by each circuit is shown in a final column together with the sum total peripheral resistance that by arithmetic logic, is a smaller figure than any of the individual components. These resting values change remarkably as the organism adjusts for exercise and other physiological states.

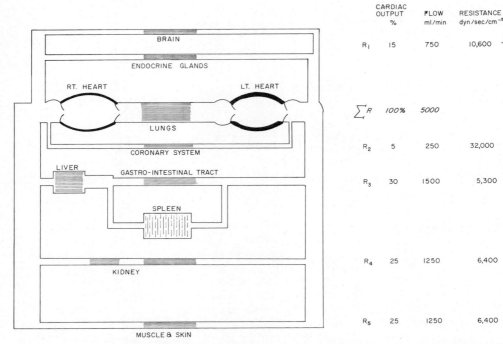

Fig. 4-1.—The parallel resistances of the circulation. The table on the right indicates the total peripheral resistance and the approximate value of the various components when in the resting state. Flow and per cent of the total cardiac output are inversely proportional to resistance. (The brain and neck-thyroid circuits are treated as one unit.) (From Gauer, O. H.: Kreislauf des Blutes, in Landois-Rosemann: *Lehrbuch der Physiologie des Menschen,* 28th ed. [Munich: Urban & Schwarzenberg, 1960], Fig. 77.)

Branching of the Arterial Tree

The length of the major arteries leaving the heart can be measured in fractions of a meter, but those of the fourth to fifth order from the heart are no more than a fraction of a centimeter long. The sum of the cross-sections of the branches greatly exceeds that of the main trunk, so the result is a very rapidly rising over-all cross-section of the vascular bed (Fig. 1-1). In a dog whose aorta may have a cross-section of 0.8 cm^2, that of the capillary bed will be of the order of 600 cm^2. The result is an enormous increase in the surface exposed in the capillary net, thus meeting the essential precondition for an effective diffusion bed. Figure 1-1 presents this concept in diagrammatic form and Table 4-1 gives the data in a form that, although it uses many simplifying assumptions, still permits a number of important conclusions. Despite the enormous cross-sectional area of 4,000 cm^2 in an average-size man of 70 kg, the capillary bed contains only some 6.5% of the total blood volume. This is because the individual capillaries are so short, i.e., 0.1 cm. Hence, if the total blood volume of the man is estimated as 6,000 cc, the volume in the capillaries will be 4,000 × 0.1 = 400 cc, or only 6.6% of the total. The volume in the arterioles, 160 cc, is even smaller. So that even when completely constricted or strongly dilated, they have little effect on the blood volume held in the capacitance vessels. It is their power to decrease their cross-section that is critical, for it has the controlling influence on the peripheral resistance.

Since the same cardiac output flows through the arteries, the diffusion bed, and the veins, the velocity of this stream in any particular region depends on its cross-sectional area. An illustration is a river flowing through a gorge. It does so rapidly, often with turbulence, and yet the same volume flow when the water opens into a broad valley may be placid and gentle. Although the cardiac output is of the order of 5 liters/min, i.e., 80 cc/sec, the rate of flow in the capillary bed is of the order of 1 mm/sec. This is because the number of capillaries is so great, 1.2 × 10^9, that their total cross-sectional area is enormous, despite the fact that each has a diameter of only 8/1,000 of a millimeter.

TABLE 4-1

	Diameter mm	Number	Cross-Sectional cm² Area	Length cm	Total Volume cm³
Aorta	10.0	1	0.8	40.0	30
Large Arteries	3.0	40	3.0	20.0	60
Major Branches	1.0	600	5.0	10.0	50
End Arteries	0.6	1,800	5.0	1.0	5
Arterioles	0.02	40,000,000	125.0	0.2	25
Capillaries	0.008	1,200,000,000	600.0	0.1	60
Venules	0.03	80,000,000	570.0	0.2	110
Terminal Veins	1.5	1,800	30.0	1.0	30
Major Branches	2.4	600	27.0	10.0	270
Great Veins	6.0	40	11.0	20.0	220
Vena Cava	12.5	1	1.2	40.0	50

Applicability of Poiseuille's Law to the Circulation

As has already been discussed in Chapter 1, the flow of liquid in a small tube is determined by the radius to the fourth power, the length of the tube, the viscosity, and the driving pressure. Therefore, because of the strong dependence on caliber, if the diameter were to increase only 20%, flow rate would be doubled, and a doubling of the radius decreases resistance to one-sixteenth. If the pressure-flow relationship of isolated organs such as the lungs and kidneys is studied, it is found to deviate very sharply from the Poiseuille rule. One reason is that the vessel wall is elastic and stretches under pressure, increasing the radius. It may even actively relax and expand depending on the activity of the muscle in it. Instead of a linear relationship between pressure and flow, the flow at low pressures will be much greater than expected if the walls are very flaccid, yet they will readily reach the limit of their expansibility. On the other hand, with active contraction, flow will be less than expected. The vessels may stay closed with no flow at all (critical closing pressure) until the pressure within is sufficient to open up the bed. In the kidney, it is suspected that the flow through the organ is kept constant by the contraction of the smooth muscle in the vessel walls in response to increased pressure within the vessels. This "Bayliss effect" is also thought to occur to some degree in the brain and in the arteries of the hands and feet. This automatic stabilizing influence on the flow through the region persists in spite of denervation and is a local reflex. The measurement of pressure-flow relationships permits no simple conclusions as to the influence of drugs on peripheral resistance. Changes in flow in response to small changes in pressure, or a constant flow rate with varying pressure can be due to local responses of smooth muscle in the vascular bed.

Elements in the Vascular Wall

In addition to the endothelium, which prevents loss of blood and yet serves as a semipermeable membrane for the diffusion of material between

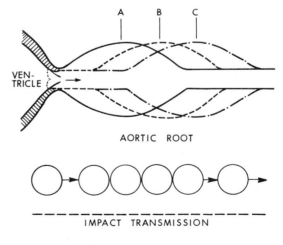

Fig. 4-2.—Diagram illustrating that the rate at which the pressure wave is transmitted (interaction of the banging balls) considerably exceeds the actual movement of the blood column. (From Selkurt, E. E.: *Physiology*, 2d ed. [Boston: Little, Brown & Co., 1966], chap. 16, p. 338, Fig. 3.)

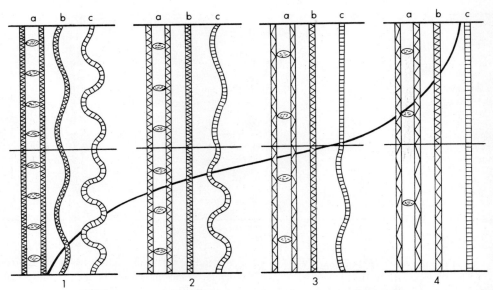

Fig. 4-3.—Schematic presentation of the behavior of the different tissues in the wall of the elastic-type vessels at different degrees of extension. The stretch is in the vertical direction. The S-shaped line is the pressure-volume curve of a young human aorta (See text.) (From Bader, H.: The Anatomy and Physiology of the Vascular Wall, in Hamilton, W. F. (ed.): *Handbook of Physiology: Circulation* [Washington: American Physiological Society, 1963], Vol. II, p. 876, Fig. 9.)

blood and tissue, the delivery and collecting ducts of a closed circulatory system must have certain structural characteristics. The arterial side must serve as a buffering chamber, storing energy that by elastic recoil drives the blood along during diastole, maintaining the pressure differential needed for sustained capillary flow. The next contraction usually starts before the pressure has fallen much more than one third from the peak. Consequently, as stated, the pulse fluctuation is not more than ±20 mm Hg about a mean of 90 mm Hg. This is transmitted down the arterial tree as far as the division into the controlling arterioles with no more than a 2–3 mm Hg loss of mean pressure. Figure 4-2 illustrates the mechanism of the pulse transmission. The injection of blood into the distensible vessel causes bulging and a rise in pressure at point A. Pressures farther along the vessel will not rise until the elevated pressure at point A causes a small quantity of fluid to pass along the vessel. This causes it to distend to point B, while elastic recoil shrinks it at point A. Pressure at B builds up because of the momentum given to the blood, while that at A continues to fall. This process is repeated in sequence at point C, and so on. The velocity of this pulse wave is far faster than the actual movement of blood down the vessel. The row of billiard balls illustrates this idea. The impact is rapidly transmitted down the chain of balls whose actual movement is only a fraction

Fig. 4-4.—The plethysmograph: If venous outflow is blocked with a pressure cuff, the accumulation of blood in the region distal to the cuff will be equal to the arterial inflow. By placing the part in a fluid-filled indistensible container, a graphic record can be made of the rate and extent to which this occurs. (From Weale, F. E.: *An Introduction to Surgical Haemodynamics* [Chicago: Year Book Medical Publishers, Inc., 1967], p. 22, Fig. 13.)

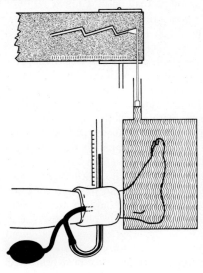

of the distance covered by the wave in the same time. Thus the pulse wave velocity in the aorta is 3–5 meters/sec while mean blood velocity is 0.5 meters/sec. This pulse wave velocity increases as the vessels get smaller, yet the actual velocity of blood flow decreases. To achieve the needed elasticity the artery must have special tissue components in addition to endothelium and muscle. These are of two types: so-called elastic tissue, a rubberlike material that gives the stretch for normal pressures, and a relatively inextensible collagen jacket, like the nylon woven into a rubber garden hose. The proportions of elastic tissue and tough collagen protecting from blowout are important and vary from vessel to vessel.

The elastic tissue has high extensibility and is composed of protein fibers arranged at random. It will stretch twice its original length but has a tensile strength $1/25$ that of collagen. It is found in the large proximal and, to a lesser extent, in the peripheral arteries and veins. It deteriorates with age, becoming calcified with the onset of arteriosclerotic changes. Collagen, the basic material for tendons, is far stronger than elastic tissue but $1/15$ as extensible. It is found in all vessels, appearing in the unstretched wall as wavy bundles that straighten out only if pressure is raised above normal values. The collagen then comes into play, serving as inextensible tough bands that permit the imposition of enormous overloads without rupture.

The interaction of the three wall elements in the elastic arteries is illustrated in Figure 4-3. Sections 1 through 4 represent different stretch phases. Element A represents two elastic fibers that are connected by smooth muscles fastened onto the membranes at right angles. Contraction of the muscle elongates the fibers, but the circumference of the vessel is not changed. This arrangement also permits raising the tension of the elastic fibers with relatively little work on the part of the muscles. Element B is an elastic fiber that is unstressed, and element C is a collagen fiber. The progression from phase 1 to 4 in the diagram illustrates that first the elastic, then the collagen fibers take up the pressure. Thus the pressure volume diagram, at first concave to the abscissa, becomes convex as the point is finally reached at which the wall distensibility depends solely on the collagen tissue.

Practical Aspects of the Laplace Relation

The Laplace relation points to the fact that the force pulling the vessel wall apart in a tangential direction is proportional to the pressure and the radius of the vessel.

If the stiffness of the system increases as a

Fig. 4-5.—Pressure-volume diagrams of the vessels of the hand—an in vivo experiment. *A* temperature in the plethysmograph 25.5°C, vessels contracted; *B* temperature 31.5°C, vessels normal; *C* temperature 36.0°C, vessels relaxed. (From Bader, H.: The Anatomy and Physiology of the Vascular Wall, in Hamilton, W. F. (ed.): *Handbook of Physiology: Circulation* [Washington: American Physiological Society, 1963], Vol. II, p. 878, Fig. 12.)

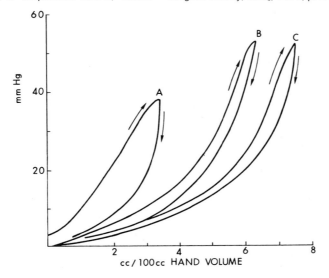

result of muscle action in the walls, then the small vessels will actually empty into the larger ones because, for the same tension, a smaller vessel produces a higher pressure. If there is a deficiency or weakness in the wall of one of the larger vessels, e.g., the aorta or a cerebral artery, then an aneurysm or bulging may develop in this region under the influence of momentary sharp rises of intravascular pressure. The greater the bulge, the greater the tension in its walls for a given internal pressure. Thus in a capillary with a radius of 4/1,000 of a millimeter, the wall tension is only 1/10,000 that of a vessel the size of the aorta, whose radius is more than a centimeter. Therefore, in the bulging vessel, a vicious circle develops in which only the collagen in the wall counters the increasing stretching. Such dilations may end with rupture of the aneurysm.

Pressure Volume Diagram of the Vessels

METHODS

To determine the storage capacity of a biological reservoir with distensible walls, it is necessary to make a pressure volume diagram for each condition of contraction of the muscles in it. This is not too difficult for isolated organs, such as the ventricle of a cold-blooded animal. The various pressures needed to fill it to different volumes can be readily determined, and the same can be done with an aorta removed from the body. For the veins of the hand or the foot, the same end can be accomplished by encasing the extremity in a plethysmograph and causing venous pressure to rise by use of a cuff on the wrist or ankle. As the blood is dammed up behind the cuff, its pressure can be determined by a needle in a vein and the volume changes registered by the plethysmograph (Fig. 4-4).

The instrument can be used to study the volume changes that accompany the local application of hot and cold water to the hand or foot. Heat leads to relaxation and cold to a constriction of the muscle in the vein walls. As the diagram (Fig. 4-5) shows, the curve with the relaxed vessels of the hot hand runs out swiftly with a great volume increase for small increases in pressure and then turns up sharply as the elastic tissue and collagen take over. In contrast, the cold-constricted hand shows a much steeper curve. Also, it does not return upon itself, but exhibits the characteristic of hysteresis. This is because the smooth muscle that forms a major

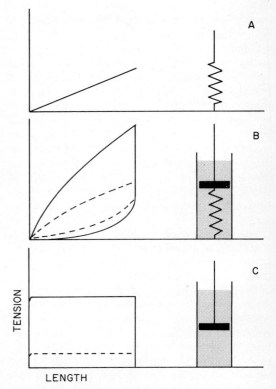

Fig. 4-6.—Illustrating the behavior of an elastic **A**, viscoelastic **B**, and viscous **C**, material with stretch. The zigzag line represents a spring element, the horizontal bar a braking disc, and the shading a fluid element providing viscous drag. *Ordinate:* tension. *Abscissa:* length. (From Bader, H.: The Anatomy and Physiology of the Vascular Wall, in Hamilton, W. F. (ed.): *Handbook of Physiology: Circulation* [Washington: American Physiological Society, 1963], Vol. II, p. 866, Fig. 2.)

part of the vessel walls is viscoelastic. The aorta, which contains far more elastic tissue, does not behave in this way. Figure 4-6 illustrates this peculiar property with a combination of figures and diagrams in which tension and length are assigned arbitrary values. In A, a spring illustrates an elastic material with its identical extension and release curves. A viscoelastic material is demonstrated in B by a spring that has a braking disc on the top and moves up and down through a liquid. The extension and release curves describe a loop, i.e., they show the hysteresis effect. The separation between the curves is determined by the velocity of the extension and release, i.e., the outer curve represents a fast and the inner, a slow stretch. An infinitely slow movement will follow the same curve as in A. The viscous component of the above visco-

THE HIGH-PRESSURE SYSTEM

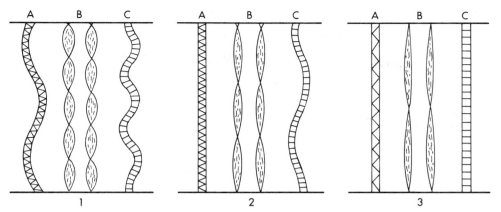

Fig. 4-7.—Schematic presentation of the behavior of the different tissues in the wall of muscular vessels with different degrees of extension. (See text.) (From Bader, H.: The Anatomy and Physiology of the Vascular Wall, in Hamilton, W. F. (ed.): *Handbook of Physiology: Circulation* [Washington: American Physiological Society, 1963], Vol. II, p. 879, Fig. 13.)

elastic combination is represented in C by a braking disc that moves in a liquid. It will assume any position to which it is brought by an external force, but the force required to move it to this position depends upon the velocity of extension.

The behavior of the vascular bed is determined by the successive recruitment of the three basic elements in the vessel wall. At first, the dominant consideration is the viscoelastic smooth muscle, then the elastic tissue plays a role, and, finally, the relatively indistensible collagen fibers are responsible for the resistance of the muscular vessel to further stretch. As a result, in contractile vessels, the curve is S-shaped and initially concave (with volume the most rapidly changing parameter), then relatively linear, and finally turning in the opposite direction as the collagen fibers take up the strain, yielding little volume for large pressure increments. The action of the three wall elements in such a muscular vessel is presented in Figure 4-7. The three sections depict different degrees of stretch. Element A is an elastic fiber, the two elements B are smooth muscle with the individual muscle fibers in series, whereas element C is a collagen fiber. At the beginning of stretch (stage 1), the elastic and collagen fibers are wavy and only the smooth muscle bears the stress. If the muscle fibers are relaxed, first the elastic (stage 2) and, finally, the collagen fibers become involved in the stretch (stage 3). Arteries with intermediate amounts of elastic tissue would have a correspondingly intermediate composition of muscular, elastic, and collagen elements.

Volume Elasticity Coefficient

The physicist defines the elasticity coefficient of a material by the length that a 1 mm^2 section extends when exposed to a pull of 1 kg. The elasticity modulus is the weight in kilograms needed to extend an elastic body of 1 mm^2 cross-section by its own length. The term volume elasticity coefficient

$$E = \frac{\Delta P}{\Delta V} \text{ dyne cm}^{-5}$$

was introduced to give practical, intuitively perceptible form to a most important cardiovascular parameter. It tells how easily a portion of the vascular bed will take up a given volume by defining the pressure change needed to induce a particular stretch. An arterial vascular bed in which the muscle is contracted shows a smaller E, i.e., it is more distensible than a system in which the muscle is flaccid. As the vessel reaches the limit of its stretch, this distensibility factor diminishes. In the venous system, this occurs at pressures in excess of 30 mm Hg; in the arterial tree, the pressures must be considerably greater. The sum of the volume elasticity coefficients for different segments of a long tube taken together with the volume will give information as to the velocity at which a pulse wave will travel down the tube. It is thus possible, given a measurement of the pulse wave velocity and the volume of the arterial segment under consideration, to determine its volume elasticity coefficient.

Elastic Reservoir Function of the Aorta

In considering the action of the heart with its abrupt filling and emptying, it is clear that the mechanics of heart contraction are significantly affected by the elasticity of the aorta. This region can be readily distended to three times its volume at zero pressure. If the vessel were rigid, systole would have to move forward, not merely the stroke volume, but also the entire contents of the vascular bed. As a result, pressures would fluctuate violently between zero and very high values. But thanks to the elastic properties of the vessel, after valve closure the volume held under pressure in the aorta can empty into the vascular bed, giving a continuous flow during diastole. A demonstration of this action is given in Figure 4-8. Water flows from a reservoir down two tubes—one rigid and one with an elastic side chamber. Given the same resistance in the two tubes, the flow will be the same. If, however, the flow is interrupted rhythmically, that through the elastic tube will significantly exceed that through the rigid one.

The aorta serves as just such an expansion chamber. It permits a pressure wave to pass down it so that at any one time only a part of the wall is stretched. There is more elastic tissue in that part of the aorta closest to the heart, so that the reservoir function is chiefly confined to this part of the vessel. By removing the aorta from a cadaver and tying off all the small vessels to it, it is possible to make a pressure volume study of the organ, and in Figure 4-9, some of the conclusions are shown. During growth and development, the vessel is at first so small that the extent to which the pressure rises as the result of a given volume change, i.e., $\frac{\Delta P}{\Delta V}$, is correspondingly high. So, although the walls are thinner and stretch more readily, the curve relating pressure to volume in the aorta of the newborn and 1-year-old is very steep. In accordance with Laplace's law, it flattens out as the size of the vessel increases. By 10 years,

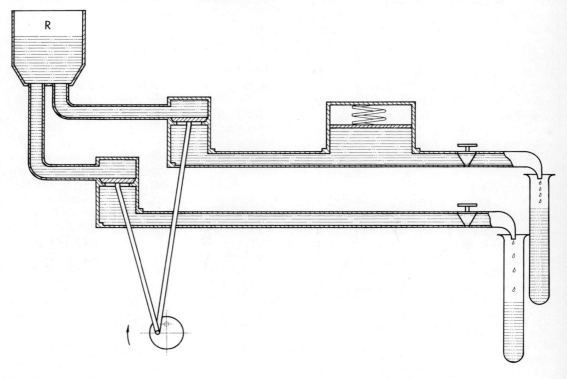

Fig. 4-8.—Demonstration of the action of an elastic reservoir. Water flows out of a reservoir through two tubes of equal size. One tube is rigid; the other is elastic. When the resistance to flow is set to the same value in each tube, the amount flowing into the measuring cylinders is the same. If the flow is rhythmically interrupted by use of the lever, then the flow through the elastic tube will be greater.

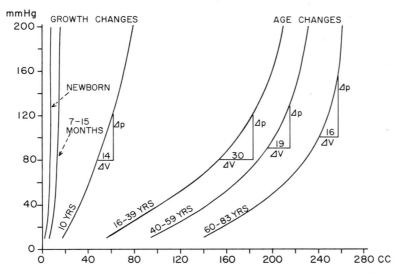

Fig. 4-9.—Influence of age on the pressure-volume curve of the human aorta. With the increase of aortic volume with maturation, there is a decrease of $E = \frac{\Delta P}{\Delta V}$ and the vessel becomes more readily distended. Later the distensibility decreases in part because, with the increase in blood pressure with age, the pulse pressure is working on a steeper part of the elasticity curve. (From Gauer, O. H.: Kreislauf des Blutes, in Landois-Rosemann: *Lehrbuch der Physiologie des Menschen*, 28th ed. [Munich: Urban & Schwarzenberg, 1960], Fig. 88.)

the effect is significant; at 16–39 years, development of the vessel is complete and the curve is at its flattest.

With old age, the elasticity of the aortic reservoir will decrease in many people as arteriosclerotic changes progress. Elastic tissue deteriorates, and the increased rigidity leads to an increase in pulse wave velocity in such vessels. They may fortuitously continue to perform almost the same function because these changes are compensated for by an increase in diameter of the deteriorated vessel as it ages. In fact, despite the greater rigidity, there is not much decrease in distensibility, since the increased diameter exposes the vessel to greater wall tension and hence to greater stretching. As Figure 4-9 shows, the ratio of dp/dv is not altered as much as might be anticipated. Another factor that effectively decreases distensibility in the aged is the frequent increase in blood pressure that forces an ascent to the steeper portion of the pressure volume curve.

An unexpected effect of the decrease in distensibility that may occur in the deteriorating smaller vessels of the aged is a failure of the pressure wave to bounce back as effectively as it does when it reaches the end of the young man's arterial tree. As a result of this wave reflection, the amplitude increases progressively toward the periphery in the normal child. In arteriosclerosis, this alteration during transmission becomes progressively less, and, in severe cases in older people, the wave remains virtually unchanged throughout the tree (Fig. 4-10). An effect of this decreased distensibility is an impairment of the efficiency of the artery in accepting the pulsatile flow, so increasing the work of the left ventricle.

The capacity of the adult aorta is about 170 cc and that of the whole arterial tree some 850 cc or 15% of the estimated blood volume. The elasticity of the aorta

$$E = \frac{\Delta P}{\Delta U} = \frac{40 \text{ mm Hg}}{30 \text{ cm}^3} = 1.3 \text{ mm Hg}$$

per cubic centimeter volume increase. In order to convert this into the absolute units of the centimeter gravity-constant second system, this value must be converted to cms, i.e., 0.13 mm Hg per cm³. It is then multiplied by the density of mercury, i.e., 13.6, and by the gravity constant 981 cm per sec per sec. Thus $E = 0.13$ cm $\times$ $13.6 \times 981 \frac{\text{dynes}}{\text{cm}^2}$ per cm³ = 1,730 dyn. cm⁻⁵. This means that, in the normal man, the elasticity constant of the system is so high that an

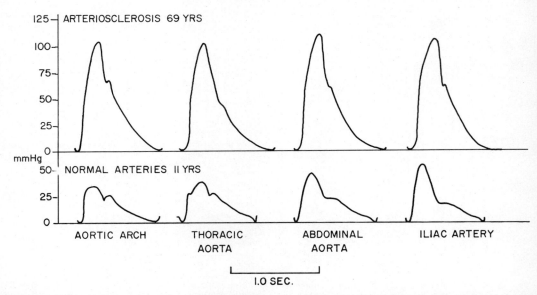

Fig. 4-10.—Pressure-wave transmission along the human aorta. In the normal child, the amplitude increases progressively; but in arteriosclerosis, it is virtually unchanged. (From O'Rourke, M. F., et al.: Pressure Wave Transmission Along the Human Aorta—Changes With Age and in Arterial Degenerative Disease, Circulation Res. 23:567–579, 1968. By permission of the American Heart Association, Inc., New York, N. Y.)

increase in pressure of 100 mm Hg will increase the volume of blood in the arterial tree by no more than approximately 100 cc.

The Arterial Pulse

Pulse Wave Velocity

Each contraction of the heart generates a pressure wave in the ascending aorta which travels away from the heart at a speed which is directly related to arterial distensibility. Pulse wave velocity c is given by the formula

$$c = \sqrt{\frac{\Delta P}{\Delta V} \cdot \frac{V}{\rho}}$$

where V is the absolute volume of the aorta and ρ the density of blood (1.05 gm/cc.). From the above formula it can be shown that wave velocity in the aorta is

$$\sqrt{1{,}730 \times \frac{170}{1.05}} \text{ or } 5.3 \text{ meters/sec.}$$

Wave velocity in the most proximal part of the aorta of a young man is approximately 4 meters/sec and this increases to 7–12 meters/sec in peripheral arteries, reflecting low distensibility of these vessels. Arterial wave velocity increases with age as the vessels degenerate. Thus the relationship between pulse wave velocity and distensibility permits conclusions about alterations in distensibility of the blood vessels. Wave velocity may be measured from the time taken for the foot of the wave to travel from a proximal to a more peripheral vessel as $c = L/\Delta t$ cm/sec where L is distance traveled and Δt the time taken. It takes some 2/10 of a second for the pulse wave to reach the dorsalis pedis artery from the heart; in this time the freshly ejected aliquot has only reached the arch of the aorta. This brings out the difference between pulse wave velocity and blood velocity.

Pulse Contour

The pulse wave that is felt at the wrist and whose amplitude is measured with a sphygmomanometer has complex origins. It is the resultant of the interaction of waves traveling from the heart to peripheral vessels with those returning from the peripheral vessels to the heart after reflection. There are a number of conclusions that can readily be drawn from the mere act of feeling this pulse. The rate and the rhythm of the heart can be detected. The expert can make more refined observations. He can observe the rate of onset, i.e., whether it is abrupt, as in aortic regurgitation, or gradual, as in aortic stenosis. The size of the pulse is significant, i.e.,

THE HIGH-PRESSURE SYSTEM

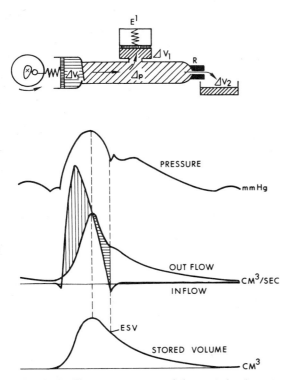

Fig. 4-11.—The pressure curve of the central pulse, as demonstrated by a model incorporating an elasticity factor. (From Gauer, O. H.: Kreislauf des Blutes, in Landois-Rosemann: *Lehrbuch der Physiologie des Menschen*, 28th ed. [Munich: Urban & Schwarzenberg, 1960]. Fig. 85.)

whether it is large and readily palpated, as after exercise in a sweating man, or small and hard to feel, as after vasovagal syncope. The low pressure and soft walls of a young person and the rigid walls and high internal pressure of a hypertensive with arteriosclerosis can be distinguished. This pulse, as it is felt in the wrist, is considerably modified from the original pressure wave, as it develops in the aorta. The changes are induced by the viscous resistance of the arterial walls and by the development of standing waves, as the wave is to some degree reflected from the termini of the great vessels in the limb. Using the simile of a pump, Figure 4-11 indicates that the pressure in the aorta is a function of the volume, V_1, momentarily discharged into the aorta. This depends on the speed at which the blood is ejected out of the heart into the reservoir, i.e., the rate of the inflow $\frac{\Delta V3}{\Delta t}$ versus the speed of outflow $\frac{\Delta V2}{\Delta t}$ through the peripheral resistance R.

The cam reproduces the velocity of inflow into the base of the aorta; i.e., it has a very rapid rise and early peak. Inflow, at first, is so rapid that outflow cannot match it, and the pressure rises. With the rising pressure goes an increasing speed of outflow. The vertical shading indicates the volume gained as a result of these differences in velocities. With the end of systole, inflow ceases. The cross-over point between the inflow and outflow curves is the maximum content of the aorta and so, also, the point of peak pressure.

Thereafter, as the horizontal shading indicates, the outflow is more rapid than inflow, and the pressure falls to the point of valve closure. The remaining end-systolic volume filling the aorta (which is not to be confused with ventricular end-systolic volume) is used to perfuse the periphery throughout the diastolic period.

The model gives some idea of the various factors influencing the intensity and contour of the central pulse. The elastic reservoir of the aorta is shown as a cylinder with a spring-loaded piston on top. In order to simulate the passive elastic element of the heart muscle during systole, another spring is placed between the cam and the main piston of the "heart pump." If the work of the pump is held constant, then the shape and the height of the pressure waves depend on the degree and nature of the factors opposing to the pump's outflow. The less distensible the reservoir and the faster the runoff (i.e., the lower the peripheral resistance), the faster the pressure returns to the resting values.

If all arterioles could be clamped off, the pressure would rise in the system right until the end of systole, and it would be possible to determine the stroke volume V_3 from the change in blood pressure Δp. If the volume elasticity coefficient E were known, cardiac output could be readily determined. Unfortunately, the opening presented by the arterioles constitutes a huge deficiency in the elastic reservoir, and the volume changes that are responsible for the pressure differences are a dynamic compromise between the volume ejected from the heart and the runoff into the periphery. Measurements of pressure and flow rates at the aortic root show that the flow out of the heart rises very rapidly, reaching a peak considerably in advance of the pressure (Fig. 4-12). Maximal filling and hence maximum systolic pressure is attained when the rate of outflow exceeds inflow. The valves soon close, and it is the end-systolic, not the peak pressure,

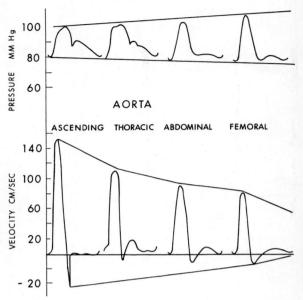

Fig. 4-12.—Comparison of pressure and flow pulses in the arteries as they travel away from the heart. Mean pressure falls slowly, but pulsatile pressure variation increases until, in the smaller limb vessels, it may be double that at the root of the aorta. Flow oscillation diminishes sharply; these changes are due to reflection of the waves in the peripheral vessels. (From McDonald, D. A.: *Blood Flow in Arteries* [London: Edward Arnold & Co., 1960].)

that constitutes the driving force that continues to propel the store of blood needed to sustain the circulation during diastole.

The foregoing reasoning is based on models like the one in Figure 4-11. This views the arterial tree as an elastic reservoir or "Windkessel" as was first suggested by Stephen Hales and used extensively by Frank and others. Although useful, theories based on such a model fail to take account of blood density and so have not provided convincing accounts of the factors controlling wave velocity and wave reflection.

WAVE REFLECTION AND VASCULAR IMPEDANCE

It has been accepted for years that wave reflection is an important factor in determining pulse contour, and Frank recognized this as an objection to his "Windkessel" model. Difficulties arose in quantitating wave reflection and in determining where it came from. A major step forward resulted from the collaboration between the mathematician Womersley and the physiologist McDonald in the 1950s. These men introduced the study of the arterial pulse in steady state oscillation, applying the techniques of harmonic analysis. They developed experimental methods which established the validity of the technique of relating corresponding frequency components of arterial pulses. This work was extended by McDonald's pupil, Taylor. Taylor introduced the concept of vascular impedance to describe the relationship between both steady and oscillatory components of arterial pressure and flow waves. He showed how this approach can be used to study the properties of the vascular bed distal to the point of measurement—such properties including blood viscosity and density and arterial viscosity, elasticity and geometry. Figure 4-13 shows impedance graphs determined from simultaneously recorded pressure and flow waves in the femoral artery of a dog. Like electrical impedance, vascular impedance is a complex quantity and is displayed as graphs of modulus (amplitude) and phase (delay) plotted against frequency. Modulus at any frequency represents the amplitude of a pressure oscillation generated by a given flow oscillation at that frequency. Phase at any frequency is the delay between pressure and flow oscillations at that frequency. The resistance of the femoral bed is the impedance modulus at zero frequency. The impedance graph yields a quantitative measure of the total opposition to pulsatile flow within the bed under consideration. Using realistic models of transmission lines, it has been calculated from impedance plots such as that in Figure 4-13 that 80% of the wave traveling into the femoral bed is reflected and that in man the average of all reflecting sites is some 20 cm from the groin—just below the knee. Since reflection results from abrupt alterations in vascular properties and since reflection can be eliminated by

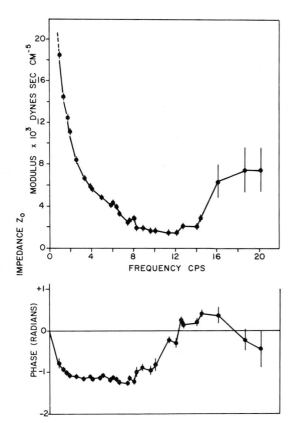

Fig. 4-13.—Vascular impedance in the femoral bed of a dog. Modulus *(above)* and phase *(below)* are plotted against frequency. Data points were obtained by relating corresponding harmonics of pressure and flow waves recorded simultaneously in the femoral artery. The dog had heart block and its ventricle was paced at different rates. Linearity is suggested by the regularity of results. The resistance of the bed (mean pressure ÷ mean flow) is the impedance modulus at zero frequency, in this case approximately 140 dyne sec cm^{-5}. The vertical bars represent four times the standard error of the mean. (From O'Rourke, M. F., and Taylor, M. D.: Vascular Impedance of the Femoral Bed, Circulation Res. 18:126, 1966.)

paring harmonic components of the waves, but one does not have to do this to recognize the influence of wave reflection. Thus the diastolic waves clearly represent reappearance of the original wave after reflection.

Recent studies have shown that the whole complicated network of arteries in the body behaves as though it has two functionally discrete reflecting sites—one representing the resultant of all individual reflecting sites in the head, neck and upper limbs and the other the resultant of all individual reflecting sites in the trunk and lower limbs. The pressure wave is reflected back and forth between these sites, causing blood to slosh to and fro in a damped diastolic oscillation. Predictably, as can be seen in Figure 4-12, diastolic flow oscillations are maximal at the center of this system (the descending thoracic aorta) and minimal at its ends, whereas pressure oscillations are maximal at the ends and minimal at the center. The changes that have been noted in arterial pressure wave transmission with age (Fig. 4-10) can readily be explained on this basis. Degeneration of arteries results in both an increased pulse wave velocity and a decreased peripheral reflection coefficient (due to decreased impedance mismatch at the arterioles). With faster travel of the pulse, incident and reflected waves come closer together in time and so cannot be distinguished separately, whereas lowered reflection results in less increase in amplitude of the peripheral pulse (Fig. 4-10). Changes in the pulse with alterations in arterial blood pressure can be similarly explained (Fig. 4-14), for with an increase in mean arterial pressure, wave velocity is increased. As a consequence, the reflected wave from the lower part of the body returns earlier and moves from diastole into systole, causing increased amplitude of the proximal aortic pressure wave. The wave form is similar to that seen in arterial degeneration, and the mechanism is identical. With a decrease in mean pressure, wave velocity is slowed, and the caudal reflected wave is seen much later in diastole. Pressure waves similar to those in arteriosclerotic humans and in hypertension are often seen in normal birds and reptiles. Again the mechanism is the same—wave velocity is fast and arterial dimensions short in relation to the duration of ventricular ejection so that the reflected wave returns during systole and is not recognized as a distinct entity.

vasodilators injected intra-arterially, it has been inferred that the high resistance elements, the arterioles, are the most important reflecting sites in a vascular bed.

Figure 4-12 shows pressure and flow waves recorded between the ascending aorta and femoral artery of a dog. Amplitude of the pressure wave is greatly increased toward the periphery, whereas the amplitude of the flow is decreased. These changes are what one would expect in a system of tubes with a high peripheral reflection coefficient. They are more accurately delineated, as McDonald and Taylor have shown, by com-

There is evidence that the wave reflection that results from the pulse slamming into the high

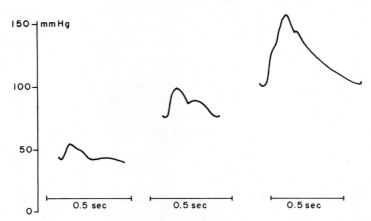

Fig. 4-14.—Pressure waves recorded in the ascending aorta of a rabbit at various levels of arterial pressure. **Center,** control conditions. **Right,** after injection of epinephrine. **Left,** after the induction of vasodilation by the injection of pilocarpine. The normal diastolic wave represents the original impulse returning after reflection in the lower part of the body. At the higher pressure this occurs early (due to the more rapid wave velocity) and it consequently merges with the systolic portion of the wave. At lower pressures the diastolic wave frequently comes later due to slow wave velocity. (Redrawn from data of E. Wetterer.) (From O'Rourke, M. F.: Arterial Hemodynamics in Hypertension, Circulation Res., Vol 32, July, 1970.)

resistance arterioles carries certain benefits with it. It helps to maintain constancy of arterial pressure throughout the heart cycle. This is advantageous, as the work done against aortic pressure during systole determines much of the heart's energy requirements.

There are two components of the energy lost by blood flowing through the systemic circulation. The first is steady work which is dissipated mainly in the arterioles as the blood flows forward. The second is pulsatile work which is lost in arterial pulsations and which is a necessary accompaniment of the intermittency of cardiac contraction. Normally, pulsatile work accounts for only 5–15% of the total external left ventricular work. This is a result of favorable design of the arterial system which results in the impedance modulus being very low over that frequency range which contains most of the energy of the left ventricular ejection wave. The magnitude of pulsatile work depends on the relationship between ascending aortic impedance and the harmonic content of the left ventricular ejection wave. The steep fall in the impedance modulus from its value at zero frequency is a very desirable feature, since it results in low values of impedance at the frequency of the first harmonic of the ascending aortic flow pulse, which, irrespective of heart rate, contains more energy than any other harmonic component. Hypertension and arteriosclerosis interfere with these favorable impedance characteristics and result in higher values over that frequency band that contains most of the energy of the flow waves from the ventricle. In these conditions more energy is lost in vascular pulsation.

The steadier the maintenance of pressure in the aorta, the better will be diastolic perfusion of the ventricular muscle mass by the coronary arteries. Unfortunately, in a passive physical system such as the arterial tree, the best that can be hoped for is a relatively small difference between mean systolic and mean diastolic pressure. Wave reflection plays an important role in maintaining this difference at its normal low value of 10 mm Hg. Placement of the heart with respect to reflection sites and the precise timing of the reflected waves are further important factors in determining optimal cardiac function. The efficiency of the arterial system is also affected by a gross elevation or by a serious fall in the mean pressure. Finally, alterations of distensibility and even more subtle factors such as changes in vasomotor tone and heart rate impair the efficiency of the arterial system in its vital function of receiving blood intermittently from the heart and maintaining nutrient flow to the pump and to the rest of the body.

Causes of Variations in the Blood Pressure

In addition to the pulse wave itself, which is a primary variation if the blood pressure is recorded over long periods, secondary variations will be found that fall into two groups. One cause is respiration. In man, inspiration is often accompanied by tachycardia and a slight fall of arterial pressure and expiration by the opposite. The changes may be attributed to the central action of afferents from the lungs and from the atria upon the efferents controlling the cardiovascular system. With inspiration, the respiratory pump accelerates flow from the great veins into the lungs, and expiration does the opposite. There are also slow changes of blood pressure having a period of 10 seconds or longer that are attributed to periodic changes in the tension of the peripheral vascular bed. The mechanism of these Traube Hering waves is not well understood.

During sleep there is increased reflex responsiveness with a resetting of reflexes that favors lower arterial pressures. The rapid eye movement (REM) phase is associated with marked pressure fluctuations, and it may rise significantly in exciting dreams. On the other hand, quiet, slow-wave sleep is associated with a fall of some 20 mm Hg from normal resting waking values, as is the relaxed post-sleep state in the morning hours in bed.

Strong external stimuli such as cold or pain (as, for example, during the cold pressor test in which the hand or feet are immersed in buckets of iced water) will lead to a rise in pressure from 10–30 mm Hg.

Visceral stimuli, as when the bladder of a paraplegic patient is distended, will lead to very considerable blood pressure rises of 100 mm Hg or more. On the other hand, stimuli to the pleura, as in thoracic surgery, will often induce vasovagal syncope and a fall in blood pressure.

Psychic stimuli, whose nature is determined by the previous experience of the individual, will lead to sharp elevations of blood pressure, especially if fear and anger are involved. Muscular exercise commonly leads to an elevation of blood pressure in proportion to the intensity of the exercise. To some extent, this is due to psychic stimuli, and the elevation is less in exercise that is not accompanied by some element of compulsion, discomfort, and emotional arousal.

Estimation of Mean Blood Pressure

The most straightforward way of obtaining an accurate measure of the mean pressure is to make a recording with a catheter of adequate size and an adequate recording device.

In the case of a reading taken from the aorta, as may be seen in Figure 4-15, the mean pressure will be almost precisely the midpoint between systole and diastole. In the case of a peripheral pulse, the horizontal line dividing the pulse contour into equal areas, i.e., the mean, goes through a point one third of the way from diastole to the systolic peak. When such accurate measures are made, it is found that, despite the increase in peak or systolic pressure, the actual mean arterial pressure diminishes by only 2–3 mm Hg in passing from aorta to the periphery. The energy loss due to the pulsatile phenomena is 8% in the young. This compares favorably with the figure of more than double this value in arterial degenerative disease and is a tribute to the efficiency of the distribution network.

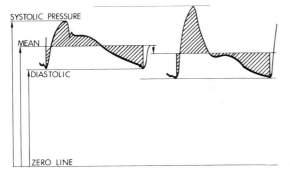

Fig. 4-15.—Determination of mean blood pressure of one pulsation of the aorta **(left)** and the iliac artery **(right)**. In the aorta the area above and below the mean line is equal and is the arithmetic mean of systolic and diastolic pressure. In a peripheral vessel, such as the iliac, despite the increase in amplitude, there is a fall of mean pressure; the pressure is estimated as diastolic plus one third of the pulse pressure. (From Gauer, O. H.: Kreislauf des Blutes, in Landois-Rosemann: *Lehrbuch der Physiologie des Menschen*, 28th ed. [Munich: Urban & Schwarzenberg, 1960], Fig. 97.)

REFERENCES

Bader, H.: The Anatomy and Physiology of the Vascular Wall, in Hamilton, W. F. (ed.): *Handbook of Physiology: Circulation.* (Washington: American Physiological Society, 1963), Vol. II, chap. 26, pp. 865–889.

Best, C. H., and Taylor, N. B.: *The Physiological Basis of Medical Practice* (Baltimore: Williams and Wilkins Co., 1966).

McDonald, D. A.: Elementary Hydrodynamics of the Circulation, in Davson, H., and Eggleton, M. G. (eds.): *Starling and Lovatt Evans' Principles of Human Physiology* (Philadelphia: Lea & Febiger, 1962), pp. 197–215.

O'Rourke, M. F., et al.: Pressure Wave Transmission Along the Human Aorta: Changes with Age and in

Arterial Degenerative Disease, Circulation Res. 23:567, 1968.

Remington, J. W.: The Physiology of the Aorta and Major Arteries, in Hamilton, W. F. (ed.): *Handbook of Physiology: Circulation.* (Washington: American Physiological Society, 1963), Vol. II, chap. 24, pp. 799–838.

Ruch, T. C., and Patton, H. D.: *Physiology and Biophysics,* 19th ed. (Philadelphia: W. B. Saunders Co., 1965).

Rushmer, R. F.: *Cardiovascular Dynamics,* 2d ed. (Philadelphia: W. B. Saunders Co., 1961).

Weale, F. E.: *Introduction to Surgical Hemodynamics* (Chicago: Year Book Medical Publishers, Inc., 1967).

5

Exchange of Substances Through the Capillary Wall and the Role of the Lymphatics

Capillary Function

GENERAL CONSIDERATIONS

INTERPOSED BETWEEN the end of the high-pressure system and the beginning of the low-pressure system is the systemic microvascular bed. In these thin-walled blood vessels, the circulating medium comes into most intimate contact with tissue fluid to allow exchange of substances across the hematoparenchymal barrier. The systemic microcirculation is a transition zone between the high- and the low-pressure systems. Active mechanisms for modifying the hemodynamic resistance before and beyond the microcirculatory bed may result in a pressure within the small blood vessels, at times, closer to that of the large arteries and, at other times, closer to that of the venous system. However, for the most part, pressure falls from high to low levels in the arterioles at the beginning of the systemic microcirculation.

Because the arterioles interpose a variable resistance between the microcirculation and the arterial tree, there is no necessary relationship between arterial and capillary pressures. For example, if the arterioles are constricted, the arterial pressure can be higher than normal, whereas the pressure in the microcirculation beyond this high resistance could be below normal. The relationship between capillary pressure and that in the veins is somewhat more straightforward, since the pressure in the capillaries must always exceed that in the veins. The gradient between the small vessels and the large collecting vessels will depend on the magnitude of the postcapillary resistance, which is thought to be of great importance by some workers and is the focus of active research.

The morphologic arrangement of the systemic capillary bed is especially adapted to foster the effective exchange of solutes. At least three geometric considerations are involved. First, their microscopic diameter assures the maximum surface-to-volume ratio for the blood they contain. Because they are so small, a unit volume of fluid within a capillary has a larger exposed surface area than in any other portion of the vascular system. The product of the cross-sectional area of the small, individual capillaries and their total number provides a very large total area that is many times greater than the total cross-sectional area at any other "stage" of the vascular system (Fig. 1-3). Second, the physics of fluid flow determines that, in a continuous liquid-filled system, the transit time for a unit volume of blood through the stage of maximum area must be the slowest. Finally, because of their small caliber, the individual blood vessels need a minimum tension in the wall to support the pressure. It will be remembered that the tension in the wall of a vessel is inversely proportional to its radius when the pressure is held constant. Thus, even though the pressure in a capillary is greater than that in the veins, the walls are much thinner. The transfer of material across this barrier is, therefore, almost unhindered and almost as rapid as free diffusion.

The exact path by which the solutes move is still unclear. Much indirect evidence indicates that most of the water-soluble small molecules or ions move along continuous aqueous pathways between the endothelial cell borders. There is evidence for gradients of permeability: the wall at the venous end of the microvessels tends to be more easily breached than elsewhere.

Because the capillary wall permits free movement of solute and water molecules, and because the pressure in open capillaries exceeds that in the surrounding tissues, water as well as solutes should leak from the capillaries continuously. This loss of fluid would ultimately embarrass the circulation. However, the tendency for water to escape is opposed by the oncotic pressure, which is the force created by the fact that the large, colloidal molecules cannot escape. When a barrier that separates two solutions permits free movement of all except a single solute, an osmotic force is set up favoring transfer of fluid into the compartment with the higher concentration of the nonpenetrating substance. At the capillary wall, movement of all solutes except the plasma proteins is unrestricted, and the osmotic force resulting from these proteins is of the same order of magnitude as the hydrostatic pressure in the capillaries. It can, therefore, serve to restrain the escape of fluid from the circulatory system.

Filtration and Absorption

The first formulation of this vital equilibrium of forces that balances the circulating fluid within the capillary against the factors tending to lead to its diffusion through the thin wall was made by Starling in 1896. Discussing the mechanism of absorption from tissue spaces, he emphasized that, while transudation is determined by the capillary pressure, yet, small though it is, the osmotic pressure of the plasma protein is big enough to determine absorption. The general relationship based on Starling's principle may be formulated as follows: fluid movement, i.e., filtration or absorption, is a constant (K) times the sum of the hydrostatic pressure in the capillary, minus the osmotic pressure of the plasma proteins, minus the pressure in the interstitial fluid compartment, plus the osmotic pressure of the proteins in the interstitial fluid outside the capillary walls.

The rate of this fluid movement is determined by the constant (K), which is proportional to the permeability of the wall to isotonic fluid, i.e., by a filtration coefficient. Each of these various factors has been extensively investigated during the past 30 years, and considerable quantitative information gathered about them. The information has been reviewed by Landis and Pappenheimer in a masterly chapter in the circulation section of the *Handbook of Physiology,* and the present material is largely drawn from it.

Hydrostatic Pressure in the Capillary

In principle, the measurement of capillary pressure is simple, but, in practice, it demands great skill and patience. This is because it involves the insertion of a fine cannula directly into the minute vessel. By choosing an appropriate region such as the thin skin on the dorsum of the finger, the capillary can be visualized

Fig. 5-1.—Curve comparing the gradient of pressure drop *(open circles)* in man with the corresponding osmotic pressure of his plasma proteins. (From Landis, E. M.: Physiol. Rev. 14:404, 1934.)

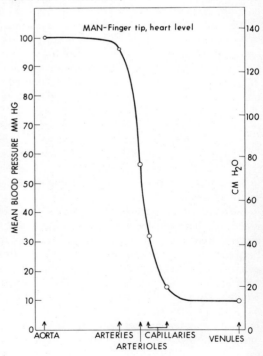

CAPILLARY WALL EXCHANGE AND ROLE OF THE LYMPHATICS

under a microscope, and a glass micropipette drawn down to a few μ at the tip can be inserted into the lumen. The pipette is mounted in a micromanipulator; it is filled with heparin-saline and connected to a manometer and syringe so that the pressure on the saline in its tip can be changed to balance the changing pressure in the capillary. With minute rods also under microcontrol, the tissues can be kept steady. The pressure readings are determined at a moment when there is flow into or out of the capillary, and the accuracy of readings confirmed by showing that venous congestion of the region induces a corresponding rise of pressure in the capillary.

Curves obtained by Landis demonstrated the low pressure in the capillaries at the fingertip. It was shown that the approximately 25 mm Hg osmotic pressure of the plasma proteins was of a value just such that filtration was favored at the (approximately 30 mm Hg) arterial end and that absorption predominated at the (12 mm Hg) venous end of the capillary net (Fig. 5-1).

In the glomerular loops, pressures are higher, ranging from 50 to 60% of the full arterial value. These pressures of 50 mm Hg, together with a great effective pore area of the membranes, will account for the rapid filtration rates typical of the region. The pressure in the renal peritubular capillaries that receive the effluent from the glomeruli is lower, i.e., of the order of 20 mm Hg.

This means that the osmotic pressure of the plasma proteins, especially when accompanied by a raised renal interstitial pressure, will help to draw fluid from the tubules back into the peritubular capillaries. When the filtration process is heavy, this effect is enhanced by a significant increase in the osmotic pressure of the blood due to hemoconcentration in the glomerular loops.

In the pulmonary capillaries, the situation is the opposite of that in the glomeruli. Here the pressure is extremely low, i.e., of the order of 5–15 mm Hg. It is thus well below the osmotic pressure of the plasma proteins, and so the reabsorption of fluid is favored. It is important that this be so, for the lungs must have a minimum thickness of interstitial fluid on the alveolar walls to permit the most rapid possible exchange of gases across them. The critical importance to this region of the plasma protein osmotic pressure is shown when pulmonary edema develops in heart failure. This occurs when central venous and, hence, pulmonary capillary pressure rises above the critical 25 mm Hg mark (Fig. 5-2).

Morphology of the Fluid Exchange Network

There are several morphologically distinguishable categories of blood vessels in the microcirculation. The arterial system ultimately ram-

Fig. 5-2.—Rate of edema formation (filtration) in lungs of dogs subjected to prolonged elevations of left-atrial pressure. Significant filtration did not appear until left-atrial pressure exceeded 25 mm Hg, i.e., the osmotic pressure of the plasma proteins. (From Guyton, A. C., and Lindsey, A. W.: Effect of Elevated Left Atrial Pressure and Decreased Plasma Protein Concentration on the Development of Pulmonary Edema, Circulation Res. 7:653, July, 1959, Fig. 6. By permission of the American Heart Association, Inc., New York, N. Y.)

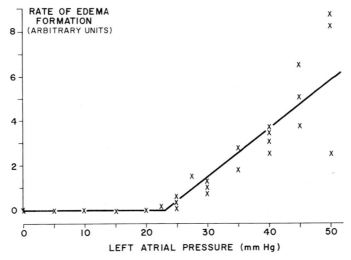

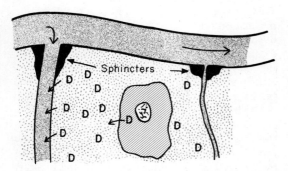

Fig. 5-3.—As the dilator produced by a metabolizing cell accumulates, it causes the precapillary sphincter to relax, opening the vessel and increasing the blood flow in that area to carry away the material and restore the original concentration. (From Winsor, T., and Hyman, C.: *A Primer of Peripheral Vascular Diseases* [Philadelphia: Lea & Febiger, 1965], p. 67, Fig. 6-2.)

ifies into terminal arterioles with a continuous, smooth muscle coat. These vessels divide into branches known as metarterioles, in which the muscle layer becomes discontinuous and ultimately disappears. The metarteriole plus its nonmuscular extension constitutes a simple, direct passage for blood from the arterial to the venous side. Even under conditions of curtailed blood flow through a tissue, these thoroughfare channels remain patent. Arising from the metarterioles and from the terminal portions of the arteriole is a complex interconnecting network of small vessels, the true capillaries, which ultimately drain into the distal portion of the thoroughfare channels and the venules. These capillaries are no more than a single layer of naked endothelium with a simple ring of smooth muscle that forms a sphincter at the point of origin from the terminal arteriole or metarteriole (Fig. 5-3 and Fig. 5-4). There is no similar muscle guard at the point of re-entry of the capillary into the distal portion of the thoroughfare channel or into the venule. The true capillary, unlike the thoroughfare channel, may be completely deprived of flow; often, in a living preparation of ischemic tissue, it is impossible to detect these vessels. Thus the precapillary sphincter can completely stop flow in the capillary, whereas the muscular coat of the metarteriole may diminish the lumen but will never obliterate it.

Actual dimensions of the vessels vary greatly, but the arterioles have a caliber of approximately 20 to 30 micra, that is, approximately 3–4 red cell diameters. The diameter of the thoroughfare channel at maximum constriction, as well as that of the true capillaries, is about 7 micra, but, under certain circumstances, the latter may be considerably smaller. Since the

Fig. 5-4.—The network into which the arterioles break down has a number of specializations, including true capillaries in which the flow may on occasion be halted, and thoroughfare channels, which form continuous connections between the arterial supply and the venous drainage. (From Winsor, T., and Hyman, C.: *A Primer of Peripheral Vascular Diseases* [Philadelphia: Lea & Febiger, 1965], chap. 6, p. 65. Fig. 1.)

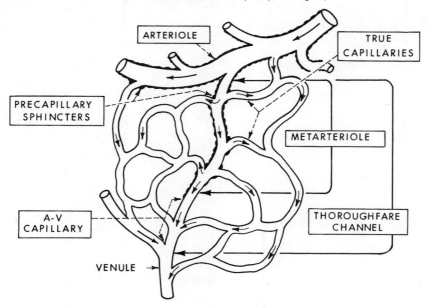

erythrocyte is very easily deformed, it can move through blood vessels considerably smaller than would be expected in view of its apparent resting diameter.

In different tissues, there are interconnections and basic patterns that differ according to local needs. Thus in skeletal muscle there are many cross-connections that compensate for local pressure rises as the muscle fibers contract, and, in the skin of the hands and feet in particular, there is a marked development of AV anastomoses. This variety of channels permits the more efficient regulation of the supply of cell nutrients to the needs of the precise locality served by a single minute vessel.

Nerve fibers can be traced to the smooth muscle of the arterioles and metarterioles but only rarely to the capillary sphincter. Rather, the spontaneous ebb and flow and the selective restriction and diversion of the blood that occurs appears to be under some kind of control by local chemical agents. When the exchange in an area is inadequate to supply the needed substrates or to remove metabolic by-products, the resulting change in local concentration of substances, whose identity remains controversial, tends to relax the precapillary sphincter with a corresponding change in capillary flow.

In vessels concerned with the exchange of metabolites, control of their function appears to be determined by the duration of perfusion rather than by an adjustment of flow. The sphincter controlling a minute vessel is either completely relaxed, permitting maximum flow, or closed, shutting off that capillary (Fig. 5-5). After flow has persisted for some time, the constrictor stimulus begins to take precedence and dilation passes off. An alternating opening and closing of the individual capillaries takes the place of the graded flow characteristic of the large vessel. The adequacy of perfusion of the local exchange vessels is determined by the rate of production of various local chemical agents. Of course, if the blood supply has failed due to a spasm or other obstruction in the larger vessels upstream, no arrangement of local flow will match local needs, even if there is complete relaxation of the precapillary sphincters.

The exact route taken by the fluid as it filters outward from the vessel in the high-pressure region of the capillary is not settled. The basic concept is that outward filtration occurs at the arteriolar end of the capillary and reabsorption is limited to the venous end. It is, however, pos-

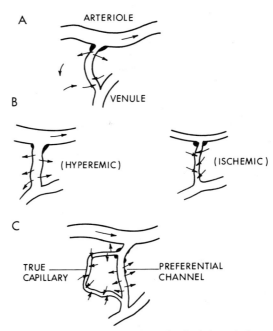

Fig. 5-5.—Alternative hypotheses for the balance between inflow and outflow of fluid from the vascular bed.

A, the classic view—hydrostatic pressure at the arterial end of the capillary vessels exceeds that at the venous end, with outward filtration of fluid at the arterial end and reabsorption at the venous end.

B, the ebb and flow—where most of the vascular bed has a hydrostatic pressure in excess of the colloid osmotic pressure during periods of hyperemia, with a generalized outward filtration of fluid. During ischemia, pressure throughout the filtration area is lower than the colloid osmotic pressure, and there is a generalized reabsorption of fluid.

C, different vessels involved in the two processes—the thoroughfare channel hydrostatic pressure may be somewhat higher than in other vessels in the bed; therefore, over the greater part of its length, fluid filters into the tissues. The true capillaries would have pressures below the colloid osmotic pressure and hence serve as areas for the reabsorption of fluid.

Each of these hypotheses can be supported by direct experimental evidence in special cases. All of these systems probably coexist in the body. (From Winsor, T., and Hyman, C.: *A Primer of Peripheral Vascular Diseases* [Philadelphia: Lea & Febiger, 1965], p. 76.)

sible that in certain localities the mechanism of ebb and flow holds, so that first there is dilation with a rise of hydrostatic pressure along the entire length of all the capillaries (Fig. 5-5). This would then be followed by a vasoconstriction such that the pressure falls below the colloid osmotic pressure, permitting a continuous overall reabsorption of fluid into the same capillary. It is also possible that the pressure in the thoroughfare channels is high enough to provide continuous outward filtration, whereas in the true capillaries the pressures are lower and they serve as areas of reabsorption (Fig. 5-5).

This balance of forces between the osmotic pressure within the capillaries and the hydrostatic pressure produces an extravasate whose function is highly specialized. It is not responsible for the nutrition of the tissue cells proper, but for the transfer of larger molecular-weight substances, including globulins, to the interstitial spaces where they can exert metabolic and antibody function, contributing importantly to the nutrition and defense of the tissues.

There is indirect evidence of the foregoing proposed intermittent fluctuation between over-all high and over-all low pressure in a segment of the microcirculatory bed. It is difficult, otherwise, to explain events such as the intermittent entry of physiologically balanced salt solutions into the skin when a fine canulla is introduced without breaching either capillaries or lymphatics.

Another factor that is important in determining the over-all pressure in the microcirculatory bed is its position relative to the heart. Thus the pressure in a capillary loop of a man's fingertip held at heart level is 32 mm Hg at the arterial end and 12 mm Hg in the venous portion. When the hand is raised 30 cm above the heart, these averages become 23 and 10 mm Hg, respectively. On lowering the forearm to 40 cm below heart level, the arteriolar and venous capillary pressure increases to 45 and 33 mm Hg.

In still more exaggerated circumstances, as in the feet when the individual is vasodilated, hot and sweating, the pressures will rise beyond the balance point between hydrostatic and osmotic pressure (Fig. 5-6). When the person is cool and vasoconstricted, the pressures are lower because, by the interaction of the valves in the veins and muscle movement, blood is steadily milked from the extremity faster than it enters through the constricted arteriolar supply vessels.

The balance between capillary blood pressure and the osmotic pressure of the plasma protein is variable. During vasoconstriction and elevation of an extremity, absorption may predominate; whereas, during vasodilation and dependency, the reverse holds. In fact, in prolonged dependency with high temperature where there has been local injury with inflammation, as after a break or sprain, the capillary filtrate exceeds the amount that can be reabsorbed. Under these circumstances, the lymphatics constitute an important safeguard against excessive accumulation of capillary filtrate in the interstitial fluid compartment.

Functional Changes of Capillary Blood Pressure

Where there are dramatic changes in the circulation, as, for example, during the vasoconstriction and virtual cessation of blood flow of Raynaud's disease, the pressure in the minute

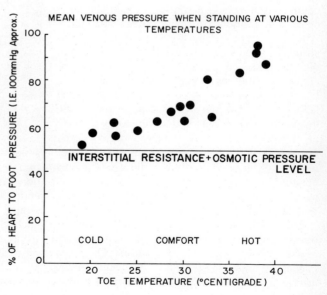

Fig. 5-6.—Depending on the temperature of the skin, blood flow through the foot will be slow or fast. Intermittent movements of the standing subject reduce venous pressure to a degree dependent upon the blood flow rate. In hot environments, the pressure in the veins will exceed the plasma osmotic pressure, and the Starling equilibrium will permit tissue fluid accumulation. (From Henry, J. P., and Gauer, O. H.: J. Clin. Invest. 29:855, 1950.)

vessels will fall to 5–8 mm Hg. When the vessels recover and vasodilation sets in, the pressure may rise to 30–40 mm Hg in the same capillary loops. In fact, when the vessels are dilated, as in inflammation, the pressure may rise to the 50–60 mm Hg range. An interesting sidelight on the effects of very marked dilation is that the flow of lymph does not necessarily increase. This may be because when vasodilation is general, involving a manyfold increase in the requirements of the region for blood, there will be a fall in the pressure in the small supply arteries; i.e., there will be a large pressure drop as the blood flows from the main artery to the dilated peripheral vessels, as from the brachial to the digital arteries. The result is that the rise of capillary pressure is limited because, even with maximal arteriolar dilation, the pressure head at the arterioles themselves is now limited. Finally, the effect of arteriolar dilation may not be enough to raise the capillary pressure if, at the same time, the veins and venules are simultaneously dilated in a similar proportion.

In the reverse effect, if venous pressure is increased, as when there is congestive heart failure, the capillary pressure is also increased. This is reflected in the development of edema in dependent regions. In general, filtration and reabsorption are far more affected by a rise in venous pressure than by the same increase in arterial pressure. This is shown by the formula for mean capillary pressure which is:

$$Pc = \frac{\frac{Rv}{RA} \cdot PA + PV}{1 + \frac{Rv}{RA}}$$

Rv and RA, respectively, are the pre- and postcapillary resistances, and PA and PV, arterial and venous pressures. The equation implies that, at given values of arterial and venous pressures, the mean capillary pressure will depend on the ratio between the postcapillary and precapillary resistance to blood flow.

Recent work indicates that these resistances are under nervous control. Öberg and Folkow have shown that, when the volume of fluid in the thoracic viscera is increased, fluid accumulates in the interstitial spaces as a result of the increase in the ratio of post- to precapillary resistance. The reverse effect accompanies a decrease in volume of the blood in the thorax. This reflex is a significant factor in the regulation of fluid volume and in the return of fluid from the interstitial spaces when it is required due to a reduction of blood volume. If arterial pressure falls and there is intense vasoconstriction, then there is a severe fall in blood flow; this, in turn, limits edema formation simply because there are not large volumes of blood plasma available for filtration. It has further been shown that the capacitance and the resistance vessels both constrict in response to sympathetic stimulation; however, capacitance vessels do so more vigorously. With such stimulation, precapillary resistance increases more than postcapillary resistance, with an accompanying reduction of capillary blood pressure of from 2 to 15 mm Hg. Epinephrine in large doses and norepinephrine, also, lead to an increase of arteriolar resistance and reduction in capillary blood pressure, the precise effect depending on the relative predominance of α and β receptors in the vessel.

Fig. 5-7.—Showing the basic principles of an osmometer with the protein-containing solution placed within a semipermeable membrane that is surrounded by a crystalloid solution. As fluid is absorbed, the pressure in the colloid container rises, displacing the manometer column. (From Starling, E. H.: J. Physiol. [London] 19:312, 1896.)

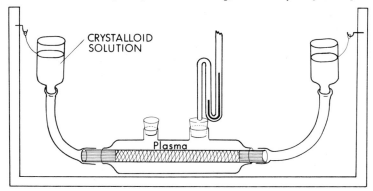

Osmotic Pressure of the Plasma Proteins

Starling's idea in 1896 that there was a balance between the capillary hydrostatic pressure and protein osmotic pressure was supported by actual measurements of the pressure required to maintain fluid balance across a semipermeable membrane separating plasma from plasma ultrafiltrate. Starting with a membrane stretched across a bell jar, he worked with progressively more efficient osmometers (Fig. 5-7), and subsequent investigators, notably Hepp, continued the improvement with the development of instruments in which volume that had to be displaced was reduced to the order of 10^{-6} ml per mm Hg of pressure. Such devices will equilibrate in minutes instead of the days required by Starling's first osmometers. Using these instruments, the osmotic pressure can be used for rough determinations of the molecular weight of the protein by the van't Hoff equation:

$$\text{Mol Wt} = \frac{10 \text{ (concn in gm/100 cc) R.T.}}{\text{Osmotic P (in atmospheres)}} \text{ (liter atmos)}$$

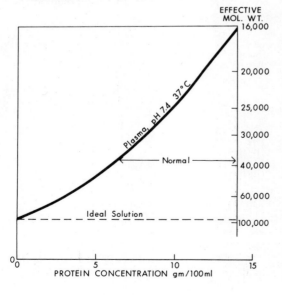

Fig. 5-8.—First derivative of protein osmotic-pressure concentration curve showing deviation from van't Hoff's law. At infinite dilution, the average molecular weight of plasma proteins is almost 100,000, but, in normal plasma, their osmotic behavior corresponds to an ideal solute of molecular weight, 37,000. (From Landis, E. M., and Pappenheimer, J. R.: in Hamilton, W. F. (ed.): *Handbook of Physiology: Circulation* [Washington: American Physiological Society, 1963], Vol. II, p. 973.)

Although the theory does not hold for concentrated protein solutions, due to interacting forces between the molecules and to other factors, the method has not only been useful to physiologists interested in the play of forces across the capillary membranes, but, until the introduction of the ultracentrifuge, it yielded serviceable estimates to physical chemists as well.

Although albumin is present in large amounts in the plasma and is the chief osmotically active protein, there are low molecular-weight globulins that also contribute significantly. The fact that only 65% of the total osmotic activity is due to albumin helps to explain the survival of persons with analbuminemia; their plasma osmotic pressure still remains nearly one-half normal. The remaining factors in the adaptation of these apparently healthy people with this excessively rare but intriguing condition may turn around a low level of mean capillary pressure and, perhaps, an active fluid return by the lymphatics.

In the fetus, the protein osmotic pressure is always less than that of the mother. Fetal globulins have a very low molecular weight, i.e., 65,000 versus the adult 96,000. These figures change immediately after birth, partly owing to the absorption and retention of the unchanged large globulin molecules from the colostrum. The mechanism of this absorption and the significance of these fetal-maternal differences remain an area for future investigation.

The interaction of the protein molecules when they are in concentrated solutions, as in plasma, has effects on the osmotic pressures that are of great practical significance. In tissue fluids where protein concentrations are low, the molecules behave as would be expected of their high molecular weight, and the osmotic pressure is correspondingly low. But at the high protein concentrations of plasma, the osmotic coefficient is almost threefold, so that the proteins exert an osmotic pressure equivalent to what would be an impractically viscous 12% protein solution (Fig. 5-8). No precise theoretical explanation of the intermolecular forces responsible for these changes is available. However, these nonlinear osmotic pressure variations with changes of the plasma protein concentration have a practical significance (Fig. 5-9). When, as in severe water deprivation, there is hemoconcentration, then the osmotic-restoring force increases. Thus when 30% of the plasma volume has been lost, osmotic pressure increases by 18 mm Hg, instead of the

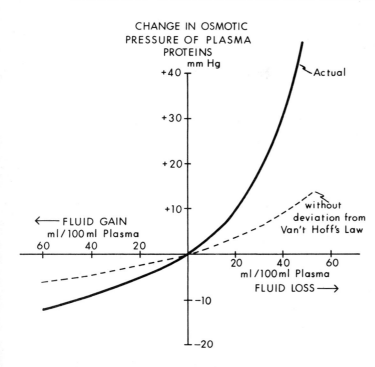

Fig. 5-9.—Physiological significance of deviations from van't Hoff's law. Fluid loss from plasma causes a disproportionately large increment in the osmotic-restoring force; conversely, hemodilution causes a relatively large diminution of protein osmotic pressure. (From Landis, E. M., and Pappenheimer, J. R.: in Hamilton, W. F. (ed.), *Handbook of Physiology: Circulation* [Washington: American Physiological Society, 1963], Vol. II, p. 975.)

6 mm Hg expected in theory. In this way, the organism that has lost effective blood volume enjoys an important compensatory increase in the restoring forces throughout the vascular bed. An additional advantage that can be seen in Figure 5-10 is that the protein osmotic pressure in efferent glomerular blood rises sharply as the filtration fraction increases. This not only limits the filtration rate, but, as was mentioned previously, a further advantage of the change in osmotic pressure with concentration is that the increased value in glomerular efferent blood will give increased force for the transcapillary absorption of fluid in the peritubular circulation.

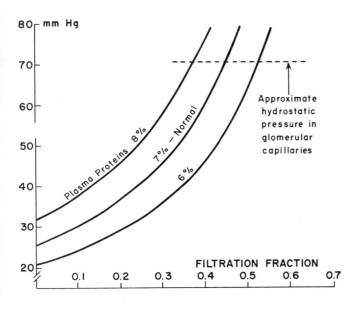

Fig. 5-10.—Illustrating the significance of protein osmotic pressure for glomerular filtration. The rapid increase of protein osmotic pressure as a function of concentration places an upper limit to the filtration fraction of the kidney. (From Landis, E. M., and Pappenheimer, J. R.: in Hamilton, W. F. (ed.): *Handbook of Physiology: Circulation* [Washington: American Physiological Society, 1963], Vol. II, p. 976.)

Interstitial Fluid

Pressure in the Interstitial Fluid Compartment

Accurate plethysmography gives indirect evidence that the pressure in tissue spaces changes during venous congestion. By pressurizing the device and so collapsing the vessels and obtaining estimates of the volume of cells plus tissue fluid, Landis and Gibbon showed that, when the venous pressure was increased, filtration into the forearm at first proceeded rapidly but then slowed as interstitial fluid pressure rose above the resting level. Figure 5-11 shows the increase in pressure as the fluid accumulation became so great that the edema level was reached. This occurs at some 10 cc per 100 cc of tissue in the limb. When so much fluid accumulates, there is a great increase in the rate of reabsorption by the capillaries, and the lymph flow rises.

Normal tissues contain vanishingly small amounts of fluid layered between the cells. In order to measure its pressure directly, a fine needle must be used. No capillaries or lymphatics may be breached, and the flow of fluid must be adjusted by manipulating the pressure in the micropipette so that there is a balance without movement in either direction. The results of numerous studies of interstitial fluid pressures show resting values of the order of 2–5 mm Hg. If there is a rapid rise of venous pressure, as in the foot when the individual stands erect and still on a hot day, then the interstitial pressure will rise to values of the order of 20–30 mm Hg. After a few hours, the tissue elements are abruptly forced apart and overt edema forms. If the rate of fluid accumulation is very slow, as in the edema developing in persons with heart failure, then the interstitial pressure may not be significantly elevated despite gross distension of the tissue spaces.

There is evidence that interstitial pressure can be negative due to increased absorption by the capillaries during vasoconstriction. In studies by Guyton using implanted perforated plastic capsules, negative pressures were observed in the tissues of the abdominal wall as well as in muscle. The negativity may be due to active and passive pumping movements of the valved lymphatics. Not only are these evacuated when the tissue pressures rise with body movements, but there may also be active movement of the muscle cells in their walls. The exact value of interstitial pressure differs from tissue to tissue. The pressure within the kidney appears to be relatively high, i.e., of the order of 10 mm Hg, rising and falling throughout the interstitium, tubules, and the peritubular capillaries in accordance with the tension exerted by the capsule.

Osmotic Pressure of Proteins in Interstitial Fluid Outside Capillary Walls and the Function of the Lymphatics

Throughout most tissues there is distributed a network of fine, closed lymphatic tubes, which are modified veins lined by endothelium. Particularly dense in the dermis, periosteum, and submucosa of the genitourinary, respiratory, and gastrointestinal tracts, they pass through lymph nodes distributed all over the body with special aggregates in the mesentery, axillae, and groin. Although some nodes appear to be directly connected with the local veins, the majority of lymphatics grow larger by convergence, forming ever-bigger channels that finally end in the right lymphatic trunk, draining arm, head, and neck, and in the thoracic duct, draining the rest of the body. The lymph then enters the blood circulation through the left subclavian vein. In addition to the well-recognized, bacterial-scavenging role of the network, the lymphatic system is a vital bilge pump that returns to the circulation the 2–4 liters

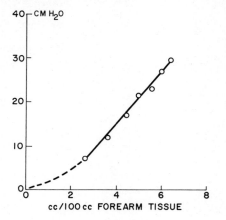

Fig. 5-11.—In this figure, calculated interstitial fluid pressures are charted against the cumulative volume of added interstitial fluid. As the interstitial compartment is distended by an increasing volume of filtered fluid *(abscissa)*, interstitial pressure in the forearm tissues rises slowly at first and then more rapidly *(ordinate)*. (From Landis, E. M., and Pappenheimer, J. R.: in Hamilton, W. F. (ed.): *Handbook of Physiology: Circulation* [Washington: American Physiological Society, 1963], Vol. II, p. 978.)

per day of fluid that normally escapes from the vascular bed, together with the protein that would otherwise form a gel in the tissues and lead to intractable edema.

Electron microscopy shows that the vessels closely resemble capillaries but seem to be more loosely put together at the cell margins. Thus they more readily permit the entry of particulate and macromolecular materials. The bigger vessels are less leaky, having quite tight walls impermeable to molecular weights in excess of 2,000. They have very delicate paired valves, above each of which are often accumulations of smooth muscle cells that could drive the lymph centrally. Pressures in the system are very low, of the order of a mm of mercury or so. Since lymph contains as much as 4–5% protein, this means that fluid may move from the tissue spaces into the vessels. However, the mechanism by which they stay open is not clear in view of their leaky nature. Certainly, movement through the lymphatics is greatly assisted by local changes of tissue pressure, such as those accompanying muscle movement, including peristalsis in the case of the gut, and the pulsation of arteries in their proximity.

An important feature of this system is its function of removing protein that has escaped from the main capillary bed. Large molecules that reach the interstitial fluid space do not appear to be able to get back out again through the venous end of the capillary bed. The lymphatic network is the only route for the return of protein from the interstitial fluid spaces. Direct measurements of edema fluids have yielded an average interstitial fluid protein content of the order of 0.4%. The same figure was obtained by Pappenheimer and Soto-Rivera by measurements of the plasma protein lost from blood passing through congested hind limbs of cats. The concordance of these sets of data gives confidence in the accuracy of the over-all value. It indicates that the capillaries are very effective in retaining protein as long as their walls remain intact.

Since the lymph from a resting extremity contains 1–3 gm of protein, the interstitial fluid must have been concentrated some tenfold as it passed into and down the lymphatics. There is more than 0.3% of protein in the extravascular fluids of the liver and intestines. Depending on the tissue, the content ranges up to 1% with the tissue fluid osmotic pressure varying from 1.0 mm Hg to as much as 9 mm Hg. Hence, the figures that can be placed in the Starling equilibrium equation cited at the beginning of this chapter are somewhat varied:

$$\begin{matrix} \text{Filtration} \\ \text{or} \\ \text{Absorption} \end{matrix} = K \begin{matrix} \text{Capillary P} \\ \text{35 mm Hg} \end{matrix} - \begin{matrix} \text{Os P Plasma} \\ \text{25 mm Hg} \end{matrix} -$$

$$\begin{matrix} \text{Interstit P} \\ \text{1–9 mm Hg} \end{matrix} + \begin{matrix} \text{Tissue Os P} \\ \text{1–5 mm Hg} \end{matrix}$$

The equation expresses the fact that, depending on the location in the capillary, there is fluid flowing into the interstitium or back into the

Fig. 5-12.—Schematic diagram of "an average limb capillary" to indicate approximate pressure and movement of filtrate in different sections. (Modified from Landis, E. M., and Pappenheimer, J. R.: in Hamilton, W. F. (ed.): *Handbook of Physiology: Circulation* [Washington: American Physiological Society, 1963], Vol. II, p. 985.)

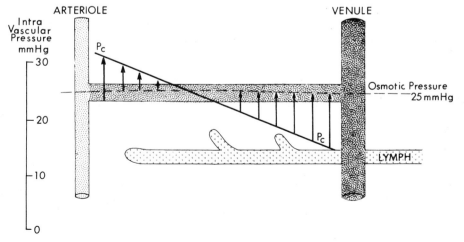

capillary (Fig. 5-12). The protein content of the lymph in the resting limb is high, i.e., 1-3 gm. But with venous congestion, this falls to less than 1%. In burns when permeability rises due to injury to the capillary wall, the protein concentration in the interstitial fluid is high; indeed, it does not differ greatly from that for the lymph, for the flow is rapid and the interstitial compartment is well irrigated by capillary filtrate.

In lymphedema with obstructive fibrosis of the bigger lymphatic vessels, the flow of interstitial fluid almost ceases. This leads to an accumulation of extravascular fluid with a high concentration of protein that may become invaded by fibroblasts, leading to a hard, intractable edema. Because malignancies invade the lymphatics, cancer of the breast is treated not only with simple mastectomy but with a block dissection of the axillary lymph nodes as well. The same block dissection will be applied in conditions such as a melanoma on the leg. Chronic edema is a frequent, long-term, postoperative accompaniment of the reduction by such techniques of the lymphatic drainage of a limb to a few remaining skin vessels. This edema is made worse by any inflammation of the limb that involves the overloaded lymphatics, causing their obstruction by fibrous tissue. These limbs frequently swell during states of emotional arousal. A possible mechanism may be spasm of the few remaining lymphatics under the influence of sympathetic stimulation.

The treatment of chronic lymphatic deficiency conditions is difficult. Patients are warned to avoid burns, scratches, and skin punctures. Infections must be treated at once. An attempt is made to reverse the physiological circumstances. The arm is kept raised and used at work above heart level whenever feasible. It is exercised to keep as much tissue fluid pumped away by muscular action as possible. Carefully fitted elastic sleeves designed to exert some 20-40 mm Hg counter-pressure are used to displace the Starling equilibrium in a favorable direction by increasing the effective interstitial pressure. Finally, the arm or leg can be placed in a rubberized nylon massaging bag and the pressure intermittently elevated briefly to still-higher levels, i.e., 60 mm Hg. This can be done at home for several hours a day using a pump, cycling approximately once a minute with a pressure phase of some 20 seconds. Procedures such as these assist in the reduction of edema, and inadequate lymphatics may hypertrophy to take over the function of the lost drainage system.

CIRCULATION OF INTERSTITIAL FLUID

There are a number of physiological roles played by the protein that leaves the capillaries and enters the interstitial spaces. Not only does it contribute to the defense against infection, but it is also involved in normal cell metabolism. Hormones and fatty acids attached to it are carried through the capillary wall. The greatest movement of protein occurs in the liver where albumin is synthesized and metabolic requirements are high.

Thus, in addition to the circulation of 8,000 liters every day from the heart through the

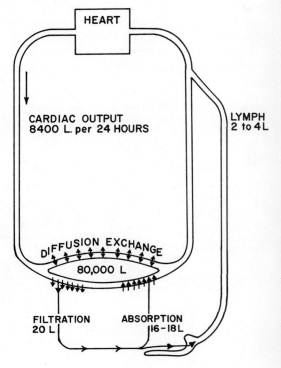

Fig. 5-13.—In 24 hours, the heart of the average adult pumps 8,400 liters; of this, 20 filter out from the high-pressure end of the capillaries. Some 16 to 18 liters are reabsorbed at the venous end, while the remaining 2 to 4 liters are returned to the circulation via the lymphatics. Meanwhile, a prodigious 80,000 liters of fluid are exchanged by diffusion across the highly permeable capillary walls. (Modified from Landis, E. M., and Pappenheimer, J. R.: in Hamilton, W. F. (ed.): *Handbook of Physiology: Circulation* [Washington: American Physiological Society, 1963], Vol. II, p. 987, Fig. 5-2.)

capillaries and back, there is, as the diagram indicates (Fig. 5-13), a further filtration of some 20 liters out of the high-pressure end of the capillary with a reabsorption after passage through the tissues at the low-pressure end of 16–18 liters. Yet another circulation occurs with the passage of 2–4 liters out of the 20 liters of filtrate from the high-pressure portion of the capillary that is not reabsorbed but goes on to enter the lymphatics and thence returns to the venous circulation. These figures, which are derived from studies of forearm fluid shifts, give a filtration fraction of $\frac{20}{8,000}$ or 0.25%.

It is probable that the liver and intestine contribute even greater amounts of filtrate. As stated, lymph flow in a fasting man at rest is 2–4 liters per day, rising to 3–4 liters if allowance is made for effects of meals and activity. Actually as much protein normally passes in 24 hours through the capillary wall as is present in the circulating blood volume. Giving large volumes of intravenous fluid will increase that rate of protein passage and, with it, the rate of thoracic duct flow. The amount of protein involved is very considerable, i.e., the 20 liters of filtrate contains 0.2–0.4 gm per cent or 40–80 gm/diem of protein. This must find its way back from the interstitial spaces to the circulation via the returned lymph.

When blood volume is lost, as after an acute hemorrhage, the continuing flow of lymph into the blood stream can effectively replace the protein in the lost plasma and speed the restoration of a normal blood volume. In the forearm, Landis and Gibbon found a value of 0.0033 ml/min/100 cc blood (Fig. 5-14), and, in experiments inducing an over-all rise of venous pressure by repeated Valsalva maneuvers, Brown *et al.* have determined the filtration coefficient for the body (except for the abdomen and thorax). It is 0.0036 cc/min/100 gm body weight for every cm rise of venous pressure. With a mean venous pressure increase of 20 cm water for a period of 30 minutes, some 400 to 700 ml is lost from the circulating blood volume. This change in filtration process has been shown to be 5 to 10 times more sensitive to an alteration of pressure of the venous end of the capillary than it is to the same change at the arterial end.

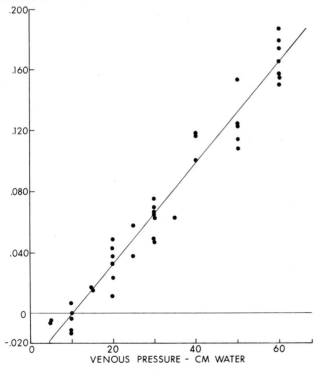

Fig. 5-14.—Rates of filtration measured by pressure plethysmography in the human forearm during graded elevation of venous pressure for 10-minute periods. The slope of the line corresponds to a filtration coefficient of .0033 ml/min/100 ml forearm tissue per cm H$_2$O increase of venous pressure. (From Landis, E. M., and Gibbon, J. H.: J. Clin. Invest. 12:118, 1933, Fig. 3.)

In the lungs, the average capillary pressure is far lower than in the systemic circulation and is only half the osmotic pressure of the plasma proteins (Fig. 5-2). Filtration and an increase of interstitial fluid volume do not occur until the atrial pressure is increased to the plasma osmotic pressure level of 25–30 mm Hg. At this point, gross filtration commences as the pulmonary capillary pressure becomes excessive. The lung is a very dry tissue, having only a thin fluid layer to satisfy surface tension requirements. In the lung, as well as in the human forearm and in the dog's leg, the requirements of the Starling filtration absorption principle are met; it is the difference between the hydrostatic and osmotic forces acting across the membrane that determines the net rates of filtration or absorption.

The work of Pappenheimer has permitted the derivation of values for the (K) of the original Starling equation:

membranes shows that the rate at which water and lipid insoluble substances including protein pass through the capillary wall is so slow that other effects must be taking place. It has been concluded that diffusion is not the only process involved in the passage of materials across the capillary, but that a combination of diffusion with the flow of fluid through pores or channels leading out of the vessel into the interstitial spaces is involved. As Figure 5-15 indicates, if the pore radius is large enough, the dominant effect will be this hydrodynamic flow and vice versa. Damage to the capillary wall appears to increase the effective pore size and, so, in circumstances such as acute hypoxia, the fraction of plasma filtered rises from some 2–4% to much higher values, and the corpuscles begin to pack together as plasma is progressively lost. In severe cases of capillary stasis, a solid plug of cells

---

Filtration = K (Cap Pressure−Plasma Osmotic P−Interstitial Pressure + Tissue Fluid Osmotic P)

This constant is a measure, not of gaseous diffusion, but of the hydraulic or hydrodynamic conductivity of the capillary wall and defines its capacity to pass large and lipid insoluble molecules. The term may be contrasted with capillary permeability, which refers to the capacity to permit diffusion of small, lipid soluble molecules, specifically oxygen and carbon dioxide. A comparison of the filtration coefficients for cell membranes, capillary walls, and artificial

forms at the venous end of the vessel and flow ceases.

There is some evidence that the platelets help to restore a relative impermeability to protein by helping to close the distended pores in the capillary wall as it recovers from the injury. There is a diminution of fluid loss to normal values and a return of absorption at the venous end. With the renewed balance of activities, the osmotic pressure of the tissue fluids decreases and normal

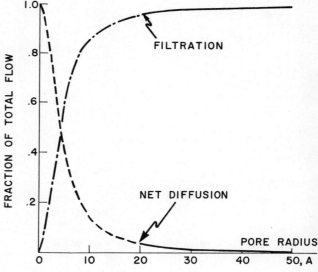

Fig. 5-15.—Net diffusion and hydrodynamic flow of water as a function of pore size during flow induced by hydrostatic or osmotic forces. For membranes with effective pore radii greater than about 20 Å, the net flow of water by diffusion is negligible compared to filtration. (From Pappenheimer, J. R.: Physiol. Rev. 33:395, 1953, Fig. 1.)

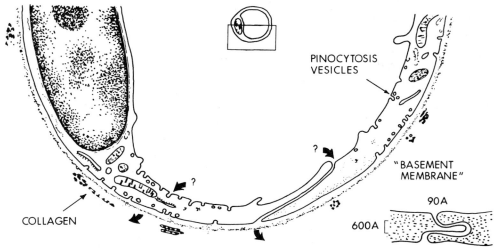

Fig. 5-16.—Diagram illustrating current concepts of fine structure in muscle capillaries. Small figure above represents area of capillary that has been enlarged. The nucleus of a single endothelial cell is shown at left. The capillary cross-section may be formed by a single cell rolled into a tube or may be made up of several cells. The interendothelial region appears as a thin slit pore with direct connection from inside to outside of capillary. (See arrows to right of diagram and inset at lower right.) It occupies only a fraction of 1% of the total endothelial surface. The cytoplasm contains numerous small vesicles and inpocketings of the surface that are characteristic of microphagocytosis or pinocytosis; this mechanism may be involved in the transcapillary passage of particles that are too large to traverse interendothelial openings (arrows to left of diagram). The outer surface of the endothelium is enveloped by an amorphous basement membrane about 600 Å in thickness and with histochemical properties indicative of a mucopolysaccharide. (From Landis, E. M., and Pappenheimer, J. R.: in Hamilton, W. F. (ed.): *Handbook of Physiology: Circulation* [Washington: American Physiological Society, 1963], Vol. II, p. 1011, Fig. 9-3.)

flow recommences through the vessel. The capillary blood pressure which rises during stasis to arteriolar levels begins to fall as the permeability of the wall returns to normal and the column of aggregated red cells starts to move again. Although it is true that oxygen lack affects capillary permeability in the foregoing way, nevertheless, such hypoxia must be exceedingly severe; a systemic oxygen lack compatible with life has no significant effect on capillary permeability or plasma flow.

This does not mean that oxygen lack due to a local deficiency in blood flow may not have the most severe effects. Histamine and other agents that seriously affect capillary permeability appear to increase the size and number of the larger openings in the wall by increasing the slit-like separation between endothelial cells. The amount of protein going through the wall increases, but the mechanism is not yet conclusively established. Proteins pass with fluid through minute channels between the cells, whereas lipid soluble molecules like CO_2 and O_2 diffuse through the lipid plasma membranes of the endothelial cells. It was facts such as the observation that lipid insoluble molecules like sucrose, which cannot pass through the membranes of normal tissue cells, can pass quite freely out of capillaries that led to this conclusion. It is now directly supported by electron microscopic studies that clearly show there are, indeed, appropriately sized channels between cells.

As Figure 5-16 indicates, in a muscle capillary, the junction between two endothelial cells may be a thin slit or a pore making a direct connection from the inside to the outside. The slit is about 90 Å wide and 0.5 to 1 μ long; it thus occupies much less than 1% of the total endothelial surface. In addition, there are many small vesicles and surface impocketings that suggest pinocytosis, the active mechanism by which particles too large to get through the interendothelial openings may cross the capillary wall. There are differences between the capillaries in different vascular beds. Thus the visceral organ capillaries are probably far more permeable than those in muscle, whereas there is much-diminished exchange of lipid insoluble molecules between the central nervous system and the blood. However, the permeability of the capillary bed as a whole to serum albumin is about the same as that of the isolated muscle. This is partly because muscle accounts for 65% of the body weight, exclusive of bone and fat, which are not greatly involved in capillary exchange.

The important fact is that pores do exist in the normal healthy capillary wall and that they provide for the very rapid transcapillary diffusion of small, lipid insoluble molecules. The rates at which this occurs are amazing. It is estimated that water, Na, Cl, urea, and glucose diffuse back and forth 10 to 40 times as fast as they are brought to the tissues by the blood. These high rates of exchange occur because, in spite of the small pore area, the actual path length through the capillary wall is in fact very short. The effective size of the pore in the wall is sufficient to allow even large plasma protein molecules to pass. Small molecules diffuse rapidly down fluid columns filtering through the pores from the capillary to interstitial space; they also go back up them, depending on the concentration gradient. The bigger molecules diffuse far more slowly and depend on the rate at which fluid filters down the channel. Hence, the protein molecules leave at the arterial end but cannot return at the venous end of the capillary, whereas water and small molecules are rapidly diffusing out of the capillary and back again by the very same pores.

The net rate at which fluid leaves the vascular bed to return via the lymphatics is, as noted, only 2% of the total plasma flow down the capillary. It is for this reason that the clearance of I^{131} from the skin, which is a measure of total plasma flow, is not appreciably affected by edema formation, which depends on the rate of flow of lymph out of the tissue space.

There is evidence that, in addition to the previously described minute pores between the endothelial cells, there are larger capillary leaks corresponding to holes some 200–350 Å in radius. At these areas, which are sometimes detectable by microinjection, the fluid leaks out rapidly in streams that are more frequent at the venous end of the capillary. These big pores may be present in greater numbers in the liver and intestine and account for the passage of high molecular-weight compounds.

The very high permeability of the renal glomerular membrane is probably not due to large pores but rather to a special arrangement of the epithelial cells covering the glomerular capillaries. Here interdigitating slit pores are found that are 80–100 Å wide and occupy a relatively extensive 2–3% of the total surface.

Capillary Permeability to Lipid Soluble Molecules., i.e., Respiratory Gases

The very high rates at which oxygen and carbon dioxide traverse the capillary would suggest that these lipid soluble molecules diffuse through regions in the capillary wall that are impermeable to lipid insoluble materials. They pass straight across the plasma membranes of the capillary endothelial cells instead of transversing the water-filled pores used by the insoluble molecules. The permeability of the pulmonary capillary for oxygen is some 500 times that of a muscle capillary for water. The pulmonary capillaries in particular are relatively impermeable to small, lipid insoluble molecules, but are adapted so that the lipid soluble oxygen and carbon dioxide pass through easily.

In muscle, there is another mechanism to assist oxygen passage. During maximal activity, the capillary surface may increase 2- to 4-fold by the opening up of fresh channels. In general, the permeability for oxygen and carbon dioxide is so high that the capillary wall is not a factor limiting net rates of blood-tissue exchange. More critical are the distribution and rate of flow of capillary blood, the volume of the extravascular compartments, and the rates of chemical reaction in the tissues. Only with molecules the size of insulin or larger is capillary permeability a limiting factor in the exchange in well-perfused tissues; i.e., the oxygen pressure head needed to supply the diffusion volume around each capillary is normally fully met by the capillary blood. In resting muscle, as few as 25 capillaries/mm^2 suffice to maintain metabolism. At maximum muscle activity, 500 capillaries/mm^2 are available, while brain and liver continuously provide some 200 and 100 capillaries/mm^2, respectively.

Using lipid soluble molecules labelled by Rb^{86}, Na^{23} or I^{131}, it can be shown that their distribution is blood-flow-limited and that they can, consequently, serve as measures of relative regional blood flow on the basis of their clearance rate as determined by a counter placed over the tissue.

Nonuniform alterations of blood flow in the microcirculation will determine the relationship between total blood flow and blood-tissue exchange rates. The fraction of total blood flow passing through nutrient capillaries varies greatly according to metabolic demands of the tissues.

In the skin, for instance, and in the liver and intestine, there is a nonnutrient fraction that passes through quite large arteriovenous anastomoses or, in the case of mesentery or muscle, through arteriovenous capillaries. This nonuniform distribution occurs between regions having different functions and metabolic rates as, for example, the cortex versus the medulla of the kidney and the gray versus the white matter of the brain. In the hands, the nonnutrient flow through AV shunts serves the purpose of temperature regulation. In muscle, when the sympathetic vasoconstrictor nerves are stimulated, nutrient flow through the capillary bed may nearly fail, leaving blood to flow through arteriovenous channels. This diversion is so intense in diving mammals that respiratory gas exchange is reduced to a minute fraction of normal for periods of many minutes. The division of blood into nutrient and nonnutrient flows is controlled by vasomotor nerves. I^{131} clearance, which reflects nutrient flow, may actually decrease at a moment when flow through AV channels is greatly increased.

Summary

It is the function of the circulation to provide for the exchange of materials between blood and tissues. This is the importance of the development of isotope techniques that permit function to be studied in terms of local tissue exchange rates. The material presented in this chapter indicates the strides that have been made toward the development of a quantitative background for assessing the different roles played by transcapillary diffusion and by flow through pores in the exchange of various materials between blood and tissue.

REFERENCES

Brown, E., et al.: Loss of Fluid and Protein From the Blood During a Systemic Rise of Venous Pressure Produced by Repeated Valsalva Maneuvers in Man, J. Clin. Invest. 37:1465–1475, 1947.

Guyton, A. C., Armstrong, C. G., and Crowell, J. W.: Negative Pressure in the Interstitial Spaces, Physiologist 3:70, 1960.

Henry, J. P., and Gauer, O. H.: The Influence of Temperature Upon Venous Pressure in the Foot, J. Clin. Invest. 29:855, 1950.

Landis, E. M.: Capillary Pressure and Capillary Permeability, Physiol. Rev. 14:404–481, 1934.

Landis, E. M., and Gibbon, J. H.: The Effects of Temperature and of Tissue Pressure on the Movement of Fluid Through the Human Capillary Wall, J. Clin. Invest. 12:105–138, 1933.

Landis, E. M., and Pappenheimer, J. R.: Exchange of Substances Through the Capillary Walls, in Hamilton, W. F. (ed.): *Handbook of Physiology: Circulation* (Washington: American Physiological Society, 1963), Vol. II, chap. 29, pp. 961–1,034.

Pappenheimer, J. R.: Passage of Molecules Through Capillary Walls, Physiol. Rev. 33:387–423, 1953.

Starling, E. H.: On the Absorption of Fluids from the Connective Tissue Spaces, J. Physiol. (London) 19:312–326, 1896.

Winsor, T., and Hyman, C.: *A Primer of Peripheral Vascular Diseases* (Philadelphia: Lea & Febiger, 1965).

6

The Low-Pressure System, Orthostasis, and the Return of Blood to the Central Reservoir

Introduction

THE LOW-PRESSURE SYSTEM consisting of the great veins, the right heart, the pulmonary vascular bed, and the left heart in diastole is highly distensible, and the components of this system will change markedly in volume in response to relatively small changes in pressure. Yet, the pressure changes can be large. When, for example, a man stands upright, they range from 100 mm Hg at the feet to subzero in the jugular veins, and, under the pull of gravity, enough blood may be drained from the intrathoracic compartments to jeopardize proper cardiac filling.

It is, therefore, important to determine what adjustments are made by a man who is holding the erect posture. In view of the fact that active, healthy men spend two thirds of the day on their feet or at least sitting, it is reasonable to consider orthostasis as a normal resting physiologic posture. Linked with this assumption is the inquiry into how man's blood volume and the tone of his blood vessels are so adjusted that he is able to maintain adequate heart filling in spite of the erect posture. The feat is all the more remarkable because the volume elasticity coefficient of the low-pressure system is so modest. This coefficient can be estimated by giving a blood infusion or removing a corresponding amount, for example, taking some 6.5 cc/kg and, four days later, reinfusing the stored blood together with the citrate used to prevent clotting, i.e., 8.1 cc/kg. As Figure 6-1 shows, when the pressures for 12 people were plotted, the small infusions caused the central venous pressure to rise and to maintain that level for as long as half an hour. The blood removals resulted in a fall in central venous pressure. The return to normal was delayed for at least the same length of time. This data can be presented in a diagram showing the changes in right atrial pressure for various changes in blood volume (Fig. 6-2). From this, the volume elasticity coefficient of the total circulation can be estimated.

$$E = \frac{P}{V} = \frac{7 \text{ cm } H_2O}{1,000 \text{ cc}} = 7 \text{ dyne cm}^{-5}$$

It shows that the total circulation is 200 times as distensible as the arterial elastic reservoir, which, as previously described, had a total distensibility of approximately

$$\frac{1 \text{ mm Hg}}{1 \text{ cc}} \text{ i.e., } 1,400 \text{ dyne cm}^{-5}.$$

This means that if 1,000 cc of blood are infused, then 995 cc are to be found in the low-pressure system, and only 5 cc in the arterial tree. Hence in observations that are concerned with the distribution of blood within the cardiovascular system under the influence of gravity, the volume given or taken by the arterial reservoir can be neglected. On the other hand, the distensibility of the low-pressure system raises the question as to how the total blood volume is distributed throughout this reservoir, especially under the influence of the formidable force of gravity.

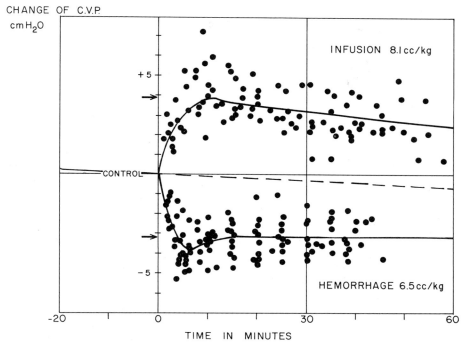

Fig. 6-1.—Change of venous pressure in 12 hemorrhage and 10 infusion experiments. In these quietly resting subjects, the control pressure fell slightly, as indicated by the dotted line. For infusion, the mean volume change per kg body weight was 8.1 cc and for hemorrhage, 6.5 cc. (From Gauer, O. H., Henry, J. P., and Sieker, H.: Changes in Central Venous Pressure After Moderate Hemorrhage and Transfusion in Man, Circulation Res. 4:79–84, 1956. By permission of the American Heart Association, Inc., New York, N. Y.)

Blood Volume and its Divisions

General Considerations

The blood volume of a well-built man is about 77 cc/kg ± 10%, which for a 70-kg subject means a volume of about 5.4 liters. Variations occur in connection with physical training, climate, and other circumstances such as high-altitude acclimatization, pregnancy, and pathological changes in the circulation such as damage to the heart valves or heart muscle.

In clinical studies, a distinction is often drawn between the absolute and the circulating blood volume. This is not legitimate unless there is a true storage of blood and unless certain regions of the circulation can actually be closed off by sphincters. In the dog, the spleen serves as such a reservoir; but in man, true blood reservoirs have not been demonstrated. The difference that is observed between effective or active blood volume and the total volume depends upon the measurement technique. If one of the usual dye dilution methods is used, then the degree of dilution is to some extent dependent upon dilution time. The earlier the sample is taken, the higher the concentration and the less the estimated volume. Now if the rate of blood flow through all parts of the circulation is equally brisk, then mixing will be rapid and complete. If, however, there are regions in which considerable amounts of blood linger, i.e., in canals with very sluggish blood flow, then it cannot be expected that the method will give a true blood volume.

In spite of increases of body fluid volume with drinking, and losses by sweating and via the urine, and in spite of vasomotor changes modifying vascular capacity, the total blood volume stays relatively constant due to the regulatory action of the kidney and the thirst mechanism. The long-term changes that develop as a result of training and climatic influences probably arise as a reflex response to expansion of the vascular bed. Because the arteries are rigid, all changes in blood volume resulting from blood loss or transfusion are intimately concerned with the highly distensible low-pressure system. When 10% of the blood volume is removed, the arterial

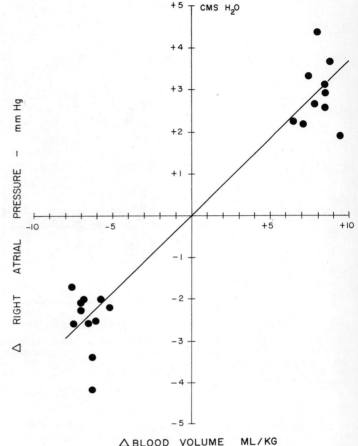

Fig. 6-2.—Effect of alteration in blood volume on right-atrial pressure in normal recumbent subjects. (From Gauer, O. H., Henry, J. P., and Sieker, H.: Changes in Central Venous Pressure After Moderate Hemorrhage and Transfusion in Man. Circulation Res. 4:79–84, 1956. By permission of the American Heart Association, Inc., New York, N. Y.)

pulse pressure falls somewhat, but mean arterial pressure is maintained and there is a compensatory rise in pulse rate. Cardiac output is not significantly impaired until at least 20% is lost. With more severe hemorrhage in excess of 30%, there is a decrease in cardiac output and a sharp increase in peripheral resistance. At 40%, serious symptoms develop; if nothing is done, one half of the subjects die. These symptoms are due to the impaired blood flow through the various organs that leads to severe tissue oxygen lack. In certain cases, despite apparent recovery, after a day or so death supervenes because previous long, drawn-out, intense vasoconstriction has led to irrevocable ischemic damage of the kidney.

The estimated capacity of the major components of the circulation together with an illustration of the components of the low- and high-pressure systems is presented in Figure 6-3. The volume elasticity or resistance to stretch is indicated by the thickness of the walls, i.e., that of the low-pressure system is 7 dyne cm^{-5} and the high-pressure system, over 1,000 dyne cm^{-5}. The arterial system contains about 900 cc or only 15% of the total blood volume. The function of this distributing network is to conduct the cardiac output to the organs and to distribute it appropriately. Because of its great rigidity, it is hardly affected by changes in total blood volume. Cardiac output may be sustained by a tachycardia, and there need be no serious change in peripheral resistance in the face of a moderate, i.e., 15 to 25% loss of blood volume. In fact, mean blood pressure may even rise slightly instead of falling.

The Central Blood Volume

The intrathoracic blood volume consists of the central blood volume, i.e., the pulmonary circulation and the end-diastolic volume of the left ventricle together with that volume within the right heart and the portion of the great veins located in the thorax. This comprises over 50% of the total blood volume. Because blood volume shifts induce corresponding changes in the gaseous content of the lungs, changes in the amount of blood within the thorax can be roughly assessed by a spirometer. Special precautions permit quite accurate evaluations.

The intrathoracic vessels are not surrounded by a solid mass of tissue but hang free in the elastic network of the lungs. They show very little vasomotor activity and are essentially surface vessels. Because of this peculiar location they can expand readily, explaining why the intrathoracic circulation serves as a pressure-equalizing network accommodating large volumes of blood. This occurs when the peripheral vascular bed is narrowed by external mechanical compression, or by vasoconstriction, or is enlarged by the action of gravity on dependent regions. Thus much of a blood transfusion is immediately taken up by the vessels in the thorax; and, on the other hand, a deficiency in the peripheral blood volume is very rapidly compensated from this same area. For example, measurements show that one half of a volume loss of 400 cc came from the thorax. In fact, the distensibility of the total vascular bed is as great as that of the tissue spaces themselves.

The functional unity of the capacitance vessels of the systemic circulation and the pulmonary vascular bed can be demonstrated by simul-

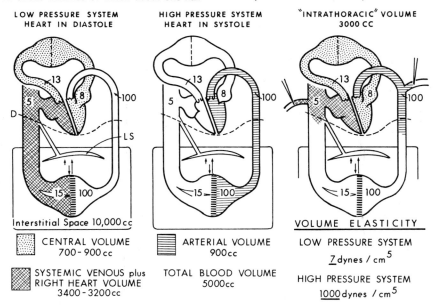

Fig. 6-3.—Estimated capacity of the major compartments of the circulation with an illustration of the components of the low- and high-pressure systems.

The volume elasticity or resistance to stretch is indicated by the thickness of the walls: 7 dynes/cm^5 for the low-pressure system and 1,000 dynes/cm^5 for the high-pressure system. The numbers in each of the sections represent the mean intravascular pressures in mm Hg. In diastole, the left ventricle is part of the low-pressure system, and, in systole, it belongs to the high-pressure system. (D is diaphragm.) The arterial volume constitutes only 15% of the total blood volume.

The central volume, consisting of the pulmonary circulation and the left-heart volume in diastole, holds approximately 10 to 12 stroke volumes of which about one-half can be ejected by the left ventricle regardless of venous return. The size of this reservoir is in some degree a measure of the cardiovascular reserves. The systemic venous plus right-heart volume is the total blood volume less the central and arterial volumes. The exchange of fluid between the circulatory system and the interstitial, including the lymphatic system (LS), is indicated by arrows.

The "intrathoracic" volume, usually determined as "needle-to-needle" volume, is about 60% of the total blood volume. It comprises the central volume proper as well as the right-heart volume, plus the volume of the adjacent great intrathoracic veins. It also includes an ill-defined additional arterial volume that changes greatly with changes of arterial hemodynamics. (From Gauer, O. H., and Henry, J. P.: Physiol. Rev. 43:423, 1963.)

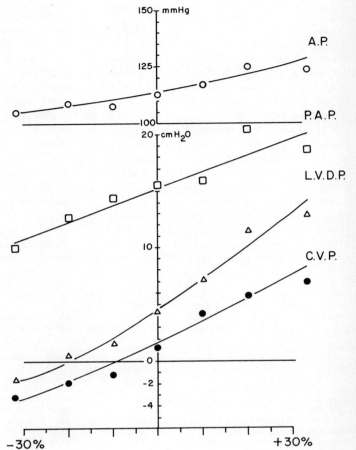

Fig. 6-4.—Multiple curves showing the relationship between changes of estimated blood volume *(abscissa)* and mean intrathoracic vascular pressures in 15 cases.

Reading from below upward: central venous, left ventricular diastolic, pulmonary arterial, and systemic arterial pressures.

The decreasing pressure differential between pulmonary artery and left atrium with increasing blood volume suggests a decreased flow resistance in the pulmonary vascular bed. (From Henry, J. P., Gauer, O. H., and Sieker, H.: The Effect of Moderate Changes in Blood Volume on Left and Right Atrial Pressures, Circulation Res. 4:91–94, 1956. By permission of the American Heart Association, Inc., New York, N. Y.)

taneous pressure measurements made in different sections of the circulation during blood loss and transfusion (Fig. 6-4). When changes are less than ± 30% of the estimated total blood volume, the mean pressures in the central veins, the pulmonary artery, and the left atrium rise and fall in unison. In the range of +15 to −15% alteration of blood volume, central venous pressure and pulmonary arterial pressure run strictly parallel, changing by approximately 2 cm H_2O for a 10% volume shift. Outside these limits, the two pressures still follow each other. The central venous and the pulmonary arterial pressure lines remain equidistant throughout. Although the right ventricle anatomically separates the systemic venous bed from the pulmonary circulation, the small hemorrhages and transfusions have so little effect on the activity of this chamber that the pressure-volume relationship is undisturbed. The slope of the pressure line of the left atrium is steeper than that of the right, and the pressure differential between the pulmonary artery and the left atrium decreases as the blood volume increases. The explanation is a decreased flow resistance as the pulmonary bed becomes more distended.

The flow resistance in the low-pressure system is so low that the right heart produces a mean pulmonary arterial pressure of only 14 mm Hg, while the mean pulmonary capillary pressure is only 6 mm Hg. Nor does the pulmonary arterial pressure increase dramatically with a quadrupling of the cardiac output—even then, it only rises by a mere 4 mm Hg. The secret of the very low resistance is that the pulmonary arteries are short, thin-walled vessels branching repeatedly into a diffuse network. They are very thin, have few muscle and elastic elements, and do not resist distension. The arterioles that are so important in the control of flow to the main diffusion network are not found in the pulmonary bed, and there is a striking absence of the smooth muscle that is so conspicuous in the small vessels of the main network. The result is that the small pulmonary vessels change caliber passively rather than actively, accommodating different volumes of blood.

The capillaries of the pulmonary bed are slightly larger than those in the systemic circuit, and their total area is about 70 square meters. The entire network has a minimum of fluid outside it; for, with a mean capillary pressure of no more than 6 mm Hg, there can be no outward drift of fluid against the inward "suction" of the plasma osmotic pressure of 25 mm Hg. This absence of a fluid layer is important for a diffusion network that is designed solely for the exchange of lipid soluble gaseous oxygen and carbon dioxide with the surrounding atmosphere.

According to a number of estimates, the central blood volume contains from 700 to 1,200 cc or some 10–15 stroke volumes. Hence, even in the event of a radical slowing of the venous stream into the right heart, the left ventricle can continue to exert as many as half a dozen normal beats. Usually, this emergency extra volume in the great vessels of the lungs and in the left atrium remains intact. It is so placed that in the event of sudden cessation of venous inflow, as when a man rises into the erect posture after lying prone for some time, the output can be briefly maintained. Various compensatory reactions can be initiated during the time consumed by the six heart beats needed to exhaust the reservoir, and venous filling can be rapidly increased to meet the requirements of a raised minute volume. The upshot is a new equilibrium state in which adjustment has been made to the changed distribution of central blood volume.

In this connection, the comparison of the left ventricle with the pump on a fire engine may be useful. The engine is always ready for any action; its reserve water tank is kept full by a connection to the fire hydrant. But suppose there is no hydrant, and the return to the tank must come from a hose sucking up the water that has been pumped by the engine and is now running down the street. Then there will be a decrease in the reserve water in the tank by the amount that is flowing down the street to the pool from which the collection hose is returning it to the engine.

Position of the Left Ventricle in the Low-Pressure System

The left ventricle is the link between the low-pressure system and the high-pressure elastic reservoir. It is the pump of the arterial tree during systole, but a part of the central blood reservoir during diastole, for it holds about two stroke volumes at the commencement of any particular stroke. The volume remaining in it after systole makes it possible for the ventricle to help compensate for a sudden drop in peripheral resistance with its resultant loss of pressure in the elastic reservoir. By greater systolic emptying, the stroke volume can at once be doubled just in going from one stroke to the next, all without having to wait for an increase in venous filling. As has been discussed in Chapter 3, the mechanism underlying this dramatic change is an increase in rate and contractility of sympathetic origin and not the Starling relationship between diastolic size of the heart, stroke volume, and minute volume.

In hemorrhage, orthostasis, and positive pressure breathing, x-rays show a more or less sharp reduction of heart size. Various approaches have given a variety of results that indicate that the heart volume constitutes about one third of the total intrathoracic blood content. Starling's law will hold and stroke volume will diminish when the end-diastolic ventricular volume falls until only one stroke volume or even less can be mustered at the peak of diastolic filling, for then the ventricle will empty completely with systole. Under these circumstances, changes in contractility can do no more, and there will necessarily be a linear relationship between stroke volume and diastolic heart size. This shift to a Starling relationship takes place when the intrathoracic volume falls from a normal of 25–30% to 15% or less of the total blood volume. Up to that point, the decreasing diastolic filling pressure has been compensated by a force velocity and rate increase of nervous origin that effectively maintains the cardiac output.

Blood Volume of the Extrathoracic Circulation

The extrathoracic circulation holds approximately 50% of the total blood volume. It can be measured by dye indicator methods or from anatomical data. The estimate of the volume of both legs and one arm as 12% of the total in a recumbent man is reasonably reliable. This value can be doubled by venous stasis. The mesenteric circulation including the liver holds some 25% of the total blood volume. With vigorous muscular exercise, this is decreased by two-thirds in man. The torso (the shoulder girdle, trunk, and pelvis) comprises about 25% of the blood volume. The skin holds 5 cc/100 cm^2 which, in the case of a total skin area of 1.5 square meters, gives 750 cc or 15% of the total. Of special interest are the changes in the blood content of the muscles in going from rest to work. As much as 10 times the normal blood content can flood a full half of the body's total muscle mass in a man at work. Since the flow and volume in resting muscle are far smaller, this means that a volume of 1,500 cc must be derived from other parts of the circulation. During the actual exertion, the rhythmic contractions help to forward blood and tissue fluid to the heart by narrowing the venous bed and cyclically decreasing the volume of blood in the muscle bed.

Relation Between Blood Volume and Interstitial Fluid Space

Small volumes of blood can be completely replaced from the interstitial fluid spaces for these are twice the size of the blood volume. Fluid is rapidly returned through the capillary wall. This space will also take up fluid quite freely if there is a sudden excess of blood volume. There are two mechanisms at work here. The first appears to be a reflex response of the muscle vascular bed and is attributed to a receptor-governed influence on the ratio of pre- to postcapillary resistance. If central blood volume decreases, there is a decreased flow of impulses from the receptors. This leads to an increased resistance at the arterial end of the capillaries, together with some decrease in the resistance to outflow from the network. The result is a decrease in the average pressure in the capillary bed; less fluid leaves at the high-pressure end while more is returned by the osmotic pull at the venous end. Öberg and Folkow regard this as a potent and sensitive device tending to keep the volume of circulatory fluid constant and helping to avoid drastic changes in intravascular pressure.

The second mechanism is a mechanical one, depending on the changes in pressure that occur in the vascular bed. As a result of the fall in venous pressure that follows a loss of blood volume, there is an inflow of fluid low in protein from the tissue spaces. The lowered colloid osmotic pressure in the plasma eventually leads to a new Starling equilibrium in which this osmotic pressure is balanced against the lowered intravascular pressure. This close coupling between the low-pressure system and the interstitial fluid space limits the extent to which the intravascular volume will be disturbed in the event of a sudden gain or loss of fluid in the system.

The compliance of the interstitial fluid space has recently been measured by implanting perforated capsules in various tissues. Using a needle to measure the pressure in the fluid accumulating in the lumen during the 2–4 week healing process, Guyton found a surprising sub-atmospheric pressure of the order of −7 mm Hg. The reason for this negative value appears to be that the mean capillary filtration pressure is far lower than the 20–25 mm Hg osmotic pressure of the plasma. Thus the balance of the factors comprising the Starling equilibrium draws fluid into the capillary lumen leading to approximately 10 mm Hg negative pressure in the interstitial space. If fluid is added to the interstitial space, the pressure there will at first rise by as much as 1 mm Hg for the addition of only 4 cc/kg body weight. After the interstitial fluid pressure has attained atmospheric level, the compliance of the tissue drops sharply and edema commences. With gross edema, as much as 100 ml can be added for a further pressure increase of only a mm or so. But under normal circumstances with modest tissue fluid accumulation, the compliance of the interstitial space is of the same order as that of the low-pressure system, i.e., the pressure of the latter increases by 0.7 to 1.5 mm Hg for a volume increase of 4 ml per kg. The fact that these two compliances are of the same order means there is, in effect, a tight coupling between the interstitial and the intravascular fluid volume so that control of blood volume and of the volume of fluid in the extracellular fluid space can be effectively monitored by the same stretch receptors in the low- and the high-pressure systems. (For further details, see Guyton, *et al.*, and Gauer, Henry, and Behn.)

Venous Pressure Gradient

The pressure difference over the entire length of the large veins is very small. But there is a measurable reduction when the tip of a catheter that is being drawn in a headward direction out of the abdominal vena cava emerges from the liver and enters the thorax.

As a result of the pull of right-ventricular systole, there is a fall in pressure with each heart beat because the blood cannot flow rapidly enough through the restricted veins as they pass through the diaphragm. Thus mean venous pressure within the thorax is 3–4 cms H_2O less than that in the abdomen (see Chap. 2). If the heart is suddenly arrested, then the venous pressures in the thorax and abdomen equalize, showing that the fall in venous pressure on entering the thorax is due to the activity of the heart and is related to the negative intrapleural pressure. An increased pressure differential between the heart and the peripheral veins is not a sign of an increased "venous return" causing a greater flow of blood from the periphery to the heart. Rather, it is an indication that the heart itself is exerting more suction to get blood back into the central reservoir.

The venous pulse is largest in the atrium where it originates. From this point, it extends headward and footward with some progressive change of form. After passage under the diaphragm, it is virtually lost since the intra-abdominal pressure effectively collapses the walls.

Influence of Respiration on Venous Circulation

The pressure changes within the thorax that result from breathing are transmitted to the central veins. With inspiration, the surrounding pressure falls and the stretch on the vessels increases. The increased inrush of blood into the thorax does not occur without resistance; for, with a very deep inspiration, there is actually a partial collapse of the veins leading into the thorax. Thus there are phasic changes in pressure within the central veins. With each inspiration, the diaphragm increases the intra-abdominal pressure so that the changes in the inferior vena cava are in the reverse phase to those in the thorax. Thus breathing works as a pressure-suction pump and serves as an accessory heart that under certain circumstances can actually exceed the performance of the right ventricle.

In contrast to the arteries, whose contour and size are primarily determined by the pressure within them, the veins are to a large extent dependent for their cross-sectional area upon the mechanical circumstances in the surrounding tissues. Even quiet breathing and certainly any effort involving closure of the glottis and straining will radically change the pressures surrounding the heart and great vessels. Many normal and pathological circulatory conditions can be understood only when the transmural pressure, i.e., the difference between the intravascular and extravascular pressure, is considered. For it is this transmural pressure taken in combination with the distensibility of the wall that determines the cross-sectional area of the vessel. Thus if the pressure in the right atrium is $+5$ cm H_2O and, with a deep inspiration, intrathoracic pressure falls to -7 cm H_2O, then the transmural pressure will be $+12$ cm H_2O. The velocity of inflow into the ventricle will depend on the intraventricular pressure, but it can be seen that the fluctuation of extravascular pressure will play an important role in determining the cross-section, hence resistance to inflow. When combined with venous valves, the rhythmic changes in transmural pressure due to respiration, compression of the veins by contraction of muscles, and pulsatile pressure increases induced by arteries that lie alongside the veins together constitute major factors in determining the onward flow of blood to the central reservoir and portals of the heart.

Influence of Orthostasis on Distribution of Blood Volume

The Hydrostatic Indifference Point

Since the pressures in the dependent parts of the body rise during orthostasis while those at the opposite end of the circulatory system fall, a transition zone must necessarily exist where intravascular pressures stay constant despite the change to the vertical posture. At this hydrostatic indifferent point, the intravascular pressure and the cross-section of the vessels are unaffected. Below it, the vascular bed becomes engorged by blood drained from the regions above. If the heart were located at the level of the indifferent point, changes of posture would have a minimal effect on the filling pressure, i.e., on heart size and cardiac output. These points can be illustrated by a model of the circulation consisting of a fluid-filled tube (Fig. 6-5). If it were assumed that atmospheric pressure prevails throughout the tube when it is horizontal, then the point 0 would represent the location where the pressure does not change on tilting the tube. The position of

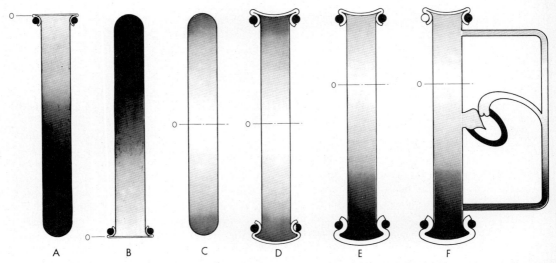

Fig. 6-5.—Hydrostatic pressures at the ends of a tube in the vertical position and the hydrostatic indifferent point (HIP). A test tube covered by an elastic membrane has zero pressure at the membrane whether it is erect **(A)** or inverted **(B)**. In the horizontal position, atmospheric pressure prevails throughout the fluid-filled tube. The point, *O*, marks the location where the pressure does not change when the tube is tilted. The position of HIP depends on the relative "give" of the ends of the tube. That is, if the elastic membrane covering the end of the tube is at the top, the pressure is zero there **(A)**; on inverting the tube, zero pressure shifts to the bottom **(B)**. If the distensibilities are equal, the HIP is located in the middle of the tube. When they differ, it moves toward the more distensible side, i.e., in **C**, where both ends are closed off rigidly, it is in the middle, as it also is in **D** when the membranes are of identical elasticity. In **E**, the lower membrane is twice as thick as the upper one, and the HIP is displaced upwards. In **F**, insertion of a pump does not change the location of the indifferent point. (From Gauer, O. H., and Thron, H. L.: in Hamilton, W. F. (ed.): *Handbook of Physiology: Circulation* [Washington: American Physiological Society, 1965], Vol. III, chap. 67, Fig. 3.)

this hydrostatic indifferent point depends on the relative "gives" at the ends of the tubes. If the distensibilities are equal, then the zero pressure point is located in the middle. When they differ, it moves to the more distensible side. If we prevent air from entering the tube and turn it upside down, the weight of the whole fluid column will be suspended from the "ceiling," exerting there a negative pressure ρh where ρ is the density and h the length of the tube. If we close the tube at both ends with elastic membranes, then, by changing the relative "give" of the membranes, i.e., by using two on one side and only one on the other, we can shift the hydrostatic reference point up or down at will. The conclusion is that, in a closed hydraulic system with distensible walls like the blood vessels, the hydrostatic pressure at the lowest point represents only a part of the pressure that could have been expected if this system were a fluid-filled tube open at the top. Part of the column is suspended from the closed top, creating a negative pressure there and, consequently, only a part of the potential hydrostatic pressure is effectively exerted as a positive pressure at the bottom.

This important principle applies directly to the human venous system in the erect posture. The heart-to-foot distance is approximately equivalent to 130 cm of water, producing a pressure difference of 97 mm Hg. In the headward direction, the difference in pressure between the aortic arch and the brain is some 23 mm Hg. Between the positive pressure in the feet and the negative subatmospheric pressure in the cranial sinuses lies the hydrostatic null point where the pressure changes from positive to negative. This point is determined solely by the pull of the columns under gravity and the elasticity of their vascular containers. In a man who is lying down, it is located about 5–10 cm footward of the diaphragm. Because of the elastic recoil of the lungs, the pressure around the heart is about 15 cms H_2O below atmospheric. Since venous pressure at heart level is slightly positive, the two cancel out and, relative to the atmosphere outside, the pressure at atrial level is approximately zero. Above the heart, the vessels are collapsed.

In an erect man, the vessels below the heart expand under the increased hydrostatic pressure and the null point moves further footward. The vascular bed is poorly filled, the null point sinks far below the heart, and its filling is grossly impaired. The critical importance of the pressure volume characteristics of the central reservoir is brought out by these considerations.

These characteristics become immediately apparent if the heart is suddenly stopped. It has been seen that the arterial tree is only expanded 1 cm^3 for a 1 mm Hg pressure increment. So when the heart stops, the arterial pressure will fall from 100 mm Hg to venous levels with the flow of a mere 100 cc of blood into the venous side. This minor accession of blood will have a negligible affect upon the central venous pressure, raising it by less than 1 mm Hg. The pressure rises in an elastic container either when fluid is added or when the tonus of the walls is enhanced. In severe congestive heart failure, both these conditions are fulfilled for there is an increase both in the volume of blood and in the tonus of the vascular bed.

Figure 6-6 is a schematic representation of the changes in the distribution of blood volume as the hydrostatic pressures are altered by progressive immersion in a water bath. There is a great shift in volume between the intrathoracic compartments and the legs as the shift is made from the erect man in orthostasis (A), through an intermediate state (B), to the man immersed up to his neck in a tank (C). In orthostasis, which is the normal condition of man for some 16 hours a day, the upper parts of the pulmonary circulation and the intrathoracic veins are collapsed, whereas the vascular bed of the legs is distended. The hydrostatic indifferent point (HIP) is considerably below the heart, and the filling pressure and the size of the heart are appreciably reduced (A). When immersed, the venous volume of the legs can be readily accommodated in the intrathoracic compartment, and the hydrostatic indifferent point shifts cranial to the atria so that the filling pressure and heart size are greatly increased. Water up to the level of the diaphragm cancels the intravascular hydrostatic pressure gradient by providing an identical external gradient. The effect of gravity is neutralized, and the volume distribution is not much different from that in recumbency (B).

If the subject is immersed up to the neck, the increased water pressure actually forces more blood into the thorax, producing a state of plethora or hypervolemia. If the pressure differential is increased still further, as by sinking below the surface of the water and breathing through a tube in the classic Indian escape maneuver, then the heart and pulmonary vessels can be overfilled; indeed, collapse of the cardiovascular system can ensue if you go deep enough.

Fig. 6.6.—Water immersion as an antagonist of orthostasis. **A,** during orthostasis, the vascular bed of the legs is distended. The necessary volume is taken from the intrathoracic region. **B,** immersion up to the diaphragm cancels the intrathoracic hydrostatic pressure gradient by an identical external gradient. Volume distribution, therefore, is not much different from that in recumbency. **C,** with immersion up to the neck, the increased water pressure forces more blood into the thorax. (From Gauer, O. H., and Thron, H. L.: Postural Changes in the Circulation, in Hamilton, W. F. (ed.): *Handbook of Physiology: Circulation* [Washington: American Physiological Society, 1965], Vol. III, p. 2,418.)

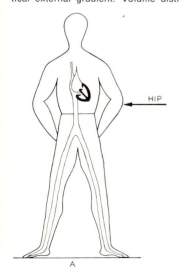
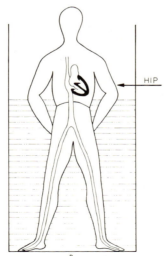
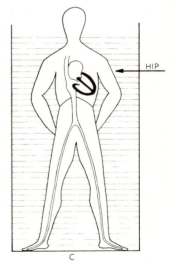

The importance of the foregoing rests in the fact that in our society the vast majority of working activities and the better part of the day is spent either standing or seated with the legs dependent. A heavy strain is placed on the cardiovascular system's protective reflexes by this continuous exposure to the earth's gravity field of an organism poorly designed to tolerate it. The primitive man either squats, sits with legs level with the buttocks, or lies when he is still. For the most part when erect, he is in motion and protected from some of the effects of orthostasis by the action of the muscle pump.

Acute Changes and Redistribution of Blood Volume in Orthostasis

In the resting or recumbent man, more than 50% of the total blood volume is in the systemic veins, about 30% is in the intrathoracic vessel compartments, and less than 15% in the systemic arteries. The result is that the large shifts in blood volume that occur on assumption of the upright position are almost entirely confined to the low-pressure system. On standing upright, the largest pressure change occurs in the big veins. The intravenous pressure will measure 120–130 cm H_2O at the ankle, and the average distending pressure in the various tissues of the thighs and lower legs may be estimated at about 80 cm H_2O. The amount of blood pooling in this mass of muscle and skin, when the pressure rises from 15 cm H_2O during recumbency to this level, may be derived from the pressure volume diagram for both legs up to the groin; it is approximately 500 ml. (Fig. 6-7). Changing the local temperature by heating or chilling the limbs will have a considerable effect on the amount of blood pooled.

With prolonged quiet standing, the high filtration pressure leads to an additional slow rise of leg volume that may go on for many hours. This appears to be in part due to a further relaxation of the vein walls and in part to extravasation of plasma filtrate. The decrease in blood volume may be deduced from the changes in hematocrit and plasma protein concentration. It may be as much as 10–15% after prolonged quiet standing.

By spirometry and use of the plethysmograph, it has been found that about three quarters of

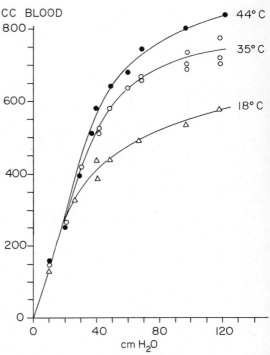

Fig. 6-7.—Pressure volume diagram of both legs up to the groin at various temperatures of the plethysmograph. In a vertical tilt, the mean venous pressure rises from approximately 15 cm H_2O to 80 cm H_2O. The concurrent volume increase at 35°C is about 500 ml. (From Henry, J. P.: J. Aviation Med. 22:31, 1951.)

the blood displaced to the dependent parts while standing comes from the intrathoracic vascular compartments, reducing the amount in the heart and pulmonary circuit by some 25%. The sum total of the evidence that the intrathoracic vessels serve as a blood reservoir is now very strong. This store in the central circulation is especially important when the individual suddenly stands erect and still after lying prone for some time in the warm sun. For several beats, the output of the heart will temporarily exceed the inflow into the thoracic pool until the capacity vessels in the legs have filled up and flow through the abdominothoracic pump is resumed.

As stated, there is evidence that one third of this blood being pumped out of the intrathoracic blood store comes from the heart, where for the most part it is located in the atria, and that the rest comes from the great veins and the pulmonary vascular bed. In the inverted, head-down position, there is no distension of the heart; rather, it may decrease in size. This is because the majority of the very distensible lung bed will then be "below" the heart. This also fits in with the behavior of the filling pressure, which is maximum in the supine posture. Thus changes of posture move large volumes of blood between the extreme ends of the circulation while leaving the abdominal region practically unaffected. The splanchnic vascular bed does not contribute to orthostatic blood volume displacements in a vigorous man because the abdominal viscera are in a water-filled jacket held firmly in place by the tone of the muscles of the abdominal wall. Pressure measurements inside the abdominal cavity in an erect man show a linear pressure gradient from pelvic floor to diaphragm. This counter-pressure from the viscera cancels out the intravascular pressure gradient in this region and means that there is no distension of veins in the pelvis as a result of an unsupported hydrostatic head of pressure.

The effects of gravity can be reproduced while in the supine position, by sealing the lower extremities in an oil drum by means of a rubber flap around the torso. By creating some 40 to 60 mm Hg negative pressure in the drum with a vacuum cleaner, much the same effect as standing in the erect posture can be obtained. Such a device will induce the syncope that commonly occurs with the pooling of more than 30% of the effective blood volume in the legs and lower abdomen.

The reverse effect of neutralizing gravity is achieved by immersion of the body in water (Fig. 6-6).

A convenient partial substitute for the counter-pressure of water is the use of a leotard made of elastic material that is fitted to the patient's measurements so that the pressure at the ankles is very much greater than that at the buttocks. Such leotards may, for example, provide 40 mm Hg pressure at the ankles but only 10–15 mm Hg in the abdomen. They are particularly useful in severe venous valvular insufficiency and in pregnancy when the pressure of the uterus on the iliac veins causes added congestion in the legs. Fatigue and exhaustion due to loss of effective blood volume ensue in the erect posture. On lying down on the right or left side, the pressure is relieved, the extra blood dammed up in the legs is returned to the thoracic reservoir, and the woman loses the symptoms of blood volume loss.

Influence of Posture on Cardiac Performance

Depending on the severity of the exposure, i.e., the duration, and heat applied to the subject, the shift of blood out of the thorax during orthostasis can be minor or very serious. With a cool environment and for brief periods, there may be some reduction of end-diastolic ventricular volume and a slight fall in cardiac output, but the blood pressure will not change. With progressive increase of the severity, the cardiac output is sustained, as is mean systolic pressure, but significant adjustments are occurring. One early compensatory factor is the sharp increase in pulse rate that keeps the cardiac output constant. As the orthostatic exposure persists, especially in a warm environment, cardiac output falls off as pulse pressure and eventually mean systemic arterial pressure fall and stroke volume diminishes. These changes can be prevented if the downward movement of blood and fluid is avoided by permitting leg activity or by counter-pressure to the legs. The evidence points to the fall in central blood volume as the prime cause of the changes in the circulation in orthostasis. In effect, it is a state of functional hemorrhage into the dependent vascular bed.

Venous Tone

The displacement of a large volume out of the intrathoracic reservoir into the dependent vascular bed during moderate orthostatic strain, as with vertical immobilization for 15 minutes in an air-conditioned room, is associated with a sharp increase of heart rate. This increase is probably a reflex response to the fall in pressure in the atria that decreases the rate of afferent impulses from the receptors there. There is, in addition, an increase in cardiac contractility as well as some constriction of the arterioles so that, between the increase of heart action and the increase of peripheral resistance, the arterial pressure is sustained, despite a fall of some 20% in the cardiac output. The central blood volume is not refilled at this stage by a generalized tightening up and constriction of the peripheral venous bed. Despite the obvious strong contractions of which the veins are capable, all available evidence shows that, for moderate changes of blood volume, the low-pressure system behaves like a container with passively elastic walls. In the well-hydrated, healthy young man, only a fleeting constriction of the skin capacity vessels occurs as long as the orthostasis induces less than 20% reduction of central blood volume. If, however, the reduction exceeds 20%, it reaches the point where the systemic arterial pressure begins to be seriously affected, and then venoconstriction commences. This becomes extreme in states of shock when the blood pressure has fallen as a result of the loss of 30–40% of the effective blood volume. It is suspected that this vigorous response of the venous system is dependent upon the intervention of afferents from the high-pressure or sinoaortic area. The conclusion is that the capacity vessels of the low-pressure system show a predominantly passive behavior during moderate reduction of the central blood volume, as by brief periods of orthostasis. This means that the anatomical size of the vascular bed is relatively constant for each individual, within the limits of passive distension due to hydrostatic pressure changes of the type that normally occur on shifting position from relaxed lying to sitting and to standing at ease.

Effects of Weightlessness and Bed Rest Upon Blood Volume

It appears that the repeated stimulation of episodes of orthostasis in the course of daily living is important for the maintenance of adequate blood volume. In weightlessness due to the absence of gravity, there is no movement of blood towards the legs in any posture. But in the standing and sitting position of normal daily work in the earth's gravity field, the chest area contains some ½ to 1 liter less blood than in the recumbent sleeping position. Normally blood displaced from the chest by gravity accumulates in the lower part of the body; the veins distend with blood, and there is, in addition, a movement of fluid into the tissue spaces. On the other hand, in the weightless state, there is an excess of blood in the chest, and the organism responds by decreasing blood volume and excreting salt in excess of intake to such a degree that, after several days of weightless flight, astronauts show a reduction of their blood volume sufficient to lead to orthostatic difficulties on re-exposure to the earth's gravity. In addition, there is a decrease of tissue fluid pressure in the extremities that leads to a more rapid and greater accumulation of fluid than normal when they are exposed to a passive standard tilt. In effect, the weightless state is the equivalent of strict maintenance of the horizontal posture. Since the blood volume decreases by as much as 20% on prolonged confinement to bed, it is to be expected that there would be a similar loss during weightlessness.

This loss can be directly determined by making measurements of blood volume, and it was indeed found to be decreased in the weightless state. It can also be tested by evaluating the pulse rate and blood pressure responses to the upright posture on a tilt table. First, the tilt table is placed horizontal for control measurements. Then the subject is tilted and told to relax. His weight is supported by a saddle, and he is secured with a harness to prevent falling off. The standard test lasts for 15 minutes. It is carried out in an air-conditioned room at 72° F. During this period, the blood rapidly leaves the chest and fluid slowly accumulates in the legs. The subject is then tilted back for post-tilt control measurements. Figure 6-8 shows records from a man who had been exposed to weightlessness for 4 days. He was a trained pilot, and his responses were reliable. Before flight, the blood pressure was well sustained during the 15-minute tilt, and the pulse rate rose only 15 beats/minute. After 4 days of weightlessness, he had lost over 4 pounds and had drunk only 3 liters instead of the 8 liters normally taken on earth during such a period. This failure to drink may have been partly due to an absence of thirst because the circulation in the chest was well filled in the weightless state and the receptors there were signaling a more than adequate blood volume. After return to the earth's gravity and re-exposure to orthostasis, he drank over 2 liters during the first 4 hours. The figure shows that on tilting 2 hours after landing, the blood pressure fell to critical levels 50 mm Hg below normal and the pulse increased to 120–130/min: the subject was on the verge of fainting. But the next tilt 6 hours later showed the effects of the fluid uptake. The blood pressure was sustained above 100 mm Hg, and the pulse rise was far less dramatic. Tilt two days after landing showed restoration to normal. The results of a number of flights suggest that cardiovascular changes occurring after weightlessness up to a period of a week or more are reversible in healthy men within a few hours and do not differ in kind or

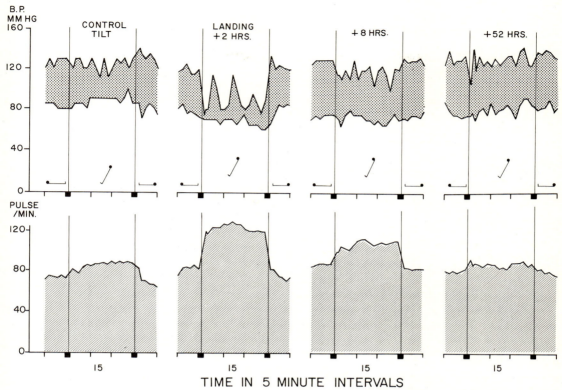

Fig. 6-8.—Tilt-table and blood-pressure responses of Gemini 4 command pilot. From left to right: Control, 10 days before launch, pressure is well sustained during 15 minutes of tilt up to 70°; 2 hours after return from 4 days of weightless flight, the blood pressure repeatedly falls close to the point where syncope frequently occurs—with this, there is a dramatic rise of pulse rate; 8 hours after landing, there is marked improvement; 52 hours postlanding, the responses have returned to control levels, showing the transient nature of the changes during 4 days of weightlessness. (From Henry, J. P.: *Biomedical Aspects of Space Flight* [New York: Holt, Rinehart & Winston, Inc., 1966], p. 87, Fig. 3-5.)

severity from those changes following bed rest for the same time period. Such studies point to the care that must be taken in restraining normal, healthy people to the recumbent posture and to the significant physiological adjustments that occur when a patient is committed to "bed rest."

The Muscle Pump and Orthostasis

Factors Regulating Venous Pressure in the Foot

When a subject stands absolutely quiet, the pressure in the veins at the ankle reaches the full value that could be expected in view of the difference between the location of the hydrostatic indifferent point (in the region of the heart) and the foot. Since this distance is a matter of some 130 cm, there is a pressure of 100 mm Hg in the foot veins of the average man standing at rest. The exact value depends on the extent of vasoconstriction or vasodilation in the vessels of the foot. This, in turn, is dependent upon the environmental temperature.

Each muscle contraction leads to a compression of the veins, sending the contents towards the heart. Because of the valves, there can be no reflux during relaxation of the muscles. The pressure in the foot thus depends on the effectiveness of the emptying of the leg veins. The rate at which they refill and the slope of the corresponding increase in pressure depends on the rate at which the arteries feed blood into the system. The veins of a warm, perspiring man with a toe temperature of 39° C fill up within 3 seconds (Fig. 6-9). But at cooler normal room temperatures, the return of pressure is far slower.

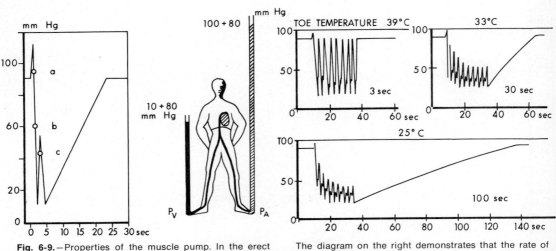

Fig. 6-9.—Properties of the muscle pump. In the erect posture, the arterial (P_A) and venous pressure (P_V) at the ankle are about 80 mm Hg above recumbent transmural pressure. (From Gauer, O. H., and Thron, H. L.: Postural Changes in the Circulation, in Hamilton, W. F. (ed.): *Handbook of Physiology: Circulation* [Washington: American Physiological Society, 1965], Vol. III, p. 2,430, Fig. 16.)

The diagram on the left shows the pressure changes in the ankle vein during a single step: *(a)* heel starts off the ground; *(b)* leg swings free; *(c)* heel again on the ground. (From J. Appl. Physiol. 1:649, 1948–49.)

The diagram on the right demonstrates that the rate of rise of venous pressure after each step is a function of arterial flow resistance, and hence of temperature. The time necessary for a full return of pressure after the step is indicated. Due to this relationship, the mean venous pressure during stepping at 39°C is approximately 90 mm Hg; at 33°C, 60 mm Hg and at 25°C, 50 mm Hg. (Adapted from J. Clin. Invest. 29:855, 1950.)

A pressure drop occurs in the foot veins with each step, as can be seen in the section on the left of the diagram, which shows pressure changes at the ankle with each step. The bottom right diagram shows that, in the cold foot of a man who is shivering, the rate of return of the pressure to resting values is slowed down to a minute or more because blood enters the area so slowly through the constricted arterioles. In relaxed normal standing, the venous pressure is depressed by every unwitting contraction of the legs that the subject makes as he shifts his position. This occurs in the normal person about once or twice a minute. In men who are dressed appropriately and comfortably in air-conditioned rooms at 72° F, there is usually some constriction of the arterioles, and foot skin temperatures are of the order of room temperature, i.e., 70–80° F. Under these circumstances, with each movement there is a depression of the venous pressure in the foot that lasts long enough to lead to a significant fall of mean venous pressure. When the man is perspiring from higher environmental temperatures, the pressure at ankle level and hence the capillary filtration pressure can be of the order of three times the colloid osmotic pressure. It is for this reason that edema of the ankles develops so readily in hot humid weather. A completely innocuous swelling may develop, especially after prolonged sitting during traveling. It may even bring the patient to the doctor in a state of anxiety about heart failure!

ACTION OF THE CALF AND THIGH PUMPS

The calf pump chamber is filled by blood coming from its powerful muscles and also up from the foot muscles and in from the shin. The pump discharges into the femoral vein which, in turn, forms part of the thigh pump (Fig. 6-10). There, the blood enters the great veins of the low-pressure reservoir system proper. The chamber of the calf pump is made up of the intramuscular veins and the other vessels of the calf that lie within the deep fascia of the leg. A number of plethysmographic studies have led to the conclusion that about 130 cc of blood are held by the lower leg when moving from the recumbent to the quiet standing posture. There are numerous and efficient valves, and the whole system constitutes an effective pump that, in exercise, will move some 75 cc of blood per stroke into the thigh area. In a running man, this can represent the return of several liters of blood per minute. During vigorous exercise in the erect posture, there is a sharp reduction of venous pressure in the calf muscles, whereas arterial pressure is enhanced by the addition of the hydrostatic head of pressure. This results in a 50% increase of the recumbent calf muscle perfusion pressure differential to some 150 mm Hg. Thus the venous pump may contribute to the efficiency of a highly stressed, much-worked muscle that is critical to man with his erect posture.

The thigh pump has large valved veins that work in the same way as the calf. It is estimated that about 200 cc are present in the femoral veins and its deep tributaries in a relaxed, quietly standing man. The valves protect this pump chamber from the reflux of blood out of the abdomen during periods of raised intra-abdominal pressure, as during weight lifting. Pressures generated by the thigh muscles are, in general, lower than in the calf. However, the gravity-determined pressure against which the blood must be discharged into the abdominal veins is correspondingly lower. Despite the greater capacity of the pump chamber, its stroke volume appears to be no greater than that of the calf. However, the evidence suggests it does effectively move on the blood delivered to it by the calf pump. Thus the active legs with healthy valves alternately pump the blood on to the abdominothoracic region where the respiratory pump takes over. One advantage of the system is the gravity-induced increase in the head of pressure supplying the active calf muscles vital for man's erect posture and locomotion.

Venous Pressure Measurements

In the upright position, as a result of the action of gravity on the blood columns and the location of the hydrostatic indifferent point near heart level, the veins above the heart collapse and are only held open by the blood flowing down them. The pressure in these collapsed segments is atmospheric, but, at the base of the brain at the orifice of the jugular vein, the pressure becomes slightly subatmospheric. Farther up in the cranial cavity, the rigid-walled dural sinuses cannot collapse, and the pressure in them when sitting or standing is subatmospheric. The degree of negativity is proportional to the vertical distance above the top of the collapsed neck veins and, in the superior sagittal sinus, runs at approximately 13 cms H_2O. The result is that neurosurgery carries hazards of aeroembolism for, if a vein is opened while the patient is tilted upright, air will be sucked into the vascular system.

If a man sitting upright is gradually tilted backwards, the pulsating upper border of the central reservoir will creep up to the neck. When the subject is lying with head up at an angle between 20–30° to the horizontal, pulsations appear in the jugular vein in the middle of the neck. A typical recording of this pulsation derived from the atria is shown in Figure 6-11. The atrial contraction wave, a, is seen just prior to the first heart sound. The c wave that rises at the moment of isometric contraction of the heart can also be seen, as can the v that corresponds to the opening of the tricuspid valves. A dominant characteristic of this curve is a systolic collapse that represents the sudden drop in pressure in the

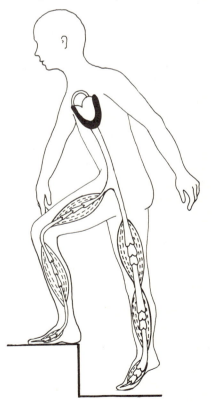

Fig. 6-10.—As the leg tenses, three separate muscle compartments enclosed by fascia compress the veins, forwarding as much as 100 cc of blood to the abdomen. On relaxation, the veins fill from below upwards, the valves holding the blood ready to be sent on by the next contraction.

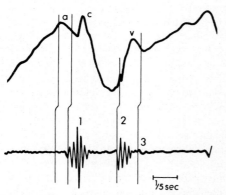

Fig. 6-11.—Pulse in the jugular vein and its relationship to the three heart sounds. Notice the marked systolic "collapse." This pulse wave shows all the characteristics of a directly recorded central venous pulse. (From Gauer, O. H.: Kreislauf des Blutes, in Landois-Rosemann: *Lehrbuch der Physiologie des Menschen,* 28th ed. [Munich: Urban & Schwarzenberg, 1960], p. 141.)

vein as the ventricle contracts, pulling downward the opening in which the valves are implanted. This drop in jugular venous pressure corresponds closely to the movement of ventricular ejection. Hence, although the jugular pulse has little value from the viewpoint of absolute pressure changes, nevertheless, when registered in conjunction with the heart sounds, it can be a useful clinical measure of the function of the valves and gives clues of departures from the normal in the timing of the heart's action.

The preceding account indicates that the pressure in the peripheral veins depends upon a large number of factors: the height of the hydrostatic column, the tonus in the vein wall, and the rate of blood flow through the region. This peripheral venous pressure as measured in the antecubital fossa or in a vein of the foot gives no reliable indication of the central venous pressure. In the case of the foot, this is obvious. In the case of the antecubital fossa, even if an effort is made to hold the manometer at heart level, false readings will be obtained from a seated patient or one reclining on pillows because the venous column must attain sufficient pressure to cause the blood to climb up the axillary vein before finally spilling over the first rib into the thorax and joining the collapsed veins at the top of the thoracic cavity above the intrathoracically located hydrostatic indifferent point. The most direct approach is to place a catheter in the right atrium, and this procedure is the method of choice in the seriously ill who need monitoring of central venous pressure. In the situation in the clinic, accurate diagnostic values can be obtained if the subject is placed on his right side with the arm hanging down. Under these circumstances, a pressure taken in the antecubital vein will be taken in a large vessel that is broadly expanded by a hydrostatic column that runs without pressure drop due to points of constriction straight from the elbow to the atrium. If the proper correction is made for the distance of the point of measurement below the right heart, this technique will give an accurate measure of central pressure.

Summary

1. In addition to the action of the heart itself, and the boost given to the circulation by the breathing apparatus, the legs constitute a third peripheral accessory pump.

2. By reducing venous pressure in the periphery, this pump reduces the filtration pressure in the capillaries and hence the danger of local edema.

3. The pressure in the arterioles of the foot is the same as that in the heart plus the 100 mm Hg hydrostatic head of pressure, making a total arterial pressure at foot level of 200 mm Hg. If the muscle pump reduces venous pressure, there will be an extraordinarily high arteriovenous pressure difference across the muscle. This may play a part in increasing the efficiency of the calf muscles during violent exertion.

4. By pressing on the capillary bed and by keeping the veins emptied, despite the high hydrostatic head of pressure, the muscle pump economizes on the volume of blood that must be yielded by the central reservoir to meet the needs of muscular activity in the erect posture.

REFERENCES

Folkow, B., Heymans, C., and Neil, E.: Integrated Aspects of Cardiovascular Regulation, in Hamilton, W. F. (ed.): *Handbook of Physiology: Circulation.* (Washington: American Physiological Society, 1965), Vol. III, chap. 49.

Gauer, O. H., and Henry, J. P.: Circulatory Basis of Fluid Volume Control, Physiol. Rev. 43:423, 1963.

Gauer, O. H., Henry, J. P., and Behn, C.: The Regulation of Extracellular Fluid Volume, Ann. Rev. Physiol. 32:547, 1970.

Gauer, O. H., and Thron, H.: Postural Changes in the Circulation, in Hamilton, W. F. (ed.): *Handbook of Physiology: Circulation.* (Washington: American Physiological Society, 1965), Vol. III, chap. 67.

Guyton, A. C.: A Concept of Negative Interstitial Pressure Based on Pressures in Implanted Perforated Capsules, Circulation Res. 12:399-414, 1963.

Henry, J. P.: *Biomedical Aspects of Space Flight* (New York: Holt, Rinehart & Winston, Inc., 1966).

Henry, J. P., and Gauer, O. H.: The Influence of Temperature Upon Venous Pressure in the Foot, J. Clin. Invest. 29:855-861, 1950.

Landis, E. M., and Hortenstine, J. C.: Functional Significance of Venous Blood Pressure, Physiol. Rev. 30:1-32, 1950.

Ludbrook, J.: *Aspects of Venous Function in the Lower Limbs* (Springfield, Ill.: Charles C Thomas, Publisher, 1966).

McCally, M.: *Hypodynamics and Hypogravics* (New York: Academic Press, Inc., 1968).

Murray, R. H., *et al.:* Cumulative Effects of Venesection and Lower Body Negative Pressure, Aerospace Med. 38:243, 1967.

Öberg, G.: Effects of Cardiovascular Reflexes on Net Capillary Fluid Transfer, Acta Physiol. Scandinav. 62 Supplement 229, pp. 1-98, 1964.

Sjöstrand, T.: Volume and Distribution of Blood and Their Significance in Regulating Circulation, Physiol. Rev. 33:202, 1953.

7

Local Regulation and Central Integration of Cardiovascular Function

Introduction

This section is concerned with the mechanisms by which volume and pressure are regulated so that the vital flow through the microcirculatory beds is maintained. Discussion of the partition of flow from organ to organ as needed to meet various environmental demands will be deferred to another chapter. The local regulation of the tissue capillary beds by which, given a sufficient pressure head, adequate flow is assured will be first described. Then an attempt will be made to disentangle the closely interlocked mechanisms by which the total volume of fluid in the system, the capacity of the vascular bed, and the pressure head across the capillary network are sustained and regulated. It will be shown that, although volume and pressure have separate regulatory mechanisms, they are very closely coordinated.

Local Regulation

The smooth muscles of the smallest arterial vessels, the precapillary sphincters, regularly show automatic contractions. They have a basic tone which is independent of influences from the brain. Indeed, in regions such as the deep cerebral vessels, there are few vasomotor nerves. Local environmental factors affect the basal tone of these vessels, with the result that the blood flow through the tissue is locally regulated in the sense that increased vasodilation compensates for any inadequacy of flow and the reverse holds for excess flow. This local regulation will be effective even if all nervous connections to the tissue are blocked off. It is suspected that the precapillary smooth muscle is itself the receptor-effector unit. The rhythmic activity that it inherently demonstrates is increased by passive stretching, implying that the muscle cells themselves serve as tension receptors. It is thought that the refractory period of the cells determines the contraction frequency evoked by a given distending stimulus so that the amount of resistance obtainable when the pressure is raised is limited. This hypothesis suggests that vessels in which the smooth muscle shows little spontaneous myogenic contractile activity would not show autoregulation. Such is the case with larger arteries, the AV shunts of the skin, and the venous system. The activity of all of these depends almost entirely on their nerve supply. These portions of the system have no spontaneous activity that can be built up and accentuated by changes in transmural distending pressure. On the other hand, those sections of the vascular bed that demonstrate inherent tone, i.e., the precapillary resistance vessels, can respond to nervous control but they are not completely dominated by it and are capable of considerable response to local conditions. There is evidence that this accentuation of spontaneous activity by transmural pressure is most marked in the viscera such as the liver, kidney, and intestine.

The local concentration of metabolites that induces vasodilation is also an important autoregulatory factor. If vasodilator substances accumulate when blood flow is reduced, this dilates the resistance vessels and restores flow. If flow increases, the metabolites are washed out and flow decreases proportionately. This type of local regulation has been noted in muscles, especially the heart muscle, and in the brain, but not in the skin. It is considered likely that there are multiple factors responsible for local regulation. Oxygen lack may play a role in reactive hyperemia, that is, the increase in blood flow that follows temporary arterial occlusion. This effect is maximal in the coronary and cerebral circulation, prominent in muscle, and less marked in the skin and liver. Decreasing the oxygen saturation of arterial blood increases the flow rate through an isolated dog limb to an extent that goes far in compensating for the loss of oxygen tension in the inflowing blood. It has been shown by experiments on isolated tissues that small arteries such as metarterioles and precapillary sphincters are very sensitive to low oxygen concentrations. Furthermore, oxygen is the most flow-limited substance that is transported in the blood stream. A decrease in blood flow that drops below 50% will cause a serious oxygen deficiency in most tissues. Muscle is not so sensitive to local hypoxia, and an increase of blood flow with exercise may be due to adenose triphosphate (ATP) or, possibly, acetylcholine.

Another factor responsible for vasodilation is a rise in carbon dioxide tension. This will dilate skin and brain vessels. Local regulation based on carbon dioxide has been shown to be extremely powerful in the brain. When the pCO_2 increases, the brain vessels dilate, allowing more rapid blood flow and hence a return of the pCO_2 toward normal values. Conversely, a reduction in pCO_2 can cause a cerebral vasoconstriction so severe that loss of consciousness can occur.

A gradual change in the degree of vascularity in the tissues can occur over a period of weeks. An example would be an arterial occlusion that causes the arterial pressure to fall to, say, 60 mm Hg and to remain at this level for weeks. In such circumstances, the number and size of the vessels in the tissues increases. Similarly, if metabolism increases, vascularity also increases and vice versa. It is believed that the cause of these slowly acting changes is oxygen deficiency, which has been shown to promote a new growth of vessels in the tissue. The marathon runner's heart that has been subjected to repeated very high output loads shows an extensive collateral circulation; such hearts may survive coronary occlusions that would otherwise be fatal. It is likely that this self-regulatory response of the heart muscle to chronic hypoxia is also the explanation why the heart of a nonathlete who survives a coronary occlusion will eventually show extensive collateral vessels and why angina pectoris is often a self-limiting condition, gradually improving as the months go by.

Other substances which accumulate locally and may have a dilator action include lactic acid and adenylic acid and related compounds. In injured tissue, histamine released from the damaged cells dilates capillaries and increases their permeability. Finally, the vasodilator peptide bradykinin is receiving increasing attention. Like histamine, it stimulates visceral smooth muscle, relaxes vascular smooth muscle, dilates capillaries, and increases the permeability of the capillary endothelium. There is some evidence that this product of sweat gland activity plays a role in local vasodilation of the skin due to heat and "blushing" or emotional flushing of the face and shoulders. Finally, the temperature rise in active tissues due to the heat of metabolism may contribute to vasodilation.

Stretch Receptors in the Low- and High-Pressure Systems

The foregoing discussion relates to the most basic and phylogenetically the earliest method of regulating the circulation through the tissues. As Figure 1-1 indicates, in a complex organism, it is also necessary to have elaborate central control because the effective maintenance of flow is predicated upon two basic requirements: an adequate pool of blood in the central reservoir from which the pump can draw fluid for each successive stroke volume and a proper adjustment between force of stroke, elasticity of the arterial tree, and rate of runoff in the diffusion beds so that the perfusion pressure is maintained. Thus a reflex feedback is needed whereby the volume available for the heart and the mean pressure feeding the arterioles is constantly monitored. Control of volume means control both of the size of the vascular bed and of the rate at which fluid and sodium enter and leave it. Control of pressure demands a proper balance between the output of the heart and the resistance to flow from the various parts of the arterial tree. The regulation of volume appears to be determined by subendocardial receptors strategically located in and near the atria, the most distensible part of the low-pressure system. The regulation of pressure is achieved by receptors in the adventitia of the elastic arterial walls that, by determining variations of stretch, can evaluate pressure in the system. In addition, receptors in other locations such as the ventricular endocardium may transmit information relating to the force of the beat and the size of end-systolic volume (Fig. 2-3).

Stretch Receptors in the Low-Pressure System

The preceding chapters have shown that there is a critically important pool of blood in the lungs and heart that is constantly changing in volume in response to the demands of exercise and gravity. It was shown that when, as in orthostasis, some of this blood leaves the heart and lungs to fill the legs it induces changes in the low-pressure system that will persist for upwards of an hour. Receptors in the pulmonary veins and atria are well suited to convey information concerning this amount of blood available to the heart, i.e., the effective blood volume. These receptors are particularly numerous in the superior and inferior

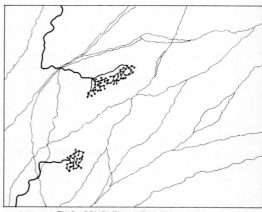

TWO COMPLEX UNENCAPSULATED ENDINGS SUPERIMPOSED ON A SENSORY END NET IN SUBENDOCARDIUM

Fig. 7-2.—Diagrammatic representation of an end net, contrasting it with two superimposed complex unencapsulated endings (CUE) of Nonidez.

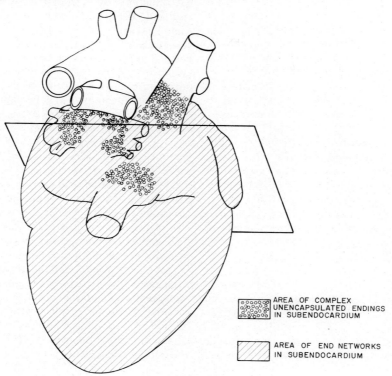

Fig. 7-1.—Posterior view of a heart showing the location and approximate extent of the areas where the CUE of Nonidez are to be found. The shading over the rest of the organ indicates the general distribution of the end networks, which are present in the ventricular as well as the atrial subendocardium. (From Nonidez, J. F.: Am. J. Anat. 61:203, 1937, Fig. 1.)

REGULATION AND INTEGRATION OF CARDIOVASCULAR FUNCTION

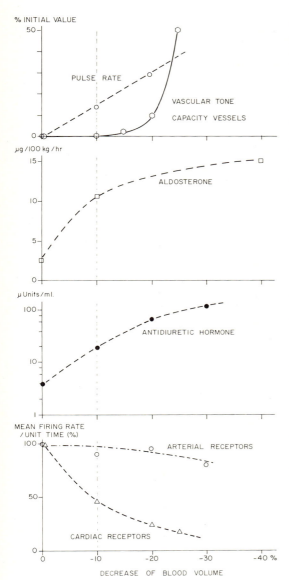

Fig. 7-3.—Data showing from above downwards the measured responses of dogs to a graded hemorrhage in terms of: the autonomic drive expressed as measured changes of the compliance of the capacity vessels of the forearm and as pulse rate increases; volume-regulating hormones expressed as μ units of aldosterone released into the plasma and μ units of ADH; and receptor drive expressed as mean firing rate per unit time.

With loss of the first 10% of the blood volume, the drive from baroreceptors in the low-pressure system increases sharply as the firing rate of the atrial receptors falls to one-half. As the loss exceeds 20%, there is an increasing influence from the arterial system. Meanwhile, the plasma aldosterone and antidiuretic hormone concentrations increase, effecting water and salt retention. The pulse rate shows a steady acceleration up to the point of impending syncope, i.e., the loss of some 20–30% of the blood volume. There is no appreciable change of the tone of the capacity

vena cava and the pulmonary veins just before they enter the atria, i.e., in the intrapericardial portion that is invested by myocardium (Fig. 7-1). Endings are not found in the extrapericardial portions of these veins, but they are found in large numbers in the subendocardium of the atria. Their subendothelial, repeatedly branching aborization among the loose elements of connective tissue and their specialized endings make them appropriate to measure the minor changes in stretch of the walls of the central reservoir (Fig. 7-2). In addition to these complex unencapsulated endings (CUE) that are confined to the atria and in general to the atriovenous orifices and the posterior regions, there is the recently described end-net system of nerve fibers. This net is to be found thickly distributed throughout the atria. It is also found in the auricular appendages and in the ventricular subendocardium. The role of these end nets has not been definitely established; however, they appear to be sensory. Afferent impulses from the CUE are primarily routed through the vagi. It is possible that future work will demonstrate that the end-net fibers are part of a more primitive volume-regulating system and that they, too, play a role in cardiovascular sympathetic responses to volume loss including renal effects. It is certainly intriguing that the CUE are only to be found in mammals, whereas, the more primitive end net is to be found in all vertebrates.

By examining fibers of the vagus nerve, it is possible to demonstrate that the Nonidez CUE are responsible for large numbers of impulse volleys running up to the brain stem. The sensitivity of these atrial receptors is very high. If the atrium is isolated and then filled under pressure, their response can be shown to be linear. They fire in time with the v wave of the atrial pressure curves and not with the a wave or atrial systole (Fig. 2-3) because they are for the most part activated by the distension of the atrium during diastole.

Figure 7-3 shows how small changes in blood volume that increase or decrease central venous pressure by only a few centimeters of water will radically change the firing rate of these receptors. Influences that change the volume of blood in the thorax, such as pressure breathing, will lead

---

vessels until collapse threatens. At this point it increases, effectively moving blood towards the central region. (From Gauer, O. H., Henry, J. P., and Behn, C.: Ann. Rev. Physiol. 32:547–595, 1970.)

to corresponding changes in atrial firing rate. The distension of a small balloon in the atrium will lead to a violent discharge. Cooling the vagus nerve prevents passage of these impulses. Their control role will be considered after a description of the receptors in the high-pressure system.

Stretch Receptors in the High-Pressure System

In both carotid sinus regions above the bifurcations of the common carotid arteries and in the arch of the aorta there are stretch receptors that appear as a very fine network of neurofibrils, showing the same repeated branching and specialized endings as the CUE. They are mainly located in the adventitia of the carotid sinus and in the adventitia and outer part of the media of the aortic arch. In both regions, the network is attached to the elastic fibers, and they are probably running, for the most part, in parallel with them. If the smooth muscle in the vessel contracts, then, because these elements are attached to the elastic tissue, the tension in the neurofibrils will increase and with it their stimulation. Thus the sensitivity of the baroreceptor mechanism is, in part, determined by the tonus of the muscle in the region.

The aortic receptors are supplied by fibers of the vagus nerve that run in a close group in the main nerve trunk. They have the same complex structure as the carotid sinus endings, and their number is about the same as the atrial receptors. The carotid sinus baroreceptors are endings of afferent glossopharyngeal fibers that form a separate small carotid sinus nerve running to the carotid bifurcation. By the same process of dissection under paraffin and placement on electrodes that is used to demonstrate atrial receptor firing, activity of the carotid sinus and aortic arch receptors can be shown to occur with every rise in systolic pressure. Each nerve supplies several hundred baroreceptors, and they faithfully record the stretch and, therefore, the pressure changes in the vessel (Fig. 7-4). Thus, if the arterial pressure is raised significantly as by injecting adrenalin, the impulse activity in the nerve increases. A fall in pressure decreases their discharge, and a static pressure produces a steady firing. Unlike the aortic arch area, it is easy to isolate the carotid sinus, and the sinus can then be subjected to a series of steady hydrostatic pressures. The recordings from a preparation containing a single fiber show that the impulses start at a certain threshold, usually 60–70 mm Hg, and increase steadily in frequency up to some 200 mm Hg, the limiting range of the healthy animal's blood pressure. If a T-cannula is put into the carotid below the sinus and connected to an air reservoir that serves as a damping chamber, the normal pulsations can be suppressed without affecting mean pressure. On turning from steady to pulsatile pressure, the firing becomes rhythmic with a peak frequency exceeding that shown during steady pressure. Furthermore, the change to the pulsatile state at the same mean pressure brings in fresh units, as receptors with high thresholds are affected by the peak of the wave.

These mechanoreceptors are thus very well suited in terms of their location and function to serve as "buffer" nerves. That is, they minimize departures from either side of the blood pressure level to which the central nervous system has been set.

Pulmonary arterial mechanoreceptors are found in the adventitia of the wall of the main pulmonary trunk and its branches. They also run in the vagus nerve and can be recognized during dissection of the vagus in the neck. Their function has not yet been determined.

Impulses from receptors firing with ventricular systole have been observed in vagus slips. There appear to be far fewer from this region than from the sinoaortic area. They fire only during the isometric contraction of systole, and their pattern can be changed by disturbing ventricular function. Their role may be to signal excessive diastolic filling of the ventricles. It is also possible that they respond with a discharge if end-systolic volume is reduced, especially if the ventricular pressures rise as the walls of the empty cavity squeeze on each other.

Since some observers fail to find ventricular receptors within the myocardium, it is possible that the source for the impulses coinciding with systole may be that part of the previously described end net that is found in the ventricular endocardium.

Coronary receptors have been recently described along the path of the major vessels; they fire as the pulse wave passes. Stimulating them induces a fall in blood pressure and a slowing of the heart, which is similar to the response to veratridine first described by Bezold and later attributed to the heart receptors by Jarisch.

REGULATION AND INTEGRATION OF CARDIOVASCULAR FUNCTION

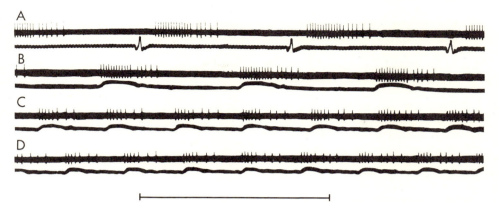

Fig. 7-4.—Aortic fiber showing the change in burst number with progressive hemorrhage. **A,** control with EKG; **B,** 10% loss of estimated blood volume with thoracic aortic pressure curve; **C,** 20% loss; and **D,** 30% loss. Note marked increase in pulse rate that cancels out decreased number of impulses per burst, so that the firing rate is not significantly changed. Time: 1 sec. (From Gupta, P. D., *et al.*: Am. J. Physiol. 211:1429, 1966.)

Chemoreceptors are found near the aortic arch in the carotid bodies and at the root of the subclavian arteries. They consist of highly vascular clumps of epithelioid cells that have a rich innervation. The carotid body is supplied by the sinus nerve and the subclavian by the vagus. Blood flow through them is exceedingly high, and their morphology would suggest they signal information via the sinus nerve of changes in the chemical composition of the blood. It can be shown by the technique of nerve-fiber separation that, if the oxygen tension in the organ is significantly reduced, these receptors are stimulated. This occurs when local vasoconstriction within the organ reduces the rate of blood flow through it, as well as when the oxygen tension of arterial blood reaching them is reduced, as in asphyxia.

AFFERENT PATHWAYS AND CENTRAL REPRESENTATION

SPINAL VASOMOTOR REFLEXES.—Although there is incontrovertible evidence that most afferent impulses from the heart run through the vagi to the medulla, there is a possibility that reflexes that rely on the sympathetic nervous system connect the heart with viscera such as the spleen and kidney. Certainly in spinal man, distension of the urinary bladder elicits an elevation of blood pressure and vasoconstriction in the fingers. In persons suffering from cholecystitis, gall bladder distension may induce pallor of the abdominal skin. In the spinal dog, an increase in arterial pressure results in an increase of spleen volume. It has been observed that, in vagotomized dogs, changes in sodium excretion can be induced by blood volume changes despite loss of afferent impulses by this pathway. Less sodium shift occurs in dogs with denervated hearts. It remains to be seen whether sympathetic connections between these viscera will be demonstrated.

MEDULLARY CARDIAC AFFERENT LOCATIONS.—The carotid sinus afferents return by the glossopharyngeal nerve and the atrial and aortic arch afferents run with the vagus nerve, both ending in the same region in the medulla. Recordings from the vagus rootlets reveal cardiovascular afferents discharging in time with the heart beat. By cutting the rootlets, it can be shown with degeneration studies that the critical region for the cardiovascular afferents is at the headward end of the tractus solitarius of the vagus and dorsal to it. Bursts of spikes related to heart rate can be recorded in this region. The carotid neuroreceptors are located slightly headward of those from the atria area, and the areas assigned to both overlap. This supports the impression that the mechanisms regulating pressure and volume are closely linked.

SUMMARY.—Cardiovascular afferents in the periphery are divided into impulses from the low-pressure system, concerned with effective blood volume, and from the high-pressure system, giving the level of blood pressure and pulse pressure. As soon as they reach the brain, they become inextricably intertwined; beyond the medulla, there is only indirect evidence of their undoubted combined input into the complex controls of the higher centers.

Efferent Pathways and Hormones Controlling the Cardiovascular System

INTRODUCTION

The preceding section indicated that, despite a quite clear initial functional differentiation into receptors serving the high- and the low-pressure system, the information pouring into the central nervous system soon escapes our current capacity to follow and analyze it. Leaving for a moment what occurs inside the brain, the following section will be concerned with the output of that complex.

The vascular responses and hormones concerned with volume regulation can to some extent be differentiated from those concerned with pressure. It should be emphasized that our presentation deliberately accents the differences of overlapping systems in order to gain clarity.

VOLUME REGULATORY RESPONSES

ANTIDIURETIC HORMONE.—The regulation of water and salt metabolism is vital for the determination of the volume of circulatory fluid. The present section is concerned with the source and function of the water-controlling antidiuretic hormone (ADH). The well-defined supraoptic and paraventricular nuclei of the anterior hypothalamus give rise to a tract of unmyelinated fibers that passes directly down the pituitary stalk to the posterior lobe of the hypophysis. The hormone released there into the bloodstream promotes reabsorption of water from the renal tubules, thus limiting the amount of water lost as urine. Urinary volume is inversely related to the amount of ADH in the blood reaching the kidney, and the secretion of ADH is dependent on the integrity of the hypothalamo-hypophyseal tract. The hypothalamic nuclei are neurosecretory and elaborate ADH, which diffuses down the axons of the tract to be ultimately stored in the posterior hypophysis. The supraoptic and paraventricular nuclei are themselves acutely sensitive to changes in the osmotic pressure of the blood, so that when the ingestion of water dilutes the blood, it leads to inhibition of ADH secretion and an increased output of water. Dehydration, as in sweating, by increasing osmolarity does the reverse. However, the ADH-secreting nuclei are also sensitive to other information coming to them by nervous pathways, as will be detailed later.

SYMPATHETIC OUTFLOW AND CONTROL OF VENOUS TONE.—The capacity of the great veins is so enormous that it is critical that their tonus should be under central control, for a failure of tone could lead to a catastrophic pooling of blood within this reservoir. Vasoconstrictor fibers from the thoracolumbar sympathetic outflow are distributed to blood vessels throughout the body. After relay in the paravertebral ganglia they run as postganglionic fibers out along the peripheral nerves and also directly along the blood vessels. There is no doubt that venous tone increases sharply as a part of the response to loss of blood volume and pulse pressure. But this does not occur in the normal man until the reduction of blood volume has been more than 20%; so the loss of 500 cc or a pint of blood is not enough to initiate a change in venous tone. However, loss of more than 1,000 cc induces tonus changes; as the animal or man slides toward a grossly inadequate blood volume with a concurrent fall in systemic arterial pressure, this venoconstriction becomes more intense. There is some evidence of the reverse process, for gross distension of the low-pressure system causes some relaxation of the capacity vessels.

SYMPATHETIC OUTFLOW AND CONTROL OF PRE- TO POST-CAPILLARY RESISTANCE RATIO.—In contrast with the relative insensitivity of the capacity veins to changes of central blood volume, the ratio of precapillary to postcapillary resistance is subject to very early and sensitive control. Changes in sympathetic outflow in response to atrial receptor influences alter mean capillary pressure and so alter the rate at which fluid is lost from or reabsorbed into the capillary bed. Increased outflow resistance together with decreased inflow resistance raises mean pressure and the reverse will lower it. (see Fig. 5-12). The delicate control thus provided over fluid loss or gain by the capillary network results in a valuable volume regulatory effect in response to changes in venous filling. This reflex closely links the extensive interstitial fluid stores of the muscle mass to the intravascular compartment.

BLOOD VOLUME AND THIRST.—There is evidence that the hypothalamus controls the important function of replacement of fluid volume by drinking and that factors that stimulate the osmoreceptors to increase their output of ADH also stimulate thirst. In addition, it has been shown that the reduction of blood volume without any change in osmotic pressure, as occurs in moderate hemorrhage, will cause animals to increase their water intake; the response may be due to the effect upon the brain of an increase in the angiotension level. Finally, when dehydration or hemorrhage has led to a sufficient loss of blood volume so that vasoconstriction affects the glands and the salivary secretion is impaired, then the resultant sensation of dryness of the mouth and pharynx will add to the sensation of thirst and further drive the animal to seek water.

RENIN, RENAL VASCULAR REDISTRIBUTION, AND CONTROL OF BLOOD VOLUME.—Control of the amount of sodium excreted is of great importance in the control of blood volume. It has been shown that small changes in blood volume that are not enough to alter mean systemic arterial pressure or even pulse pressure will, nevertheless, cause an increased renin excretion, thereby altering aldosterone levels and so affecting sodium excretion. In addition, the preliminary work by Goetz and his associates shows that the mere compression of the atria by slightly distending a pericardial pouch sewn around them will cause a sharp fall in sodium output in conscious dogs, together with no significant change in blood ADH levels (Fig. 7-5). The mechanism by which the atrial pouch produces this effect is not yet decided. As can be seen in Figure 7-6, the pericardium does not extend posteriorly far enough to invest the left atrial wall and pulmonary veins where the ADH-regulating Nonidez CUE of the left atrium are clustered. Hence, the changes resulting from distending the pouch are more likely to be due to a collapse of the right atrium and the rest of the left atrial walls. The end network is to be found throughout both atria including the appendages. A reduction of tension in these regions may change the input from the end nets and thus be responsible for an unsuspected effect on sodium excretion without parallel ADH changes.

No Nonidez CUE are to be found in reptiles

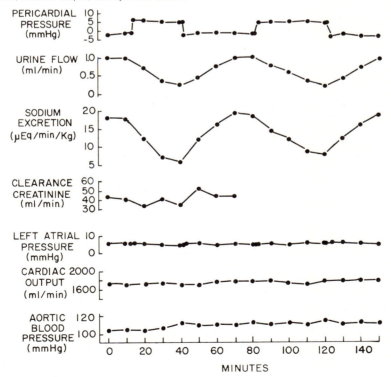

Fig. 7-5.—Distension of a pericardial pouch in a conscious dog by only 5 mm Hg induces not only a fall in urine flow but also an even sharper drop in sodium excretion. Meanwhile, creatinine clearance, cardiac output, and systemic arterial pressure remain unaffected. (From Goetz, K. L., Hermreck, A. S., and Trank, J. W.: Fed. Proc. 28:584, 1969, and personal communication.)

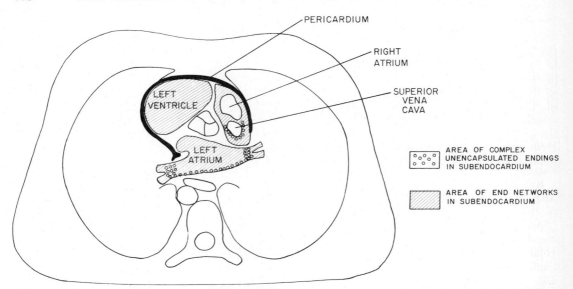

Fig. 7-6.—Schematic drawing of a transverse section of the heart to indicate the topographic relationship between the pericardium and the CUE of Nonidez in the left and in the right atria. Figure 7-2 shows the general distribution of these receptors.

and amphibia, and only the mammals have aortic and carotid sinus sensory areas equipped with these complex endings. Perhaps the recent evolution of these receptors and their location in high- and low-pressure system baroreceptor areas may be related to the responsiveness of the mammal's blood pressure to inputs from the environment, including the social group, and to their prodigal use of vital fluid volume in the regulation of body temperature by panting or sweating. These and other special needs of our line of warm-blooded vertebrates may have led to the evolution of this unique set of controls. These appear to have been superimposed upon an older system of regulation of fluid volume and blood pressure based on the end-net receptors to be found throughout the vertebrates. Certainly, modest changes in atrial dynamics, which do not change cardiac output, appear to have their effect by the stimulation of the sympathetic outflow down the renal nerves, for blocking of these nerves has been shown to eliminate the effect. Recent work suggests that the sympathetic discharge may change the rate of renin release by the direct action of the nerve fibers that can be demonstrated ending on the juxtaglomerular apparatus.

Work by Barger's group suggests that such a volume-induced sympathetic discharge will decrease the perfusion of outer cortical peritubular capillaries in relation to that of the outer medulla. This redistribution of intrarenal blood flow promotes sodium reabsorption by the tubules. The mechanisms involved are not known but may include increased sodium reabsorption by the loops of Henle as medullary blood flow lowers interstitial sodium levels. Further, the improved medullary O_2 tension may improve the efficiency with which the loops reabsorb sodium.

Finally, physical factors intervene as a result of changes in the peripheral vascular bed. Both hydrostatic and colloid osmotic pressure may decrease in the cortical peritubular capillaries as a result of glomerular vasoconstriction. The combined effect of these factors is to increase the reabsorption of sodium as the Starling pressure equilibrium changes across the capillary walls.

Pressure Regulatory Responses

INTRODUCTION.—The devices available to the central regulatory mechanisms to control the volume of blood have been outlined. This section is concerned with the regulation of pressure, which is subtly achieved by reflexes that alter arteriolar resistance and by the action of motor nerves to the heart that adjusts both the force and the rate of its contractions.

REGULATION OF ARTERIOLAR RESISTANCE.—The thoracolumbar sympathetic outflow that supplies the veins also runs to the arteries and the arterioles. These fibers arise in the medulla and pass down the cord in the lateral columns. Connector cells lie in the lateral part of the gray matter of the spinal cord. Fibers leave these cells to pass on to the ganglia of the lateral sympathetic chain and to the cervical, celiac, and inferior mesenteric ganglia. These supply the entire body with its vasoconstrictor nerve supply.

By stimulating these nerves at different frequencies, varying degrees of arteriolar constriction ensue (Fig. 7-7). Thus an increase in frequency from 0 to 6 impulses/sec resulted in a linear rise of the peripheral resistance and a vasoconstriction of 80% of the maximal effect obtainable in the muscle. In skin, an even sharper initial rise was obtained that flattened out at the higher frequencies of stimulation. If the stimulus is withheld, the constriction passes off in a few seconds. It seems probable that in normal physiological states the maximum peripheral vasomotor discharge rate is 6–8 impulses/sec. This is followed by relaxation of the vessel in some 6 sec after cessation of the stimuli. Normal discharge rates are 1–3 impulses per sec.

The response to this outflow is not the same in all tissues. The splanchnic region appears more sensitive than skin and muscle, and the brain responds very little. The action is believed to depend on the release of nor-epinephrine at the nerve endings on the smooth muscle cells of the arterioles and on the muscle of adjacent smaller vessels. The net result is that the already formidable drop in pressure as the blood flows through these resistance vessels (Fig. 1-1) can be increased even to the point, as in Raynaud's disease, of cutting off all flow despite a mean pressure of 100 mm Hg in the arteries above the obstruction. The reverse effect, the withholding of the normal flow of sympathetic impulses, leads to vasodilation as a result of relaxation of normal tonus. These vasoconstrictor fibers play a major role in the regulation of blood pressure, and a small decrease of the normal discharge rate will lead to a sharp fall. A demonstration of this is the effect of putting an anesthetic in the spinal canal. If this travels high enough to affect a sufficient percentage of the total spinal sympathetic outflow, there will be a marked fall in peripheral vascular resistance and, consequently, a fall in blood pressure. Similar but more long-lasting effects result from ablation of the sympathetic ganglion chain, an operation formerly much used in the treatment of high blood pressure.

The adrenal glands themselves appear to play little part in the normal central control of vasomotor activity. Certainly, vascular changes induced by direct stimulation of the nerves are an order of magnitude greater than those resulting from the normal release of hormone from the adrenal gland.

ROLE OF THE SYMPATHETIC SYSTEM IN REGULATING THE FORCE OF THE HEART BEAT.—The

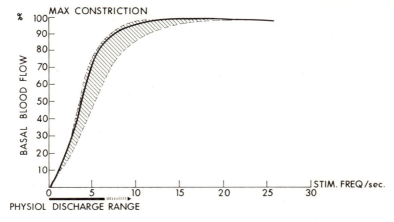

Fig. 7-7.—The correlation between stimulation rate and constrictor response. The spread between the different experiments is indicated by the hatched surface. (From Folkow, B.: Acta physiol. scandinav.) 25:56, 1952, Fig. 1.)

direct action of the cardiac sympathetic efferents can cause the ventricle to contract more or less forcefully regardless of the end-diastolic filling pressure or fiber length. The result can be a doubling or tripling of the stroke work done by the left ventricle. The increased sympathetic drive produces more complete systolic emptying and so lowers end-diastolic volume. This places the heart on a more sensitive part of its curve and means that even a low filling pressure produces a larger fiber-length increase. The stimulation also decreases the time taken for the ventricle to eject its content, so giving a longer period for ventricular diastole. This allows more adequate filling despite a low filling pressure and improves the irrigation of the ventricular muscle by the coronary blood flow. Adrenalin has the same effect as sympathetic stimulation, and both lead to an increased conduction velocity over the atrium, at the AV node, and in the ventricle. As is discussed in Chapter 3, it is probable that, in addition to the above-described influences that improve the efficiency of ventricular systole, there is a direct effect on the metabolic processes in the muscle fibers, increasing their contractility or force-velocity characteristics. Recent evidence indicates that vagal stimulation may also affect the force of ventricular contraction. Regulation of myocardial performance may then be achieved by a reciprocal action of both the sympathetic and the parasympathetic divisions of the autonomic nervous system.

Vagal regulation of the rate of heart beat.—Arising in the same dorsal nuclear region where the afferent impulses from the stretch receptors of the cardiovascular system terminate, the vagal motor fibers to the heart run down the nerve to be distributed to the SA and AV nodes and to atrial muscle, but not to the ventricles. In the normal animal, the vagus exerts a constant restraint on the action of the heart that is inversely proportional to the state of development of the cardiovascular system. Thus the athlete often has a very slow pulse, i.e., 50–60/min, and, as the demand on his system increases, heart action can be increased by a relaxation of vagal control. By starting with a slower pulse, he can go further before reaching the young man's peak rates of 180–200/min. Atropine eliminates vagal action resulting in a resting pulse of 150–180/min. These vagal effects depend on the release of acetylcholine. This hormone slows the spontaneous rhythm of the SA node and decreases the excitability of the AV junctional fibers. Thus strong vagal stimulation can induce a complete heart block. The ventricles stand still for a few seconds and then start beating at some 15–40 beats/min in ventricular escape as a result of an ectopic rhythm from a focus that is usually in the AV bundle.

Acetylcholine hyperpolarizes the junctional fibers in the AV node, and it blocks conduction by increasing the time that it takes for the membrane potential to fall low enough for self-excitation.

Sympathetic stimulation and heart rate.—An increase in the rate of firing of the sympathetic nerves coming from the stellate ganglion usually occurs simultaneously with the release of vagal restraint. In any emergency state that is associated with increased sympathetic discharge, not only are the contractility, i.e., the force-velocity characteristics, increased, but also the rate of SA nodal discharge. This, combined with the decreased conduction time and increased excitability, can lead to a tripling of the rate. These effects depend on the release of epinephrine, which, in contrast with acetylcholine, probably increases the rate of decay of the SA resting membrane potential, thus decreasing the time taken for self-excitation.

Because the systemic arterial pressure is determined by cardiac output and peripheral resistance, it can be set at any level that is needed by the organism by means of vagal and sympathetic determination of the heart rate, the force of the beat, and of the set of the resistance vessels.

Note on the Bainbridge reflex.—Over 50 years ago, the English physiologist, Bainbridge, observed a tachycardia following intravenous infusion. This was puzzling because the immediate result of a sudden stimulation of the mechanoreceptors in the low-pressure system either chemically, by the infusion of veratridine (Jarisch-Bezold reflex), or mechanically, by suddenly distending the atria with blood, is a bradycardia. However, numerous studies have confirmed Bainbridge's findings, and recent work has shown that, although there is indeed a tachycardia following an infusion in the anesthetized dog, it only develops if the resting pulse is less than 110/min. If the initial rate is higher than 110/min, a pulse slowing occurs.

It has been suggested that the reflex is due to a complex of effects and that receptors other than the CUE of Nonidez in the atrial region of the low-pressure system play a part. It is possible that the end-net receptors, which are profuse in the atria, are responsible for this effect. The same type of endings in the pulmonary artery and the ventricles may also be involved as the infusion increases pulmonary vascular pressure and disturbs the normal dynamics of the heart chambers. So far, however, this is speculation, and the problem is one needing further research.

Reflex Central Nervous Regulation of Pressure and Volume

The close proximity of the afferent and the efferent cardiovascular neurones in the medulla and the intimate overlapping and nearby location of the neurones relaying the impulses from the stretch receptors in the low- and the high-pressure systems bespeak an integrated system that coordinates volume and pressure at this primitive level in the central nervous system. The present section will briefly describe the classic method of demonstrating the effects of stimulation of the stretch receptors in the isolated carotid sinus; then an experiment will be described from which the effects of stimulating the various receptors in the left atrium can be deduced. Finally, since such isolated stimuli to individual receptor areas are highly artificial events that do not occur in nature, the results of a recent analysis of the effects of changing blood volume by increments of 10% will be discussed. Blood volume loss or gain is an event that is constantly occurring in the shift to and from orthostasis. In the course of such changes in central blood volume, receptors in both systems are inevitably affected. However, a differentiation can be made between the contributions from the low- and from the high-pressure components of the system. Viewing them separately helps to show how the two can combine to form a solid base of central regulation of volume and pressure. It is on this basis that the higher centers can develop the various flow distribution patterns needed for the effective response of the organism to the various demands imposed by the environment, i.e., by straining, digestion, heat, cold, muscular exercise, and emotional stimuli.

Carotid Sinus Perfusion Experiments

Over thirty years ago, Heymans carried out a series of ingenious cross-perfusion experiments in which the sinus of one dog (B) was isolated from the general circulation and perfused with the blood of another animal (A) (Fig. 7-8). The nerve supply to the sinus was left intact. When the arterial pressure of dog A was raised, that of dog B fell, as recorded in the femoral artery. Conversely, a reduction in the blood pressure of dog A caused a bradycardia and a rise in the blood pressure of dog B. These experiments conclusively showed that the buffer nerves are of importance in controlling the arterial pressure. There is evidence of their action in man. Thus, when a pilot is exposed to an acceleration of 4–5 g in a tight turn, the pressure in the carotid sinus region is sharply reduced. Within 6 seconds, a tachycardia and peripheral vasoconstriction develop, and an increase in the systemic arterial pressure returns the pressure in the sinus to normal despite the continued acceleration. Other work has shown that, if deformation of the arterial walls is prevented by a rigid cast, the barore-

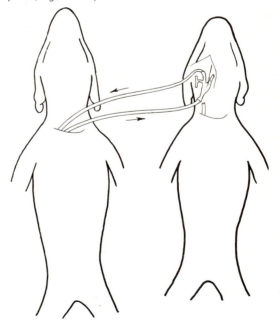

Fig. 7-8.—Scheme of perfusion of the isolated carotid sinus of one dog by another. The carotid sinus nerve is depicted as it terminates on the wall of the sinus. (From Best, C. H., and Taylor, N. B.: *The Physiological Basis of Medical Practice* [Baltimore: Williams & Wilkins Co., 1966], p. 794, Figs. 42–45.)

ceptors no longer respond to intravascular pressure changes. Also, if the smooth muscle of the wall of the artery is stimulated by applying epinephrine, there is an increase in impulses from the sinus for a given pressure and hence a reduction in blood pressure. These changes in blood pressure result from the influence of the afferent impulses from the carotid sinus upon the dorsal nucleus of the vagus in the medulla. The level of afferent impulses determines the sympathetic outflow to the heart and resistance vessels and determines the blood pressure.

These experiments were ground-breaking demonstrations of the facts of cardiovascular regulation. However, the stimulation of a single sinus in a dog, under chloralose anesthesia without concomitant change in the other sinus, the aortic arch, or in central blood volume, and hence without any change in the afferent impulses from the atria, is an event that does not occur in nature. Furthermore, it is known that in exercise, for example, and in excitement, pressures will rise very high in the arterial tree, showing that under these circumstances the carotid sinus ceases to influence the central control mechanisms in the usual way. Recent work suggests that impulses from higher centers affecting the olivary nuclei are responsible for this abeyance of the reflex.

When there is a fall in pressure, the protective reflex is not so often overridden, although there are exceptions such as vagal syncope in which the pressure will fall to critical values in the cardiovascular system without intervention from the carotid sinus mechanism.

Changes in Atrial Pressure by Use of a Balloon

Heyman's cross-perfusion experiment showed that changes in pressure in the arterial baroreceptor area induce appropriate responses in heart action and peripheral resistance that, in turn, induce a compensatory alteration of blood pressure. If a balloon is placed in the left atrium of a dog under chloralose and a tube attached to the balloon brought out through the atrial appendage and the chest wall, a distension of the balloon by fluid will lead to a rise of pulmonary

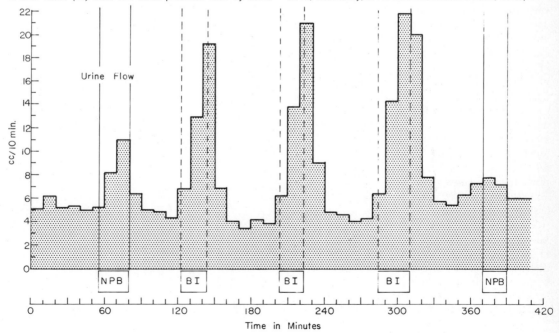

Fig. 7-9.—Effects of negative pressure breathing (NPB) for 20 minutes at −10 cm H$_2$O on the urine flow of a dog under chloralose. A small deflated balloon was placed in the left atrium several hours before the test. On distending it with water (BI) until left atrial pressure rose by some 20 cm H$_2$O, there is a sharp rise of urine flow. The onset of the diuresis is delayed by approximately 10 min and persists after removing the stimulus. This suggests that a hormonal response (ADH) may be involved. (From Gauer, O. H., and Henry, J. P.: Klin. Wchnschr. 34:356, 1956.)

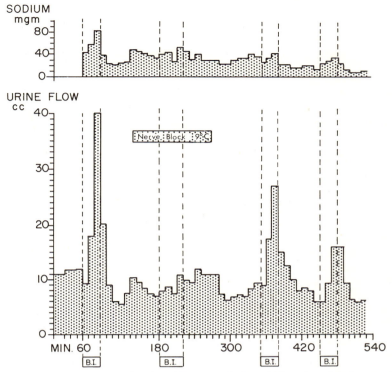

Fig. 7-10.—The relationship between urine flow in cc/10 min **(below)** and total sodium excreted/10 min. **(above)** and the inflation of a balloon in the left atrium *(BI)*. When the balloon was inflated the second time, both vagus nerve trunks had been cooled to 9° C. The response of urine flow was eliminated. There is a slight increase in sodium output in association with the first period of increased urine flow. (From Wright Air Development Center Technical Report 478.)

vascular and left-atrial pressure as a result of right-ventricular activity. By tensing snares around the pulmonary veins of the same dog and thereby raising pulmonary vascular pressure without affecting the atrium, it can be shown that an increase in urine flow will only occur when the atrium is distended (Fig. 7-9). Antidiuretic hormone assays show that a part of this increase in urine flow is due to a reduction of the ADH level in the blood. This occurs as the supraopticohypophyseal apparatus responds to the changed impulse pattern arising from the stimulated receptors. By cooling the vagus to the point at which conduction of atrial afferents is eliminated, the diuretic response is abolished, to return with warming and restoration of conduction (Fig. 7-10).

Such experiments are artificial in terms of naturally occurring events. But they help in the analysis of control mechanisms by showing that a regulatory response can be initiated by the mere distension of one stretch receptor area, this time in the low-pressure system.

In practice, when blood volume increases, both atria and especially the left atrium increase their pulsation as pressures rise throughout the low-pressure system. When the reverse procedure is carried out in the normal animal and blood volume is progressively reduced, the atrial impulse traffic greatly decreases. Then, as first pulse pressure and finally mean systemic arterial pressure fall, there will be a decrease in impulse traffic from the arterial or high-pressure system receptors (Figs. 7-3 and 7-11). These combined effects will bring on every one of the adjustments cited in the preceding pages. That is to say, a sharp reduction of blood volume will cause a rise in antidiuretic hormone level (Fig. 7-11), sodium retention, and a marked change in the ratio of pre- to postcapillary resistance. It will also cause the spleen to contract (Fig. 7-12-A) and, in the kidney, there will be a decrease in perfusion of the outer cortical peritubular capillaries, together with initiation of the release of renin. Finally, the conscious individual will experience thirst.

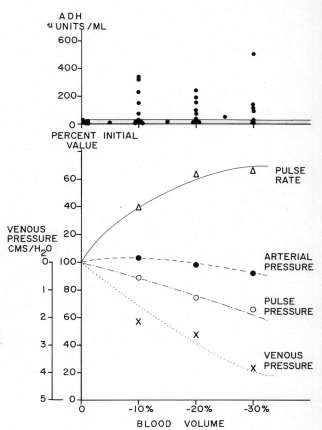

Fig. 7-11.—Conscious dogs bled progressively in 10% aliquots of the blood volume show a drop of pulse pressure and central venous pressure and, with this, an increase in blood level of antidiuretic hormone, sometimes to 200 μ units or more per cc. Maximum antidiuresis occurs when the blood level exceeds 4–6 μ units/ml. It is probable that at the higher levels, the direct vascular effects of the hormone play a significant, though as yet undefined, role. (From Henry, J. P., *et al.*: Canad. J. Physiol. & Pharmacol 46:291, 1968. Reproduced by permission of the National Research Council of Canada.)

Simultaneously, peripheral vasoconstriction will set in, first in the arterioles and finally in the veins. The heart rate will increase in direct response to the changed atrial impulse patterns, and so, despite the fall in pulse pressure, the mean blood pressure may remain unchanged. Some of these changes that have just been described contribute to the control of the volume of blood in the low-pressure system, and some contribute directly to the maintenance of systemic arterial pressure. The problem is how to disentangle the effects of stimuli that are simultaneously changing in both systems and, therefore, affecting both sets of receptors.

Responses of Atrial and Aortic Baroreceptors to Progressive Blood Loss

By making a gradual reduction of blood volume in increments of no more than 10% at a time and by recording impulses from receptors in both the low- and the high-pressure systems, i.e., from the atria and the aortic arch, it is possible to compare the flux of information from the receptors in the two systems.

In other words, moderate hemorrhage to a point short of the moment when the mean systemic arterial pressure falls has the effect of making a functional dichotomy between the receptors in the low- as opposed to those in the high-pressure system. If a comparison is made of the mean firing rate per second in the two systems, it can be shown that, with the loss of 25% of the blood volume, the atrial unit burst number drops to less than one-half (Fig. 7-3). In part because the pulse rate increases, there is no significant over-all fall in afferent impulses per second from the aortic arch. Central venous pressure will fall significantly with a moderate hemorrhage, but the systemic arterial pressure will be well maintained. As the atrial pressure and pulsation diminish with the loss of blood

REGULATION AND INTEGRATION OF CARDIOVASCULAR FUNCTION

volume, the pulse rate rises in response to sympathetic arousal. Further evidence of the tightening up of the arterial pressure defenses is the increase in contractility of the heart, despite the lowered filling pressure and the beginning increase in peripheral resistance. There is also a beginning contraction of the spleen that does not occur at these minor levels of blood loss if the nerves to the heart are cut (Fig. 7-12-B), thus showing that, up to this point, it is the receptors in the low-pressure system that are determining the responses.

The respective roles of the CUE of Nonidez in the right and the left atria and of the end net-

Fig. 7-12.—Diagrams showing the effects of hemorrhage upon a sensitive splenic size factor, i.e., contribution to the circulating red cell mass is negligible in the early stages. In normal animals, there is an immediate response that progressively increases with the extent of the blood loss. When the spleen is denervated, the response is minimal **(A)**. When the heart is denervated, it is deferred until the baroreceptors in the high-pressure system are affected, i.e., after the loss of 25% of the blood volume **(B)**.

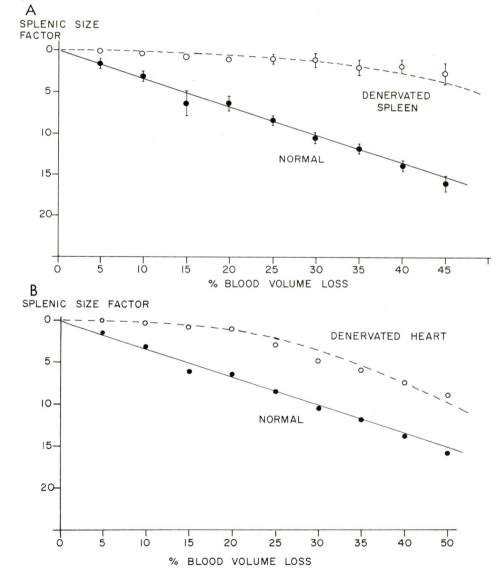

works during minor blood volume loss remain to be established. It is as yet unknown whether the CUE of the right atrium play a different role from those of the left; nor, as was previously stated, do we know whether the end net has any special effect on sympathetic vasomotor tone and sodium excretion.

Not only is water retained as a result of antidiuretic hormone activity, but, as the renin mechanism and the redistribution of blood flow from cortex to medulla progress in response to the increased renal sympathetic outflow, sodium conservation is initiated. Finally, with blood loss in excess of 20%, the tone in the great veins increases, thus decreasing the size of the venous reservoir.

Up to this point, the changes are directed at replacing the lost volume from tissue stores or from the environment by decreasing urine flow and increasing water intake. From the 25% blood loss point onward, these changes in the vigorous healthy conscious animal can only progress in intensity because the available measures for blood volume and blood pressure control have already been alerted. On the afferent side, there is an almost total loss of afferent impulses from the low-pressure system and a sharp drop in the flow from the now less-stimulated baroreceptors in the arterial tree. ADH levels, renin secretion, and renal blood flow redistribution increase further; the pulse rate rises still more; and myocardial contractility increases still further. The visceral vascular beds constrict so strongly that eventually the total renal, hepatic, and gastrointestinal blood flow are so seriously impaired that organ damage ensues. Venous constriction becomes self-evident as the skin pales and "cold" sweat develops in response to cholinergic sympathetic stimuli. The venoconstriction may become so vigorous that the central venous pressure actually rises back to normal values as the capacity of the low-pressure system is decreased until it matches the diminished contents.

Summary

This chapter has been concerned with the means by which an adequate pressure head is maintained so that the higher centers can allot to the various tissues a flow necessary and appropriate for the particular activity and energy requirements of the moment. The analogy of a pump with a reservoir is often used in connection with the circulation. In Figure 7-13, the left ventricle is simulated by a rubber bag squeezed between two hinged plates. The varying rate at which the crank can be turned (I) and its variable length (II) represent the different possibilities of stroke work and contractility. Because it is elastic, the diastolic filling of the rubber bag will vary according to the pressure in the venous reservoir above. This reservoir is depicted with movable sides, thus simulating the possibilities of a change in venous tone (A). The low-pressure system mechanoreceptors indicate to the control system the degree of filling of this system.

In the "arterial" channel leading out of the pump are the receptors for the high-pressure system. The outflow from the pump passes through a variable control arteriolar resistance before pouring into the venous reservoir. By means of "thirst" (B), the control system can induce more fluid to be fed into this reservoir. Also by a change in the pre- to postcapillary resistance ratio, fluid can either be brought into the vascular bed or lost from it. The amount of fluid leaving the system is determined by the ADH level, and the amount of salt retained or lost is determined by the renin level and by intrarenal vascular adjustments (C). By making minor changes in volume, which do not yet significantly affect the pump's output pressure, not only is a whole complex of volume regulatory responses immediately set into motion, but also the pressure is defended even before it starts to fall. These high- and low-pressure system stretch receptor reflexes appear to use the medulla as a primary coordinating center, although the antidiuretic hormone response shows that the activity of the hypothalamus farther up the chain is involved.

There is much to be found out about the role of the various cardiac receptors. Indeed, the activity of the recently discovered subendocardial end networks, which are present in all vertebrate hearts so far examined, is completely unknown. They may prove to be prime movers in a more primitive system of salt and water regulation. It is not known why the highly specialized, complex unencapsulated endings of Nonidez suddenly appeared in the mammals in the process of phylogeny. Perhaps it is because they are primarily concerned with the regulation of antidiuretic hormone. Certainly, the mammals

REGULATION AND INTEGRATION OF CARDIOVASCULAR FUNCTION

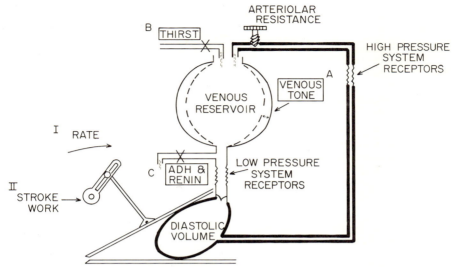

Fig. 7-13.—Diagram indicating the general principles of pressure and volume regulation. See text for details.

have greater problems with the conservation of water than the amphibia, and their sweating technique of heat regulation puts them in constant jeopardy of excessive extracellular fluid volume loss. Recent work by Öberg and White suggests that the cardiac nerve afferents make a particularly strong engagement with the vasomotor neurones controlling the heart and the renal vessels.

Certainly the receptors of the high- and low-pressure systems are very closely integrated, a fact that the anatomical juxtaposition of the relay neurones in the dorsal vagal nucleus suggests. It appears as though the arterial baroreceptors add emphasis to changes that stretch receptors in the low-pressure system have already initiated. In nature, both systems of receptors are usually affected at the same time, for a loss or gain of blood volume will affect the high-pressure system as well as the low. The sequence of events during volume loss is a simultaneous tightening up on volume and pressure controls as a disparity develops between the atrial receptor drive and the still-constant sinoaortic drive—between impulses arriving during systole, including the atrial A fibers, and the B impulses characteristically observed at diastole. With further blood loss, this tightening up with its challenge to the first line of defense becomes an emergency matter. The responses are greatly exaggerated, but they are not changed in nature when the flow of information from the low-pressure system actually vanishes, as it does with the loss of more than 30% of blood volume. At this stage, the information from the high-pressure system itself begins to falter as the blood pressure falls.

It is an oversimplification to regard these afferent systems as engaging in synaptic connections only with the medullary vasomotor and cardiac centers. They affect the activity of the entire ascending reticular system of the brain stem, and it has been shown that in doing so the carotid sinus activity directly affects the arousal state of the organism. However, in general, the medullary activities may be the dominant ones. The combination of these lower brain stem elements running to and from the low- and high-pressure receptor and effector regions can be considered the basic command system of the circulation. By assuring the maintenance of an adequate pressure head from which the blood flow appropriate to the activity requirements of each of the various tissues can be derived, this more primitive command system can sustain the competence of the organism, while higher centers go about the task of meeting the widely varying conditions and challenges imposed by the environment.

REFERENCES

Abraham, A.: *Microscopic Innervation of the Heart and Blood Vessels in Vertebrates Including Man* (New York: Pergamon Press, Inc., 1960).

Folkow, B., Heymans, C., and Neil, E.: Integrated Aspects of Cardiovascular Regulation, in Hamilton, W. F. (ed.): *Handbook of Physiology: Circulation* (Washington: American Physiological Society, 1963), Vol. III, pp. 1,787–1,824.

Gauer, O. H., and Henry, J. P.: Circulatory Basis of Fluid Volume Control, Physiol. Rev. 43:423–481, 1963.

Gauer, O. H., Henry, J. P., and Behn, C.: The Regulation of Extracellular Fluid Volume, Ann. Rev. Physiol. 32:547–595, 1970.

Henry, J. P., *et al.:* The Role of Afferents from the Low Pressure System in the Release of Antidiuretic Hormone during Nonhypotensive Hemorrhage, Canad. J. Physiol. & Pharmacol. 46:287–295, 1968.

Heymans, C., and Neil, E.: *Reflexogenic Areas of the Cardiovascular System* (London: J. & A. Churchill, Ltd., 1958).

Keele, C. A., and Neil, E.: in Wright, S.: *Applied Physiology,* 11th ed. (New York: Oxford University Press, 1965).

Öberg, B., and White, S.: The Role of Vagal Cardiac Nerves and Arterial Baroreceptors in the Circulatory Adjustments of Hemorrhage in the Cat, Acta Physiol. Scandinav. (in press).

Symposium on the Central Nervous Control of the Circulation, Physiol. Rev. Vol. 40, Supp. 4, 1960.

Uvnäs, B.: Central Cardiovascular Control, in Field, J. (ed.): *Handbook of Physiology: Neurophysiology* (Washington: American Physiological Society, 1960), Vol. II, pp. 1,131–1,162.

Vander, J. A.: Control of Renin Release, Physiol. Rev. 47:359–382, 1967.

8

Characteristics of Responses of Local Circulations

Coronary

CHARACTERISTICS OF THE CORONARY VESSELS

BLOOD IS SUPPLIED to the heart muscle mass by the two coronary arteries arising from ostia at the root of the aorta in the sinuses of Valsalva (Fig. 8-1). The right artery runs posteriorly in the groove between the right ventricle and atrium. The left divides shortly into an anterior descending branch, which passes down the groove between the ventricles, and a circumflex, which runs posteriorly in the groove between the left ventricle and the left atrium and terminates in a posterior descending branch. All are epicardial and spread out over the heart's surface, sending fine ramifications inward to penetrate the myocardium.

In 30% of human beings, the two arteries supply their respective ventricles. In 50%, the right is preponderant and supplies the entire septal wall and some of the posterior left ventricle. In 20%, the left coronary supplies the left ventricle and the circumflex supplies the posterior septum and part of the right ventricle. There is no correlation between these distributions and the severity of an attack of coronary occlusion. The SA and AV nodes are supplied by branches of the right artery; hence, disorders of rhythm such

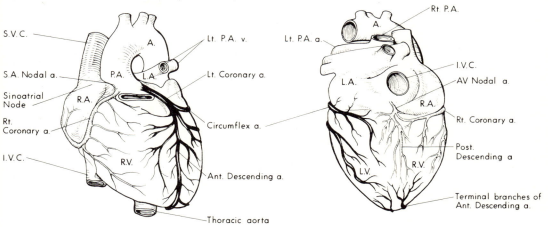

Fig. 8-1.—Distribution of coronary arteries as they most commonly occur in man. **Left,** anterior surface of the heart. **Right,** posterior surface of the heart. (From Truex, R. C.: in Likoff, W., and Moyer, J. H. (eds.): *Coronary Heart Disease.* [New York: Grune & Stratton, Inc., 1963].)

as heart block are associated with lesions in the branches of this vessel.

The large arteries escape the squeeze of the ventricle by virtue of their epicardial location. The small arteries plunge into the muscle and ramify to supply capillaries that are more numerous than in skeletal muscle. There is approximately one for each muscle fiber. The result of cardiac hypertrophy is to increase fiber diameter, but the number of capillaries per fiber stays unchanged.

There are some direct channels from the coronary arteries into the heart chambers. Some arteriolar twigs discharge directly as arterioluminal vessels and others, appropriately termed arteriosinusoidal, flow into big sinuses and then empty into the chamber. However, most of the drainage is by veins that run parallel to the arteries, ending in the coronary sinus, which empties into the right atrium; it is believed that the vast preponderance of blood returns by this route.

The coronary vessels of Western Europeans and others adopting their culture, who live on a high-fat and high-sucrose diet and who, for the past two centuries, have been in a sociocultural turmoil, are subject to the disease of atherosclerosis. It consists of accumulations of lipid infiltrated with cholesterol that form plaques that encroach on the lumen. It is combined with fibroelastic changes in the walls, and the result is a progressive and sometimes abrupt occlusion of the vessels, the latter being due to thrombus formation in the region of the plaque or to hemorrhage within the plaque. This condition is not found in culturally stable areas untouched by the industrial revolution, such as pre-World War II China or primitive Africa. Sooner or later, it results in attacks of myocardial ischemia in 20% or more of all men over 35, with the result that the state of blood supply of the heart has become a matter of major concern to the physician in our society. If the obstruction, which may also have a functional component due to spasm of the vessel walls, is acute, the result is hypoxic damage to the muscle fed by the vessel. If this area is sufficiently large, death ensues in some 25% of the victims. This may take the form of ventricular fibrillation within minutes to hours, or of heart failure that may gradually develop, or an aneurysm that eventually ruptures. The issue between death and recovery depends, not only on the size, but also on the rate of development of the lesion. Given sufficient time, the coronary arteries do not act as true end arteries. Collaterals will develop; given weeks or months, intercoronary channels will grow to the point that completely occluded major vessels can be replaced, sometimes without loss of muscle efficiency (Fig. 8-2). Thus a coronary occlusion that is survived for a month has a good chance of scar formation and recovery as long as the muscle destroyed by ischemia remains a moderate fraction of the total.

There is evidence that growth of collaterals

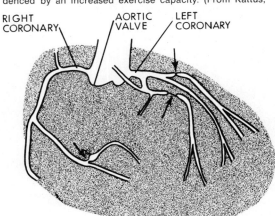
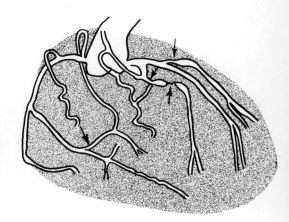

Fig. 8-2.—Coronary angiograms performed 15 months apart show that, although stenotic disease of the major vessels is somewhat worse, collaterals have developed that make the over-all picture better. The improvement was evidenced by an increased exercise capacity. (From Kattus, A. A.: Physical Training and Beta-Adrenergic Blocking Drugs in Modifying Coronary Insufficiency, in *International Symposium on the Coronary Circulation and Energetics of the Myocardium* [Basel: Karger, 1967], Fig. 3, p. 309.)

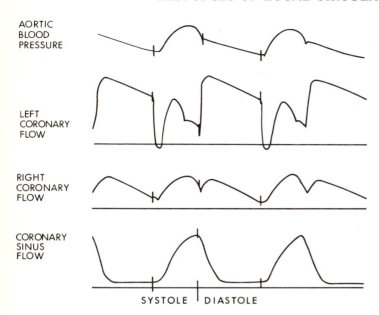

Fig. 8-3.—Schematic representation of phasic flow in the coronary vascular bed, with aortic blood pressure as a reference tracing. *Left coronary flow* is maximal at the onset of diastole and gradually falls off throughout the balance of the diastolic interval. With onset of systole, flow falls abruptly to zero or may even be temporarily reversed. Net forward flow during systole is approximately 25% of that during diastole. *Right coronary flow* pattern resembles contour of the aortic pressure pulse; because extravascular compression by the right ventricle is small, flow does not approach zero. Myocardial compression augments emptying of coronary veins during systole; phasic flow through the coronary sinus is thus accentuated during this period. (Diagram after Gregg, D. R.: in Luisada, A. A. (ed.): *Cardiology, An Encyclopedia of the Cardiovascular System* [New York: McGraw-Hill Book Co., Inc. 1959], Vol. I, pp. 2-202, Fig. 2-78.)

depends on the oxygen requirements of the tissues beyond the obstructed region. Healthy athletes who drive themselves to the limits of endurance develop collaterals as well as enlargement of their normal vessels. There is also evidence that collateral formation in the critical area may be accelerated by exercising the individual with a blood supply that has become locally limited due to a previous occlusion. Vasodilator drugs such as pyridamole may also serve the same purpose. The combination of avoidance of sustained and excessive psychosocial arousal of the sympathetic adrenal system, dietary restriction of fats and sucrose, drugs, and vigorous exercise shows hope of controlling the more severe aspects of coronary atherosclerosis.

Phasic Flow

The existence of coronary disease gives special significance to a knowledge of the dynamics of coronary flow and the mechanisms by which flow is adapted to varying demands on the heart. The development of electronic flowmeters permitting observations in normal healthy dogs is rapidly clarifying the subject. Like skeletal muscle, the heart compresses the blood vessels when it contracts. Since the pressure inside the left ventricle is slightly greater than in the aorta during systole, the innermost subendocardial layers of this chamber are only irrigated during diastole; however, there is continuous flow in the subepicardial layers. Left-ventricular coronary flow is especially impaired during tachycardia because a relatively greater proportion of the cycling time is spent in systole. As the diagram (Fig. 8-3) indicates, the flow to the right heart and the atria is better sustained because there is an excellent differential of pressure between the aorta and these low-pressure regions, even during systole. The subendocardial portion of the thick-walled left ventricle is the most subject to ischemia, and it is not surprising that it is a common site of myocardial infarction. The myocardium is at risk following a sustained depression of arterial pressure, as after an acute loss of blood volume, and in aortic stenosis when there is a prolonged and intense systole during which intraventricular pressure rises to great heights. Such conditions are liable to exaggerate pre-existing arteriosclerotic deficiencies in coronary blood supply.

The curves for coronary flow show that, whereas, the right coronary follows the aortic pressure curve, the left has an inverse relationship between flow and pressure. During the period of isometric contraction, flow through the left artery is arrested. At the same time, the squeezing of the veins ejects the blood into the coronary sinus where flow increases rapidly.

With the onset of ejection, left coronary flow recommences, but peak flow occurs early in diastole when a majority of the blood is delivered. This phasic venous squeezing is not essential to coronary flow since flow also accelerates in the arrested heart, but the fact that venous blood is massaged onwards by normal ventricular contraction is modestly advantageous in assisting coronary inflow during this period. Work with flowmeters shows that despite ventricular contraction as much as 40% of the coronary flow can occur during systole. Whether denervated or intact, the coronary flow increases two- to threefold during periods of oxygen lack. It is thought that this may not be a direct effect of hypoxia but that adenosine released by the hypoxic tissue is responsible. Carbon dioxide and changes in pH do not elicit significant responses, nor is a rise in aortic pressure necessary for an increase. Indeed there is little change in mean arterial pressure in the well-trained athlete exercising within his reserves and remaining mentally at ease, despite the fivefold or greater increase in his cardiac output.

Coronary Innervation

Recent work has finally established the great importance of the profuse innervation of the coronary vessels. They have both alpha receptors, which respond with vasoconstriction to the catechols, as well as the purely vasodilator beta receptors. Nor-epinephrine only affects the alpha receptors. It does not usually cause coronary vasoconstriction because other simultaneous vasodilator effects, such as the local hypoxia consequent upon the increased work of the muscle, are stronger. However, a measure of constriction can occur, and it has been demonstrated that direct action on the coronary vasculature by the sympathetic outflow and by catecholamines will induce either vasodilation or vasoconstriction, depending on the proportions and distribution of the alpha and beta receptors in the coronaries. In general, there are more alpha receptors in the large vessels and more beta receptors in the small ones. In addition, the presence of high levels of posterior pituitary hormones intensify vasoconstriction.

No evidence of mechanical obstruction is found at postmortem in a significant percentage of sudden deaths due to coronary ischemia. It is probable that these people were suffering from a functional vasospasm in a large coronary vessel. The beneficial effects of nitroglycerin in angina pectoris may be because it is a large coronary dilator. The clear relationship of angina to psychological stimuli, such as fear and anger, suggests the possibility of a direct constrictor response of the vascular bed. Proof, however, is lacking because the powerful inotropic effect of sympathetic stimulation simultaneously increases the work and oxygen consumption of the heart.

Studies with dogs having flowmeters implanted in the coronary vessels show that there can be a threefold flow increase with excitement. In fact, the flow changes with emotion can be more marked than those with exercise. A further problem is that an increase in total coronary flow does not necessarily mean that the flow to an ischemic area of muscle will be effectively increased. Thus nitroglycerin, which is unexcelled in the relief of the pain of angina or coronary ischemia, is not the most impressive of the coronary vasodilator agents. This appears to be because it does not affect the small resistance vessels that are responsible for autoregulation. A dilator that induces large total coronary flows by decreasing resistance will not help flow through an already fully dilated ischemic area. However, a drug, such as nitroglycerin, that has its main effect on the large vessels will increase retrograde flow up a blocked artery by increasing the supply to the collaterals feeding into the obstructed vessel beyond the point of obstruction. In this roundabout way, the nutrition of the ischemic area is improved. It is critical to know whether an agent affects large or small vessels; it is collateral not total coronary flow that determines whether there will be relief of local myocardial ischemia.

There is clinical evidence that pain, distension of the bladder or any other viscus, stimulation of afferent nerves, and experimental neurosis all will, on occasion, decrease coronary flow. These effects may be mediated by the vagus as well as by the above-mentioned sympathetic control via the alpha receptors. This latter vagal route has not yet been conclusively demonstrated.

Summary

The outstanding fact about the left coronary circulation is the rhythmic mechanical obstruction causing stop-and-go flow through the heavy ventricular muscle. An important local regulatory effect on coronary blood flow is the accumulation of metabolites. There is now proof that the rich innervation of both large and small coronary vessels, while not necessary to life, plays an important part in the physiologic adaptations and the disasters that can occur to this vital bed.

Cerebral Circulation

METHODS OF MEASURING FLOW

The two internal carotids and the two vertebrals supply the whole brain, and, in man, the major share of blood comes up the carotids. The circle of Willis connects these four vessels, and from it spring the two sets of anterior, middle, and posterior cerebral arteries supplying the cortex. Unlike the carnivora, the loss of one carotid in man cannot be adequately compensated by increased flow through the remaining channels. This becomes particularly serious in older people in whom the vessels are rigid and narrowed; arteriosclerotic disease occluding one carotid will often lead to gross ischemic damage of the cerebral hemisphere on that side. It is for this reason that so much attention is being paid today to the matter of replacement of such arteries with Dacron grafts before final occlusion occurs. Another peculiarity of the human cerebral circulation is that almost all the blood flows out through the internal jugular veins. Consequently, this blood is a fair sampling of cerebral venous blood in general. The Fick principle can be used to measure cerebral blood flow in normal people. This (Kety) technique involves increasing the volume of N_2O in the arterial and in the cerebral venous blood by inhaling a small amount of gas. The brachial or radial artery is appropriate, whereas the venous sample can be obtained by inserting a needle in the jugular bulb, a relatively safe and quite painless procedure in the proper hands.

The average cerebral blood flow in young adults is 54 cc/100 gm/min, but in children the rate is double this value (Fig. 8-4). The drop to the adult rate occurs at puberty. It is, however, unaffected by giving sex or adrenal hormones. The high value tempts speculation that it may be related to the superior learning and memorization capacity of the young.

Although the total cerebral flow can be measured quite accurately by the above method, the technique gives no idea as to the relative flow in different parts of the brain. By comparing the distribution of radioactive tracer gas in various regions with the blood level of the same gas, it is possible to make such estimates of local flow. There are marked differences ranging from 1.8 cc/gm/min for the inferior colliculus through 1.0 cc/gm/min for the thalamus down to one-fourth this value for white matter. Although the brain represents only about 2% of the body mass, its over-all oxygen consumption is some 20% of the total in the resting body. Further, its needs are imperative, and the mere cessation of flow

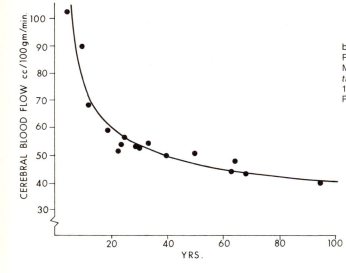

Fig. 8-4.—Changes in the human cerebral blood flow with age. (From Kety, S.: The Physiology of the Cerebral Circulation in Man; in McMichael, J. (ed.): *Proceedings of the Harvey Tercentenary Congress,* June 3–8, 1957 [Oxford, England: Blackwell Scientific Publications, 1958], p. 328, Fig. 3.)

for 5–10 sec will lead to unconsciousness. In man, this can be done by squeezing the neck and obstructing the carotids. This will not work in other animals in which vertebral blood supply is more important. If an interruption of cerebral blood flow lasts for more than 3-5 minutes, irrevocable damage is probable. There are a large number of circumstances in which such accidents occur, ranging from heart arrest to exposure to air containing insufficient oxygen, as in a coal mine or in an aircraft at great altitude. Unfortunately, the midbrain and medullary centers resist hypoxia far better than does the forebrain. Consequently, a patient who recovers from prolonged cerebral hypoxia may have residual intellectual difficulties or Parkinsonism, depending on the relative damage to cortex or to basal ganglia.

The Effects of the Rigidity of the Cranium

There is evidence of some change in blood flow in different brain regions when these are selectively activated as, for example, when the optic tract nuclei are stimulated by a light flashing in the eyes; but, in general, the changes with activity are negligible in contrast with the requirements of active muscle. Figure 8-5 indicates that the critical factors determining cerebral blood flow are the arterial and venous pressures at head level, the intracranial pressure, the degree of active constriction or dilation of the cerebral vessels, and the viscosity of the blood. The role of each will now be discussed.

The mechanical factor dominating cerebral blood flow is that it occurs in a closed box. Because the brain and cerebrospinal fluid are incompressible, the volume of blood remains relatively constant. Also, if a portion of the brain increases in size, due to tumor formation, or if there is a slow leak of blood from a ruptured vessel causing a hematoma, then the pressure within the cranial cavity will rise and it will become increasingly difficult for the blood to circulate. When the pressure rises above 30 mm Hg, this significantly reduces cerebral blood flow, and reflex responses ensue that lead to a rise in systemic arterial pressure. This feedback persists as intracranial pressure rises up to that point at which the arterial pressure can increase no more, and the cerebral circulation fails.

The fact that the brain is in a closed box also leads to certain practical results in the case of exposure to increased gravity, as when a pilot pulls out from a dive. There is a sharp decrease in arterial pressure at head level, which at 5 g may be inadequate to perfuse the brain. Consciousness may, however, be retained because there is also a pull on the veins; since the brain is a closed box, a significant suction or negative pressure develops in the region of the jugular bulb. The result is that, despite the low arterial pressure, the arteriovenous pressure difference remains more than the critical 40 mm Hg necessary for continued consciousness.

On the other hand, in situations in which intracranial and systemic arterial pressures rise, as when a man is straining, the fact that the brain is in a rigid container becomes very important. It is quite possible to increase systemic arterial, venous, and cerebrospinal fluid pressure all by 100 mm Hg with a sustained effort, as when straining to lift a heavy weight. If the brain were not in a rigid box, the capillaries would inevitably rupture; but, because this is so, and because cerebrospinal fluid pressure rises by the same amount, the pressures remain balanced and the event passes unnoticed.

Unlike the coronary circulation, the arterioles in the brain are directly affected by the CO_2 tension: a rise leads to vasodilation. A fall in CO_2 tension, as occurs during hyperventilation, can cause sufficiently severe vasoconstriction to induce symptoms of cerebral hypoxia. These effects are responsible for local regulation of cerebral blood flow. Thus, when blood flow decreases, the pCO_2, rises. This, together with a fall in pO_2,

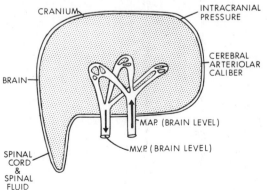

Fig. 8-5.—Diagrammatic summary of the factors affecting cerebral blood flow. (From Ganong, W. F.: *Review of Medical Physiology,* 4th ed. [Los Altos, Calif.: Lange Medical Publishers, 1967], chap. 32, p. 492, Fig. 6.)

which also has a vasodilator effect, results in dilation of the vessels, thus maintaining perfusion.

The neurogenic control of the circulation to the brain and of the pial vessels is dependent on sympathetic innervation from the stellate ganglion. That this is an innervation of practical importance in the everyday well-being of the individual is suggested by the fact that migraine headaches of extreme severity accompanied by visual symptoms are relieved by vasodilator agents and that they are related to states of autonomic arousal. Even if the sympathetic nerves are not capable of inducing in the brain the irreversible changes due to extreme vasoconstriction that they can in the viscera, nevertheless, it cannot be denied that the common headache has an uncommonly high nuisance value.

Circulation in the Skin

Environmental Factors

The circulation through the skin is characterized by its enormous variability and the extent to which this is under control by the central nervous system. The huge potential supply is used to meet the requirements of the skin's function as a radiator and an evaporator dissipating heat. This blood flow is variable because the demands vary; the organism must meet both high heat loads and the lower extremes of cold when the inner core of the organism is sheltered behind a relatively bloodless skin and a nonconducting layer of adipose tissue.

The circulation in the skin is adapted to the roles of nutrition and heat regulation by special structures in addition to the usual nutritive arteries, capillaries, and veins. There is a large subcutaneous venous plexus that can cause a considerable sheet of blood to flow within the dermis at a short distance from the ambient atmosphere (Fig. 8-6). In addition, there are arteriovenous anastomoses that open up as quite large vascular connections between the arteries and the venous plexus. They have muscular walls under sympathetic vasoconstrictor control. When dilated, they flood the venous plexuses, allowing a rapid flow of warm blood into this heat exchanger. Arteriovenous anastomoses are found in the hands, feet, lips, nose, and ears—the areas that are exposed to cooling despite the use of protective clothing. Finally, the skin contains over 2 million eccrine sweat glands to supply evaporative cooling in addition to the above radiant heat-dissipation technique.

The amount of heat lost from the skin is greatly enhanced by these glands, which are found all over the body in man, but especially in the axillae and on the face, hands, and feet. The volume of sweat can be formidable and represents a major means of heat dissipation—since from 1 to 3 liters per hour can be evaporated in acclimated men. The coiled glands are subdermal but their ducts pass through the skin to the surface. Their number is constant at birth regardless of race. However, a proportion in persons living in temperate zones suffer atrophy, whereas, in the tropics, all glands retain their activity.

The blood flow required for nutrition of the skin is only a tenth of the 400 cc/min regularly flowing in cool conditions in the average adult. However, in persistent cold, the flow may even fall below this small amount required to sustain metabolism. This is the mechanism underlying trench foot, a condition that develops in men forced to spend days on end with feet immersed

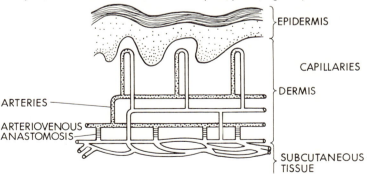

Fig. 8-6.—Diagrammatic representation of the skin circulation. Modified from Guyton, A. C.: *Textbook of Medical Physiology*, 3d ed. [Philadelphia: W. B. Saunders Co., 1966], chap. 23, p. 331, Fig. 282.)

in cold water. They swell and become numb and red. Even after weeks of painful recovery, as flow returns to the almost bloodless extremities, the vascular bed remains extremely labile and sensitive to temperature change. The reverse state of overheating leads to a vasodilatation so intense that as much as 3 liters/min will flow through the skin. In a man with a failing heart, this represents a serious increase in the load and helps to account for the higher incidence of heart decompensation in hot weather.

Nervous Control

A modest degree of control of the circulation in the skin is locally determined by the effect of heating, which increases flow, and of cooling, which diminishes it. Furthermore, if the skin is deprived of blood for 30 minutes or so, as by sitting on a hard bench, there will be an intense local hyperemia or reddening due to the accumulation of metabolites.

By far the most important control of the skin circulation is through the thermosensitive cells in the preoptic regions of the hypothalamus, which are delicately adjusted to respond to the temperature of the blood. An important adjunct is the information coming to them from receptors in the skin. This skin information is integrated with that from the central neurones, modulating it, but only in exceptional circumstances overriding it. The output of the central neurones stimulates the sympathetic vasoconstrictor fibers running to the skin. Their control over the AV anastomoses is particularly strong; at normal temperatures, these are closed off.

As the organism is heated, the first step is reduction in the sympathetic impulses with a dilation of the anastomoses and a flooding of the venous plexuses of the hands, ears, nose, and feet. The rest of the body surface follows with further warming until the point of sweating is reached. Chilling produces the reverse effect with vasoconstriction down to ambient temperatures of approximately 15° C. Below this point, an interesting reversal into vasodilation may ensue. This protects the tissues from damage for a time. Finally, however, if core temperature falls far enough, an intense and lasting vasoconstriction sets in, and, with it, cold damage ensues to the exposed extremities, particularly the digits and the ear lobes.

Vasodilator Effects of Bradykinin

A powerful extension to the direct sympathetic control of the blood vessels to the skin is the sweating mechanism, which can be called into play by the hypothalamus. In addition to water production at the skin surface, it causes still more extensive vasodilation in response to the need for heat dissipation. The 2 million-odd eccrine sweat glands scattered over the body are fairly uniformly distributed so that one half of the total sweat is given off by the trunk, the rest being distributed between the head and arms and legs. These glands are under the control of sympathetic cholinergic fibers, and their stimulation not only leads to the production of fluid at the surface, but it initiates a sequence leading to further vasodilation by the skin vessels. As Figure 8-7 indicates, during this activity a proteolytic enzyme is released into the tissues where it acts on a decapeptide bradykininogen, producing bradykinin. Bradykininogen is a plasma globulin, and the resulting bradykinin is a very potent cutaneous vasodilator that leads to an added dilation of both the dermal venous plexus and the vessels supplying the sweat glands. Interestingly, those regions that show the greatest development of arteriovenous anastomoses—the palms, soles, and forehead—are peculiar in that their sweat response is not solely determined by heat, but also by the emotional state. In the anxious, as is well known, the palms become sticky and beads of sweat appear on the forehead.

Color of the Skin

The color of the skin depends on the caliber of the surface capillaries and of the subpapillary venous plexuses. When they are both dilated and the flow through them is brisk, the color is red as long as there is no cause of cyanosis. When the capillaries are relaxed and the blood stagnates in them, the oxyhemoglobin is reduced and the skin looks blue. If the capillaries are contracted, the skin is pale. Skin temperature depends on the amount of blood flowing through it and is a measure of the state of dilation or constriction of the arterioles. On the other hand, the pallor or degree to which the subjacent venous plexuses of the skin determine its color depends on the amount of blood in the capillary bed. Thus,

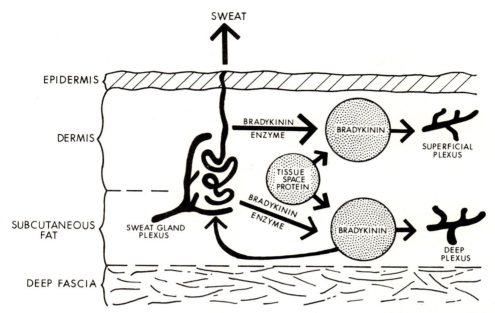

Fig. 8-7.—Schematic diagram of bradykinin formation in human forearm skin during body warming. Sympathetic stimulation of the sweat gland releases a proteolytic enzyme that acts on a tissue fluid decapeptide (bradykininogen) to form a nonapeptide (bradykinin) which has a vasodilator action on the cutaneous vasculature. (From Best, C. H., and Taylor, N. B.: *The Physiological Basis of Medical Practice,* 8th ed. [Baltimore: Williams & Wilkins Co., 1966], chap. 46, p. 843, Fig. 46-3.)

in warm weather, the skin is warm because the arterioles are dilated. However, while still remaining warm, it can be pale if the capillary bed is constricted. In cold weather, the skin blood flow is diminished due to arteriolar constriction; the color is either pale, if the capillaries are also constricted, or blue, if they are dilated with an obstruction slowing the return of blood so that it becomes desaturated. In shock, capillaries are also constricted; the blood left in the skin is strongly reduced and the dark blood in the deeper venous plexuses, visible through the superficial layers, gives an ashen cyanosis.

White Reaction of the Skin

By stroking the skin lightly with a blunt object, a white line is produced that can be shown to be due to local active capillary contraction and a direct response to the stimulation. Local anesthesia has no effect on it, so it is not due to neurogenic influences. It is not arteriolar since each arteriole supplies an irregular area of skin; if the condition were due to contraction of these vessels, it would not so sharply follow the line of the stroke.

Triple Response

If the skin is mechanically stimulated with greater vigor, a three-stage reaction develops that includes a red line, a flare, and a wheal; hence, it is called a triple response. The red line is found if an instrument is drawn firmly across the skin. In contrast to the white reaction, this represents a more intense stimulation that injures the blood vessels, causing a release of a substance inducing dilation. The flare develops after the red line forms, and the redness extends out into the region of skin around the red line. It is probably due to arteriolar increase in regional blood flow. The wheal forms a short time after the flare and extends from the area. The red line becomes raised and blanches to form a wheal representing tissue fluid at the site of stimulation. Since the plasma protein concentration within the wheal is higher than that in normal tissue fluid, the conditions may be due to release of a substance that has increased the permeability of the capillaries.

Splanchnic Circulation

Hepatic Blood Supply and Its Measurement

The liver has two sources of blood supply. The hepatic artery, which derives directly from the celiac axis of the aorta, carries oxygen-rich blood to the liver. This blood circulates at high pressure and is distributed to the parenchymal cells via a complex capillary network. The blood empties into sinusoids, lined by liver cells, both in the central and peripheral parts of the lobule. Other branches supply the liver capsule and tissue of the bile ducts.

The portal vein (Fig. 8-8) carries the drainage of the capillaries of the gastrointestinal tract and the spleen through the liver and delivers digested foodstuff directly to its cells. It also ensures the effective filtration of the blood and elimination of most of the bacteria that enter the intestinal venous blood from the gut. This portal blood flow is at low pressure and has a low oxygen saturation. In addition to its role in supplying material for the liver cells, it is an important source of oxygen; without it, there is central lobular fatty atrophy. Its volume is large, for it carries from 70–90% of the total liver blood flow.

The two circulations join at the periphery of the hepatic lobule and thence pass through the hepatic sinusoids and drain into the hepatic veins. Thus the portal vessels join together two capillary filtration networks, those of the spleen and intestine and those of the liver (Fig. 8-8). The hepatic sinusoidal pressure of some 3–4 mm Hg is between that in the portal vein (6–12 mm Hg) and that in the hepatic veins (1–2 mm Hg). These values are all far lower than the plasma osmotic pressure, which is effective in all the capillary networks. However, the hepatic sinusoids have a very high permeability and only the largest globulin molecules fail to pass through them. The resultant hepatic lymph has a protein content close to that of plasma, 6 gm/100 cc. The consequence is that the tissue oncotic pressure

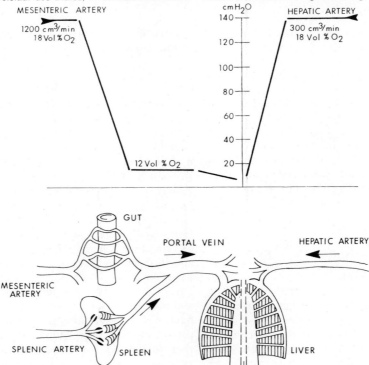

Fig. 8-8.—Schematic of the portal-liver circulation. (From Gauer, O. H.: Kreislauf des Blutes, in Landois-Rosemann: *Lehrbuch der Physiologie des Menschen*, 28th ed. [Munich: Urban & Schwarzenberg, 1960], Fig. 127.)

almost balances that of the plasma; the driving force tending to hold fluid in the capillary is very low.

The rate of flow in different parts of the liver circulation differs—with more rapid flows in the center of the organ than in the periphery.

The Fick principle that is used to measure cardiac output by the dye method and cerebral and renal blood flow by the nitrous oxide method may also be applied to the problem of hepatic blood flow. Its basis is the fact that the liver is the chief route of excretion of bromsulphonapthaline into the biliary passages. If a solution of this compound is infused until the arterial blood level is constant, then the rate of excretion will be the same as that of injection (V); the concentration in the arteries and the portal system will be the same (Ca). At this point, if a sample is taken from the portal veins, the concentration in the plasma (Cs/H) will give the hepatic flow (Q_H):

$$Q_H = \frac{V}{Ca - Cs/H}$$

By this technique, it has been established that in man the hepatic blood flow is some 1,500 cc/min or as much as 20% of the resting cardiac output. Flow through hepatic tissue is 80 cc/min/100 gm. An extra 3–4 cc O_2 is removed from every 100 cc of the already desaturated portal blood, giving an oxygen consumption of 50 cc/min/100 gm for the splanchnic region.

The portal circulation is an important segment of the low-pressure reservoir system. The return of blood into the inferior vena cava from the liver occurs at the point where the right atrium can pick up this outflow. Hence this part of the low-pressure system constitutes the segment of the reservoir from which needed increases for right-ventricular supply are the most immediately available.

In addition to the above matter of convenient anatomical contiguity, it is probable that neurohormonal influences can independently change the distensibility of this part of the low-pressure system. The precise way in which this may occur is not known, and there are several alternatives. There may be an increase in tonus of the venous walls; possibly, the support tissues of the liver itself and its capsule may contract to some degree. An important factor is control of inflow via the mesenteric arterioles or by sphincter. Vasoconstrictor fibers coming from the dorsal roots, particularly D5 to D9, are distributed to the portal system. There is some evidence of a vasodilator effect, but this has not yet been established. Other influences arise in a situation such as exercise for, in addition to the decreased rate of inflow into the splanchnic bed via the mesenteric vessels, there is an emptying effect due to the vigorous action of the abdominal muscles as they participate in the stepped-up breathing. The decreased postsystolic volume of the active ventricle is associated with a lowered pressure at the orifices of the hepatic veins. In considering its role as part of the low-pressure reservoir system, it is important to recognize that the portal circulation has as its prime function the handling of various materials deriving from the digestive tract and that this function takes precedence over any other. Thus blood volume is quite likely to increase in this region as a result of local vascular changes, despite a general passive decrease in reservoir volume due to a reduction of central venous pressure.

Stomach

Three quarters of the flow to the stomach goes through the mucosa. Epinephrine appears to be a dilator, but nor-epinephrine is a very powerful vasoconstrictor for the mucosa. There is some evidence that the flow through the mucosa is increased at times of acid secretion, and that at other times blood may be shunted through the organ via AV anastomoses. This results in an increase in oxygenation of the blood going to the liver. Such shunting may occur at later stages in digestion when absorption is occurring and the liver's oxygen needs increase.

Intestine

There are special provisions in the gut that will prevent a cutoff of blood supply in the event the bowel becomes distended and will avoid interference by peristaltic movements. This is achieved by large (arcade) cross-connections between the peripherally radiating supply vessels within the mesentery and also by the many anastomoses within the gut wall. The blood supply to the duodenum is very profuse; it takes one half of the total flow to the intestine.

There are many sympathetic fibers to the gut, and both nor-epinephrine and epinephrine decrease flow, with the evidence in favor of nor-epinephrine being the primary vasoconstricting agent. There is also evidence of sympathetic vasodilator effects.

Spleen

The splenic arterioles supply sinusoids whose walls appear to be an open lattice work permitting the passage of red cells. They thus constitute a filtering system by which the cells can be stored until they are needed. When the spleen contracts vigorously in response to stimuli such as blood loss, blood containing a very high concentration of red cells is discharged after passing back into the sinuses by diapedesis. With minor stimuli, minor contractions of the splenic capsule and trabeculae can occur without the discharge of red cells.

The contraction of the spleen is mediated by the release of nor-epinephrine by the sympathetic nerves. The action is a mechanical one, involving contraction of the smooth muscle of the trabeculae. There is evidence not only of control of inflow by arteriolar constriction, but also of storage as a result of the action of sphincters on the sinusoidal outlets. These sphincters relax during discharge while, at the same time, arteriolar inflow is decreased.

Influences causing splenic contraction range from exercise and hemorrhage to emotion. In dogs, the reservoir function is clear-cut, and the organ responds very readily to hemorrhage, contracting sharply when the blood volume is reduced by a mere 20%, an amount insufficient to cause a fall in blood pressure but enough to diminish the flow of impulses from stretch receptors in the atria. In the dog, as much as 15% of the blood volume can be supplied in this way. Since the hematocrit of this blood is high, when hemodilution with tissue fluid has occurred, the total blood volume will have been increased from 20–30%. When epinephrine is given to persons with the enlarged spleen caused by malaria, contraction has been demonstrated, but it is an open question whether this organ really serves as a significant reservoir in normal man.

Fig. 8-9.—Contrasting the two types of nephron between which blood flow is distributed. During increased adrenergic drive to the kidney, blood flow is diverted from the cortical to the outer medullary zone. In this way, the juxtamedullary nephron with its intense capacity for water conservation is favored over the cortical elements. The general morphology of the two nephron types **(left)** is related to the major components of the renal vascular bed **(right)**. (From Fourman, J., and Moffat, D. B.: Observations on the Fine Blood Vessels of the Kidney, Sympos. Zool. Soc. [London], 11:57–71, Fig. 9, 1964. By permission of The Zoological Society of London.)

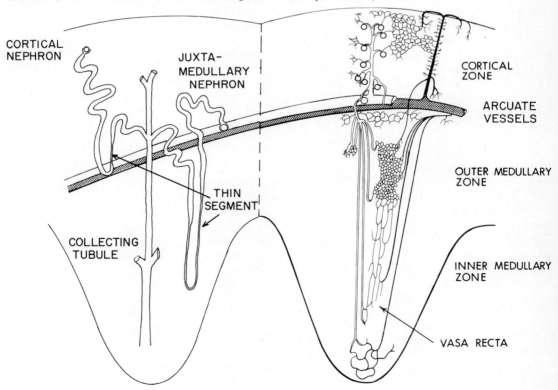

KIDNEY

The renal circulation is characterized by two capillary beds (Fig. 8-9). After the afferent arterioles have broken up into the glomerular loops, these converge to form the efferent arterioles. These, in turn, feed into a second capillary bed around the convoluted tubules from which they drain into the veins. A further peculiarity is the thickening of the media of the afferent arterioles to form spindle-shaped afibrillar juxtaglomerular (JG) cells containing renin. This juxtaglomerular "apparatus" is completed by the condensation of nuclei on one side of the distal convoluted tubule belonging to that glomerulus into an epithelial plaque—the macula densa. This plaque is closely attached to the juxtaglomerular cells (Figs. 8-10 and 11).

This aspect of the juxtaglomerular apparatus may serve as a regulating system responding to changes in sodium load in the distal tubule. In general, it has been established that the apparatus determines changes in renin production and, hence, in angiotensin and aldosterone levels affecting both blood pressure and sodium excretion.

The innervation of the kidney with sympathetic

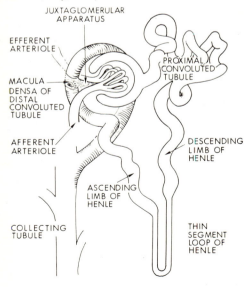

Fig. 8-10.—The distal convoluted tubule adjoins the root of the glomerulus, often between the afferent and efferent arterioles adjacent to the juxtaglomerular (JG) cells. Specialized cells in the distal convoluted tubule wall that touch the JG cells constitute the macula densa (MD). Together the JG cells and the MD form the juxtaglomerular apparatus. (From Altchek, A., Albright, N. L., and Sommers, S. C.: The Renal Pathology of Toxemia of Pregnancy, Obst. & Gynec. 31:595–607, May, 1968.)

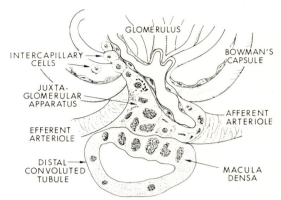

Fig. 8-11.—The JG cells are myoepithelial cells in the wall of the afferent arteriole proximal to where it reaches the glomerulus. They form a collar around the arteriole. The macula densa cells are a specialized part of the wall of the adjacent distal convoluted tubule and are associated with the JG cells that, in turn, contact the glomerular intercapillary mesangium. (From Altchek, A., Albright, N. L., and Sommers, S. C.: The Renal Pathology of Toxemia of Pregnancy, Obst. & Gynec. 31:595–607, May, 1968.)

nerves from the lumbar chain is more profuse than that of any other viscus. Fibers end in the adventitia of the arteries, in afferent and efferent arterioles, between tubular cells, and in the reticulum surrounding the glomerular capillaries. Sympathetic innervation of that part of the wall of the afferent glomerular arteriole that contains the juxtaglomerular cells has been demonstrated.

Renal blood flow can be measured by the classic Fick technique, using N_2O, or by studying the rate of removal of a substance such as para-aminohippuric acid that is cleared from the blood by a single passage through the kidney. Flow through the medulla has been shown to be one-tenth that through the cortex. The kidney is capable of a high degree of local regulation, the origin of which has been covered in Chapter 7 in the discussion on renin, renal vascular redistribution, and control of blood volume.

The evidence suggests that the over-all resistance of the organ only increases with blood loss. However, renin release and intrarenal blood flow redistribution occur in response to the minor stimulation that accompanies moderate nonhypotensive hemorrhage. This latter renin release does not occur in the denervated kidney, suggesting that it may be under direct control of the sympathetic nerves to the juxtaglomerular apparatus. There is no doubt that epinephrine, norepinephrine, and renin-angiotensin cause renal vasoconstriction. As in the case of the other viscera, there is no response to atropine, i.e., no evidence of cholinergic sympathetic control. Although an over-all reduction in renal blood flow with hemorrhage, exercise, and posture requires a severe stimulus, the influence of emotion is more subtle, as will be discussed in a later section. In this connection, recent work has finally established that the long-recognized problem of the relationship between the vasa recta system and the loop of Henle in the matter of water and salt absorption is connected with the dual circulation in the kidney (Fig. 8-9). Mild renal nerve stimulation, which may not alter total renal blood flow, may decrease perfusion of the outer cortical peritubular capillaries, thus increasing the per cent of the total perfusing the juxtamedullary regions. This redistribution of renal blood flow appears to be important in the adrenergic regulation of sodium reabsorption.

Regulation of the Pulmonary Circulation

Vasomotor Nerves

The reservoir function of the lungs and their nonreactive highly distensible vasculature has already been discussed. This diffusion network is unique in that it does not represent another parallel circuit like the kidney, muscle, etc., each of which receives its proportion of the total cardiac output, varying according to the need of the moment. Responsible for virtually instantaneous gas exchange, this network must expose all the desaturated hemoglobin returning from the other beds to a huge air-to-capillary surface area in less than a second. It is thus the only circuit to receive the entire cardiac output. It operates at a lower perfusion pressure than does the systemic circuit. Despite this low pressure, flow rates in the capillaries are sharply discontinuous, reaching a maximum during systole. The existence of a rich supply of pulmonary vasomotor nerves has been recognized for over 70 years. Yet it is still a matter for debate whether these blood vessels are under the independent control of the nervous system. Unequivocal evidence for active control is difficult to obtain because there are so many passive mechanisms that affect the caliber of the vessels. These include changes in inflation and deflation of the lungs, changes in mean alveolar pressure due to bronchiolar constriction and dilatation, and changes in cardiac output and in left atrial pressure. One experimental problem is that, because the pressures in this system are an eighth of those in the high-pressure circuits, the relationship between flow and pressure is not as easily observed. Also, the fact that the whole system is enclosed within the thorax renders it inaccessible to experimentation and measurement, particularly in the conscious animal retaining normal vascular responses.

Both vasoconstrictor and vasodilator fibers have been identified in the sympathetic and vagus supply. However, the complicated way they intermingle with each other and with bronchial and cardiac fibers makes it impossible to obtain simple effects by electrical stimulation. Anatomic study shows at once that the large pulmonary arteries and veins are more richly innervated than the small ones. Indeed, there is no muscle in the walls of the smaller vessels. The arteries have more nerves than the veins and the bronchial vessels, and the bronchi have more innervation than the pulmonary vessels. It has been shown that there is more nor-epinephrine in the large pulmonary vessels than in the small ones. This supports the hypothesis that only the large pulmonary vessels respond to nervous control, leaving to the smaller vessels with their great distensibility the role of a passive control whose resistance varies inversely with pulmonary blood flow. Thus, as cardiac output increases with exercise, pulmonary vascular resistance decreases, because the passive distension of the vessels causes an increase in cross-sectional area and also because of an increase in the number of capillaries conducting blood. Even halving the bed by removing one lung is not associated with a rise in pulmonary arterial pressure.

Violent changes in capillary pressure with an increase above the 20 mm Hg osmotic pressure of the plasma proteins would be disastrous. There are no lymphatics in the alveoli. If sufficiently rapid, exudation of fluid would not be compensated by removal. All hydrostatic pressures in the pulmonary circuit are raised by 10 mm Hg at the base of the lungs of an erect man. When the 8 mm of pulmonary capillary pressure is added, the total pressure begins to approach the plasma osmotic pressure level. Thus the rapid development of pulmonary edema when left-ventricular diastolic pressure rises still further is explicable. In severe mitral stenosis, there is evidence that there are adaptive changes to the increased pressures throughout the pulmonary vascular bed. Pulmonary artery pressure rises even higher than might be anticipated in view of the increase in atrial pressure. This increment can be eliminated by sympatholytic drugs. However, the normal role of the pulmonary vascular innervation in physiological states may not be the production of over-all changes in pulmonary vascular resistance, for, since the organ lies athwart the entire blood stream, no advantage would derive from such changes.

Effects of Hypoxia on the Pulmonary Circulation

Hypoxia causes pulmonary arterial hypertension with a gnarling and narrowing of small muscular pulmonary arteries. The same effect is obtained by the intrapulmonary arterial injection of epinephrine, nor-epinephrine, or serotonin.

In emphysema, acetylcholine causes vasodilation with an intensification of the oxygen desaturation, suggesting that the elevated pulmonary arterial pressure may be playing a compensatory role in these cases with disturbed pulmonary function. There is growing evidence that the larger human pulmonary vessels can contract and dilate. They appear to respond to local hypoxia by local vasoconstriction, thus diverting blood from the affected region to vessels in better-aerated parts of the lung. The general response to hypoxia is a pulmonary arterial vasoconstriction. This is of practical significance to those attempting vigorous exercise without an acclimatization period at altitudes of 6,000–10,000 ft. Even healthy young men may collapse and go into heart failure with pulmonary edema as a result of the temporary excessive resistance of the pulmonary vascular bed.

The Reproductive System

Erectile Tissue

Erection considered as a primarily vascular event vividly illustrates the role of vasodilator and vasoconstrictor fibers. The erectile tissue is fed by arteries that open into cavernous sinuses. These are a sponge-like system of irregular vascular spaces interposed between the arteries and veins. The intima of the arteries has longitudinal ridges that partially occlude them, restricting inflow. On dilatation of the arteries, flow into the sinuses is enormously increased, and, because of specially shaped funnel valves on the veins, outflow is impeded. In addition, distension of the vascular spaces presses the veins against the inelastic fascial investment, further restricting outflow. The result is that the pressure in the cavernous spaces rises to arterial levels. Constriction of the arteries leads to a cutting off of inflow, and the gradual escape of blood leads to a progressively decreasing passive obstruction of the veins, resulting in rapid return to the resting state.

The dilatation of the arteries is under the control of the nervi erigentes of the sacral outflow, particularly S_2. Their constriction is the province of lumbar sympathetic fibers. This rapidly occurring sequence of events is an example of the reciprocal nervous control of quite large vessels.

Menstruation

This event forcefully illustrates another aspect of the regulation of the blood vessels, that of long-term response to the appropriate hormonal levels. It is alterations in blood flow through the endometrial vessels that are responsible for menstruation. Two to 6 days before the event, the coiled arteries deep in the endometrium progressively constrict. This results in ischemic regression of the tissue. Each spiral artery, at a rate and in a sequence independent from the others, finally undergoes a sufficiently severe, hours-long contraction to lead to ischemic necrosis in its area of supply. Following this, first one then another artery relaxes, producing small hematomas in the superficial parts of the endometrium. After a few minutes of hemorrhage, each artery constricts and the bleeding ceases. An artery bleeds only once during the cycle, but successive arteries bleed at different intervals so that one area of endometrium may slough and be repaired before another has been involved. The result is the variable days-long bleeding characteristic of menstruation. The significance of the event for cardiovascular physiology in general is the fact that, as the hormones stimulating the endometrium are withdrawn, the vascular supply responds by a progressive vasoconstriction that eventually leads to regression and ischemic necrosis. The particular sequence of events in the uterus is unique, but the principle that longer-term changes in vascular tone can be induced by hormonal as well as by nervous action holds for all regions.

Placental and Fetal Circulation

The enormous increase in uterine blood flow with pregnancy is not readily explained as an example of local regulation in response to increased oxygen consumption. The AV oxygen difference is not large, and, as in the case of menstruation, some role must be assigned to the changed hormonal level. It has been proposed that estrogens act on the blood vessels. This is an interesting concept that might be extended to other tissues and other hormones. It appears probable that more cases of multiple hormonal influences will be demonstrated as increasing understanding of the control of the circulation reveals previously unsuspected complex relationships between the catechols and hormones such as vasopressin and angiotensin.

The placenta serves as a gaseous diffusion network for the fetus until such time as the lung takes over. In the hemochorial placenta of man, the maternal side is one huge blood sinus into which the fetal villi project (Fig. 8-12). Small branches of the umbilical arteries and veins expose the fetal blood to the lower carbon dioxide and higher oxygen tension of the mother. The placenta also acts as an efficient dialyzer, and solutes are exchanged across the barrier, providing the fetus with all building materials and taking away waste products.

In the fetus, the left and right ventricles work in parallel, instead of in series as in the adult. Blood returning from the body avoids the lungs and passes directly to the left heart through the foramen ovale. It is mixed with oxygenated blood from the placenta. Blood that does get into the right heart is pumped from the pulmonary artery straight into the aorta by passing through the ductus arteriosus. The blood can pass in this direction in the fetus because the resistance of the vascular bed of the collapsed lung is the same as that of the other tissues. In fact, the fetal pulmonary artery pressure is slightly higher than that in the aorta. In the sheltered, "water-immersed" intrauterine environment, there is no need for a low-pressure reservoir system; on the other hand, the arterial pressure in the fetal sys-

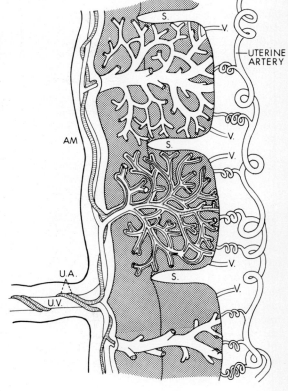

Fig. 8-12.—Diagram of a section through the human placenta. *AM:* amnion; *S:* septa; *UA:* umbilical arteries; *UV:* umbilical vein; and *V:* veins. (From Harrison, R. G.: *A Textbook of Human Embryology,* 2d. ed. [Oxford, England: Blackwell Scientific Publications, 1963].)

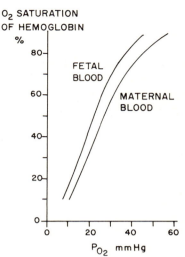

Fig. 8-13.—Dissociation curves for fetal and adult hemoglobin in the human. (From Darling, et al.: Some Properties of Human Fetal and Maternal Blood, J. Clin. Invest. 20:739, 1941.)

tem is quite low, i.e., of the order of 50–60 mm Hg.

The fetal blood returning from the placenta is as much as 80% saturated with oxygen. Because this is mixed with venous blood from the body, the fetal aorta can only supply the tissues with hemoglobin that is 60% saturated. However, the tissues of fetal mammals are very resistant to hypoxia and can operate at a lower tension of the gas than the adult, making it feasible to "shift" the hemoglobin disassociation curve "to the left." This results in a much greater saturation of fetal hemoglobin for a given pO_2. For example, at 30 mm Hg pO_2, instead of being only 55% saturated the fetal hemoglobin can carry 70% of its potential full load (Fig. 8-13). The changeover from fetal to adult hemoglobin is quite slow, and is still of this type four months after birth.

CHANGES AT BIRTH

At birth, a remarkable vascular reorganization must occur in both the mother and the new baby. The placental circulation is cut off after providing a final transfusion of some 25% of the infant blood volume as the umbilical veins contract. Peripheral resistance increases; pressure in the aorta rises and starts to exceed that in the pulmonary artery. At birth, with the loss of placental oxygenation, asphyxia sets in and eventually the infant makes a gasping action as the respiratory center is stimulated by CO_2 accumulation. With this, if the airway is clear, the lungs expand and pulmonary vascular resistance falls to one-fifth the in utero value. Left atrial pressure rises, and a valve keeps the interatrial foramen ovale closed. At the same time, the ductus arteriosus, which had been serving as a shunt from aorta to pulmonary artery, starts to constrict in response to the changes in oxygen saturation. In the normal infant, the foramen ovale, the ductus arteriosus, and the ductus venosus (which bypassed the umbilical vein blood to the vena cava) all fuse shut. In a complete system changeover, the remodeled single heart circulation is left without an external dialyser. Instead, two pumps in series, an efficient gaseous-diffusion device for exchange with the atmosphere and a low-pressure reservoir within the body, replace the placenta in a formidable set of smoothly interlocking changes whose initiating mechanisms are not yet understood.

REFERENCES

Friedman, J. J., and Selkurt, E. E.: Circulation in Special Organs, in Selkurt, E. E.: *Physiology,* 2d ed. (Boston: Little, Brown & Co., 1966), pp. 369–400.

Ganong, W. F.: Circulation Through Special Regions, in *Review of Medical Physiology,* 3d ed. (Los Altos, Calif.: Lange Medical Publishers, 1967), pp. 482–495.

Gregg, D.: The Coronary Circulation, in Best, C. H., and Taylor, N. B.: *The Physiological Basis of Medical Practice* (Baltimore: Williams and Wilkins Co., 1966), pp. 813–839.

Guyton, A. C.: *Textbook of Medical Physiology,* 3d ed. (Philadelphia: W. B. Saunders Co., 1966).

Keele, C. A., and Neil, E.: Pulmonary Circulation and Circulation Through Special Regions, in Wright, S.: *Applied Physiology,* 11th ed. (New York: Oxford University Press, 1965), pp. 139–145.

Pomeranz, B. H., Birtch, A. G., and Barger, A. C.: Neural Control of Intrarenal Blood Flow, Am. J. Physiol. 215:1067, 1968.

Selkurt, E. E.: The Renal Circulation, in Hamilton, W. F. (ed.): *Handbook of Physiology: Circulation* (Washington: American Physiological Society, 1963), Vol. II, pp. 1,457–1,516.

Trueta, J.: Kidney, Ann. Rev. Physiol. Vol. 12, pp. 369–398, 1950.

Van Citters, R. L.: The Coronary Circulation, in Ruch, T. C., and Patton, H. D.: *Physiology and Biophysics* (Philadelphia: W. B. Saunders Co., 1965), pp. 690–705.

9

Special Responses of the Cardiovascular System

Straining and Coughing and the Valsalva Maneuver

Straining and the Elevation of Intrathoracic Pressure

THE VOLUNTARY ACT of straining against a closed glottis involves a powerful contraction of the abdominal walls while the chest is fixed by a simultaneous action of the thoracic and shoulder muscles. A uniform pressure increase, which can be as much as 100 mm Hg, results throughout the chest and in the arteries leading out of the trunk. In addition, because the blood coming back from head to limbs can no longer enter the thorax, pressure increases in the large veins. The rate at which this occurs depends on the degree of dilation of the peripheral vascular bed and the rate at which blood is flowing through the limbs. In a few seconds, the veins fill up and the return of blood may recommence. However, because of their great distensibility, large amounts of blood will leave the central reservoir to fill up these peripheral veins. This loss can amount to as much as 1,000–1,500 cc. Meanwhile, there is no threat of hemorrhage in the indistensible cranial cavity because the pressure rise in the veins is balanced by one of equal degree in the cerebrospinal fluid and the arteries.

The great increase of pressure around the heart at first elevates systemic arterial pressure by

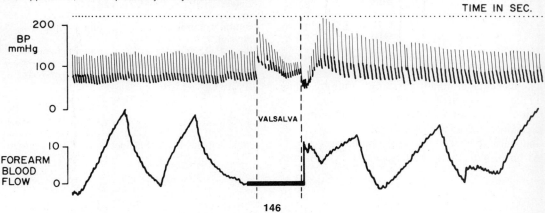

Fig. 9-1.—The response of arterial pressure to the Valsalva maneuver. The overshoot as the pressure within the thorax is released is due to the action of the baroreceptors, which are stimulated by the decreased relative pressure within the aortic arch. Note the tachycardia during pressure application, to be replaced by bradycardia and a temporary decrease in forearm blood flow when the maneuver is over. (From Sharpey-Schafer, E. P.: Effect of Respiratory Acts on the Circulation, in Hamilton, W. F. (ed.): *Handbook of Physiology: Circulation* [Washington: American Physiological Society, 1965], Vol. III, chap. 52, p. 1,878, Fig. 3.)

precisely the same extent. Then, almost at once, because of the rapid loss of blood from the intrathoracic reservoirs of the low-pressure system into the swelling veins, heart filling is impaired, and first the pulse pressure and then the systolic pressure start to decline (Fig. 9-1). If the subject is stubborn enough, this decline can be to the point where the pressure differential across the brain falls below the critical perfusion value of 40 mm Hg. Consciousness is lost if this persists for more than a few seconds. This is the mechanism underlying a variety of syncopes, i.e., the cough syncope, frequent in persons suffering from intractable bronchial irritation, as in whooping cough; syncope while straining at stool; and syncope at night when straining to urinate in the erect posture.

Coughing

There are many other circumstances in which the straining maneuver is employed by the organism. By suddenly releasing the glottis, the trachea and bronchi can be cleared of mucus or foreign substances in the vigorous cough reflex. The straining of defecation can involve the development of extremely high and prolonged intrathoracic and abdominal pressures. The same can be said of childbirth and straining to urinate, especially against growing obstruction of the urinary passages as in the case of an enlarged prostate gland. Finally, intrathoracic pressure is elevated in Valsalva's maneuver of straining against the closed mouth and nares in the attempt to equalize pressure across the tympanic membrane by forcing air through the eustachian tubes. This occurs when altitude is changed in a nonpressurized aircraft, especially when an inflammation of the pharynx causes a swelling of the tubal orifices, preventing the normal replacement of gas absorbed by the circulation in the middle ear. Some of these events are so common that every few hours intrathoracic pressure is raised by at least 20–60 mm Hg. Healthy adults can regularly achieve 60 mm Hg. Trumpet and bugle players reach 80 mm Hg; men lifting weights can raise their intrathoracic pressure to as much as 160 mm Hg for several seconds. In the cough, the transient elevations are even greater. A healthy man's single cough on request attains 50 mm Hg, but spontaneous coughing has peaks up to 100 mm Hg, and powerful males trying to allay a tickle will reach 200 to 250 mm Hg.

The pressure driving blood out of the intrathoracic reservoir region and the loss of effective blood volume may be sufficient to cause a fall in the transmural aortic pressure, thus decreasing stretch of the aortic receptors, and to cause a fall in atrial filling, which similarly affects the receptors in the low-pressure system. The balancing counterpressure of the chest is absent in the carotid sinus region and so straining stimulates these receptors, leading to a moderate bradycardia and peripheral vasoconstriction with a fall in blood flow through the muscle mass.

With the cessation of the paroxysm of coughing or of the steady straining maneuver, blood surges back into the central compartment from the distended veins. In response to this rapid increase in atrial size and ventricular filling pressure, peripheral vasodilation sets in. Experiments show this response is not due to the stimulation of the carotid sinus region but to the changes in filling of the low-pressure system. In fact, if the pressure fluctuation in the thoracic viscera is increased by breathing vigorously through a restricted orifice, thus simulating the effects of increased blood volume, vasodilation can be demonstrated in the muscle bed of the arm. This is the same vasodilation that occurs if a normal man who has been immobile in the vertical position is tilted backwards so that atrial filling is increased.

Paradoxic Lack of Effect of Straining During Heart Failure

In heart failure, the response to the increase in intrathoracic pressure imposed by a Valsalva maneuver differs from the normal. There is no decrease in stroke output or arterial pulse pressure when the volume of blood in the heart falls during the straining. Indeed, in severe heart failure, the pulse pressure actually increases and is accompanied by vasodilation. The reasons for this paradox may be that the veins are already tense and distended so that less blood is lost from the thoracic reservoir. In the normal man, an infusion leads to a rise in central venous pressure, an increase in atrial receptor firing, and a reflex vasodilation. In heart failure, the same infusion will be added to an already overfilled system. If, as is not uncommon, the central venous pressure is of the order of 20 cm H_2O, then the atria will already be grossly stretched.

In consequence, the increased intra-atrial pressure may fail to increase atrial receptor discharge. In severe heart failure, it is a known clinical paradox that, far from causing a deterioration, the arterial pressure will often actually increase during coughing. This may be because, by displacing blood from the overfilled central regions, end-diastolic pressure is reduced to more effective levels, the function of the heart improves, and arterial pressure rises.

Positive pressure breathing can be used to put the circulatory changes induced by the straining maneuver to valuable use. Intermittent positive pressure breathing is effective in the treatment of impending pulmonary edema. It reduces cardiac filling pressure and restores the balance between the pressure in the pulmonary vessels and the osmotic pressure of the plasma proteins. The pressures employed are of the order of 8–12 mm Hg, and it essentially consists of a series of short Valsalva maneuvers.

Pressure breathing can also be used to gain altitude in situations of reduced pressure, as at great altitudes above 40,000 feet where even pure oxygen alone is insufficient to saturate the hemoglobin.

If pressures of the order of 70 cm H_2O are used in a continuous-breathing technique with a special neck-sealing helmet, then temporary survival at altitudes up to 50,000 feet is feasible; however, collapse rapidly ensues. A balancing vest that distributes the breathing pressure over the thorax is a great help, but, despite this, syncope still occurs (Fig. 9-2). In addition to the loss of blood from the central region by venous distension, the imbalance of pressures is so great that fluid accumulates rapidly in the tissue spaces with resulting hemoconcentration. Hypotension and bradycardia develop as the vasovagal or fainting reflex is triggered. If, in addition to the thorax, counterpressure is applied to the arms and legs, then a certain degree of pressure balance can be attained. Equipped with such a lightweight "partial" pressure suit, a man can work for periods up to an hour in a vacuum because the rate of fluid loss into the unpressurized tissue spaces and the amount of blood forced into veins not backed up by counterpressure is small enough to be tolerable (Fig. 9-2).

Exercise

INTRODUCTION

Of all the adaptations made by the organism to the environment, those in response to the demands of exercise are the greatest and result in the most radical changes in respiratory and cardiac activity. The blood flow needed for the digestion of food and the formation of urine can be attained within the limits of the resting cardiac output of about 6 liters per minute. Sweating and vasodilatation in humid weather may increase the demand by as much as 3 more liters. However, sustained violent exertion demands an increase of oxygen consumption from 250 cc/min to some 4 liters or more per minute and an increase in cardiac output up to 20–30 liters per minute in order to carry the 4 liters to the tissues and the corresponding amount of carbon dioxide back again.

RESPIRATION

The respiratory adjustments in exercise are remarkable in that the changes in the controlling values may be negligible, despite the huge increases in gas exchange rates. An athlete may ventilate at 120 liters per minute without any detectable change in arterial pCO_2. After hours of exertion, a marathon runner can have quite normal values for lactic acid and a normal blood pH. In spite of increased carotid body sensi-

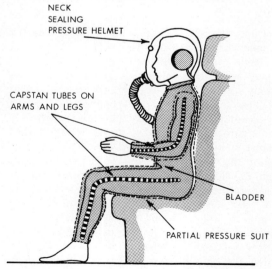

Fig. 9-2.—In the partial pressure suit, breathing pressure is applied by a neck-sealing helmet. This is balanced by an abdominal and chest bladder filled to the same pressure. Arms and legs are supported by inelastic cloth pulled tight by tapes going around expanding capstan tubes.

SPECIAL RESPONSES OF THE CARDIOVASCULAR SYSTEM

tivity, there is no evidence that arterial hypoxemia is directly responsible for the adjustments. Even in heavy exercise, the values do not fall low enough to account for the enormous ventilation. The conclusion gradually emerging from all of the available experimental data is that the respiratory gases and other factors, such as catecholamine levels, are probably all working together, each influencing the response more as a result of its conjunction with changes in other factors than it would if it were acting alone. Recent work (Fig. 9-3) has shown how ventilation rate and depth during athletic exertion are affected both by hypoxia and by CO_2 stimuli that are, nevertheless, within normal value ranges. It is thought that the clue may rest with a nervous factor, namely, with afferents from the muscle spindle receptors and possibly from the exercised joints as well. It is suggested that, with physical activity, the stream of sensory impulses from the muscles to the brain increases to such a degree that there is a general arousal of the reticular formation. This arousal may result in a sensitization of the brain stem regions concerned with respiratory regulation. The areas regulating the cardiovascular system are also affected, and the response to exercise may be determined by response systems in the medulla that are genetically preprogrammed to relay the appropriate message pattern to components of the respiratory and cardiovascular apparatus. It is hypothesized that these systems would be triggered by the appropriate information from the periphery. Neural stimuli from the limbs may be an important component of this information. The fact that the organism is receiving additional information from the muscle receptors and joints and from the higher centers (i.e., the animal or man is "aware" he is exercising) all may assist in turning the response to the exercise mode. Certainly, if there is an increase in CO_2 level or if there is some hypoxia, these stimuli meet with far greater

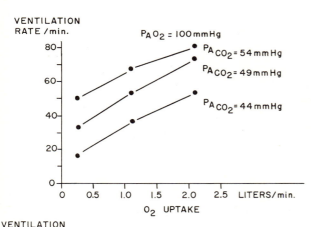

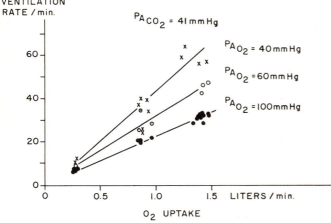

Fig. 9-3.—Above: Ventilation in relation to oxygen uptake at three different values of alveolar pCO_2 but with constant pO_2.
Below: Ventilation in relation to oxygen uptake at three different values of alveolar pO_2 but with constant pCO_2. An increase in alveolar pCO_2 acts as an additive factor to the work stimulus, and an increase in the hypoxic stimulus potentiates the work stimulus. (From Asmussen, E.: Exercise and the Regulation of Ventilation, in Chapman, C. B. (ed.): American Heart Association Monograph 15, Physiology of Muscular Exercise, Vol. 20, No. 3, pp. 1–144, Figs. 14 and 15, March, 1967, Suppl. 1. By permission of the American Heart Association, Inc., New York, N. Y.)

response during exercise than when at rest. Not all these changes originate in the central nervous system; local physicochemical factors may exert some action on ventilation by sensitizing the local mechanoreceptors, causing them to respond with a greater stream of impulses to the higher centers.

Peripheral Vascular Bed

The response of the peripheral vascular bed to exercise has been thoroughly investigated; yet, despite great effort, the local factors responsible for the sharp vasodilation that can invoke as much as a tenfold increase in flow in the exercising muscle group are not yet clearly identified. The cause of the vasodilation is apparently not the activity of the sympathetic cholinergic fibers, for the effects of sympathectomy and atropinization are both minor. It appears probable that the dilatation in the active muscles is mediated by unknown local factors. For, at the same time, there is a vasoconstriction in the nonexercising muscles and also in the skin, and there is some evidence that the tonus of the capacitance vessels, i.e., the veins, is increased. These changes in regions other than the active muscles may be a response to the general increase of sympathetic discharge.

It must be emphasized that there have been many studies of the chemical changes in the blood coming from limbs during muscular activity including O_2, CO_2, lactic acid, etc. In general, the relation of metabolites to vasodilation is obscure. It is probable that the responses to exercise involve high-level activity in the brain. Thus impulses from the motor cortex may pass through the anterior hypothalamus and permit vasodilation in the particular group of muscles at work in response to the local accumulation of metabolites and to information from stretch receptors. At the same time, a general sympathetic arousal will diminish blood flow in skin, splanchnic region, and unused muscle groups, and constrict the capacitance vessels. The release of catechols from the adrenals and of vasopressin and angiotensin also aid in the attainment of this general goal.

Heart

A series of studies of animals and men exercising freely with markers or transducers in their hearts has given a clearer picture of the adjustments made by this organ to the demands. Minor exertion can be met by an increase in heart rate alone. Furthermore, by artificially keeping the heart rate constant, it can be shown that cardiac output can be increased by changing stroke volume. In the resting state, cardiac output is not changed by changes in heart rate, and other mechanisms play an important part. However, a pacemaker-induced increase in heart rate results in an improved contractile state of the heart, increasing the stroke power of the ventricle and shortening the relative time of systole. This effect of increased velocity of contraction appears to be separate from the direct effects of sympathetic stimulation of the myocardium and apart from effects on the pacemaker. However, exercise also induces myocardial stimulation by the sympathetic system. Thus β-adrenergic blockade eliminates a component of the exercise-induced augmentation of the myocardial force-velocity characteristics that cannot be attributed to tachycardia. It appears likely that simple tachycardia and sympathetic stimulation of the myocardium are complementary influences, both of which improve the contractile state of the myocardium during exercise. Light exercise also does not increase ventricular end-diastolic size; rather, this may be reduced as tachycardia makes up the deficiency in cardiac output. If, however, heart rate remains constant, the ventricular end-diastolic size and stroke volume are greater with exercise than when at rest. During violent exertion, there is a significant increase of both factors; not only does ventricular end-diastolic size increase, but there is a tachycardia resulting from sympathetic stimulation. Indeed, in the erect posture, stroke volume may double during maximal exercise.

Thus the normal cardiac response to exercise involves the integrated effects of three factors. The first is a simple tachycardia due to pacemaker changes. In addition, sympathetic stimulation of the muscle increases cardiac contractility, which is also changed by alterations in the filling state of the ventricle. Any two of these could bring about the compensations needed for moderate exertion; but, for maximal effort, all three must be called into play.

Effects of the Supine and Erect Postures

When a man is exercising in the supine position, his heart rate and cardiac output increase as an approximate linear function. The stroke volume may increase as much as 20%. When the upright posture is assumed, the volume of blood extending from the right atrium to the root of the aorta decreases by about 20%. The stroke volume usually drops, and, even though there may be an increase in heart rate, the cardiac output decreases. If the hydrostatic shift of blood volume becomes even larger, the stroke volume may decrease to as little as 40% of the supine value due to diminished diastolic filling of the ventricles.

The oxygen uptake by the body is approximately the same in both the upright and the supine posture. However, the oxygen extraction in the upright posture is markedly increased.

During exercise in the upright posture, the cardiac output and rate increase linearly with oxygen consumption. On transition from rest to exercise in the erect position, the pumping effect of the leg muscles effectively drives the blood centrally, actually improving ventricular filling. Hence, even with mild exercise in the upright position, the thoracic blood volume and stroke volume may approach their supine values. Further increase of the exercise up to the maximum for the individual causes little further augmentation of thoracic blood volume. The stroke volume may increase, but not to more than about 90% of the supine value.

Changes Occurring During Exercise: Integrative Aspects

The uncertainties concerning the mechanisms involved in the response to exercise are finally being resolved, with the conclusion that control is neurohumoral and progressively calls into play every resource at the disposal of the organism. With maximum exertion, the organism is wide awake and thoroughly aroused. Therefore, conscious mechanisms connected with alarm or alerting come into play. Unlike the regulation of blood pressure or blood volume, we have now come to an activity that can hardly exist without consciousness, and, unlike these two more basic housekeeping parameters, much of the regulation has to occur at a level where emotion and awareness are involved. The work with cholinergic vasodilator innervation to skeletal muscles makes this very clear. In contrast with the adrenergic vasoconstrictor fibers that no longer respond after use of adrenergic-blocking agents, vasodilator nerve activity can be blocked by atropine. The tract in which these cholinergic fibers run is independent from the classical vasomotor structures in the medulla. It runs from the motor cortex, via the hypothalamus and collicular region, to the sympathetic ganglia (Fig. 9-4 and 5). Responses on stimulation lead to from three- to fivefold increases in blood flow, an increase in heart rate, release of catecholamines, cutaneous and splanchnic constriction, and, with strong stimuli, a behavioral response in the conscious animal suggesting fright or anger. These changes all seem to be part of a reaction pattern of alarm in which muscle blood flow is stepped up in preparation for "fight or flight."

When sympathetic vasoconstrictor tone to the muscle is decreased, there is increased capillary flow and enhanced clearance of radioactive isotopes, indicating opening of precapillary sphincters and increased transcapillary exchange. But when the sympathetic cholinergic fibers are stimulated, there is actually a diminished uptake of oxygen, suggesting that arterioles have opened but that the number of functioning capillaries is unchanged. The sympathetic vasodilator outflow thus seems to be part of the "defense reaction," the integration of which is controlled at hypothalamic levels. This reaction is elicited in man in response to psychic stress, e.g., difficult arith-

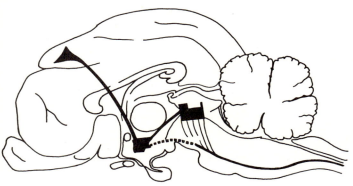

Fig. 9-4.—Intracerebral course of the cholinergic sympathetic vasodilator outflow to the skeletal muscles. (From Uvnäs, B.: Cholinergic Vasodilator Innervation to Skeletal Muscles, in Chapman, C. B. (ed.): Physiology of Muscular Exercise, Supp. 1 to Circulation Res. Vol. 20 and 21, pp. 1-83, Fig. 1, March 1967. By permission of the American Heart Association, Inc., New York, N. Y.)

152   THE CIRCULATION: AN INTEGRATIVE PHYSIOLOGIC STUDY

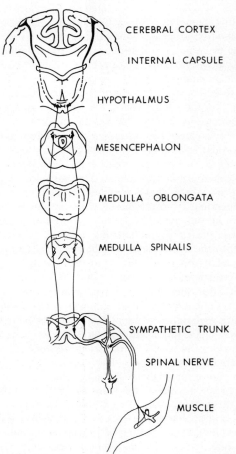

Fig. 9-5.—Schematic drawing showing the central and peripheral course of the sympathetic vasodilator pathways. (From Lindgren, P.: The Mesencephalon and the Vasomotor System [An Experimental Study on the Central Control of Peripheral Blood Flow in the Cat], Acta Physiol. Scandinav. 35 [Supp. 121]:175, Fig. 58, 1955.)

metical tasks performed under competitive conditions. It may play a part in the fainting response in which the organism, instead of fighting or fleeing, appears to be dead, with loss of consciousness, a slow pulse, and a very pale face. It has long been suspected, although not proved, that this state may involve increased muscle blood flow due to activity of cholinergic sympathetic vasodilator fibers.

Summary

The mechanisms underlying the response to exercise have eluded description for so long perhaps because this is a complex neurohumoral response that occurs in the conscious animal and is associated with quite high levels of activity in the central nervous system. Changes in the chemical parameters of CO_2 and oxygen, both locally and in the blood, have added to them impulses from the muscle afferents and from the joints. Adjustments in the nervous system at levels concerned with consciousness appear to be involved in the vasodilation of the active muscle groups, while what can be spared of the vascular bed shuts down. Exercise results in tachycardia, increased sympathetic drive of the heart muscle, increased stroke volume, and a large increase in respiratory frequency, depth, and minute volume.

Circulatory Changes During Underwater Exposure

As long as a man who ventures underwater does so in the classic diver's suit, he is subject to no particular cardiovascular stresses; the gas in the suit enclosing him exerts a uniform pressure as effectively as though he were in a diving bell. If, instead of a full diver's suit, he uses the scuba lung pressurization equipment, there is still a balance between the pressures within the thorax and blood vessels and the external pressurization by the water at depth. If, however, the man merely immerses himself in the water up to the neck and holds his breath, then a sequence of events develops in the cardiovascular system that is due to the forcing of blood into the thoracic region by the action of the water pressure on the legs and abdomen (Fig. 6-6). Under the circumstances, the atria are distended and there is a great increase in the frequency of the afferent impulses from them. Closely related studies of lower-body negative pressure, or suction from the waist down, show that, by suddenly releasing the blood that has accumulated in the lower extremities, a brief bradycardia can be induced together with a transient vasodilation of the blood vessels in the limbs.

The action of breath-holding underwater is complicated by frustrated respiratory efforts as its duration progresses and by the tendency to strain against a closed glottis. Very commonly, there is a marked bradycardia, which persists despite exercise such as swimming. The electrocardiogram suggests vagal inhibition with an increased Q-T interval and a progressively lengthening P-R interval. As the period of breath-holding persists in man beyond the thirty-second point, two factors enter in. There is a progressive anoxia that becomes increasingly significant as the one-minute mark is reached. There is also a corresponding build-up of carbon dioxide. Depending on the amount of air in the chest before immersion, on the behavior of the subject, i.e., whether he strains against the closed glottis or relaxes, and on the depth to which he dives, there will be more or less of a build-up of pressure in the thorax, inhibiting the further return of blood—as in a Valsalva maneuver. If the subject relaxes or has breathing gear, then, because of the counterpressure on the limbs and abdomen, the filling of the central reservoir may actually increase while underwater. Recent work shows that even if the immersed subject holds his breath without straining, there will be a gradual rise in central venous pressure amounting to some 5–10 cm H_2O. One cause of this increase may be a central displacement of blood as the peripheral venous bed constricts.

The bradycardia with the electrocardiographic signs of vagal inhibition and the peripheral vasoconstriction of a man doing a breath-holding dive are minor changes compared with the extraordinary adaptation of the true diving mammals. In the extreme case of the whale, the depths and pressures reached may be as much as 2,000 feet and almost 1,000 lbs per square inch. Under these circumstances, the entire air content of the lung is compressed into the trachea and pharynx. Meanwhile, the pulse decreases to one-fifteenth its normal rate. Despite this, the systemic arterial pressure is sustained. The reason is that there has been an enormous reduction of skin, muscle, renal, and gastrointestinal blood flow. The flow that continues through these organs appears to be via arteriovenous shunts, so that the metabolic or capillary bed flow is negligible. In this way, a large pool of oxygenated blood is made available for the perfusion of the capillary beds of the brain and heart alone. Furthermore, the diving animals' muscles have very large myoglobin stores, and they also work under anaerobic conditions accumulating lactic acid that does not get into the blood stream until after the dive. The result is that the seal can dive for 30 minutes and the whale for 2 hours, compared with man's maximum of 1–2 minutes. This highly differentiated central control of the oxygen supply is an example of the drastic changes in the distribution of the circulation that occur in response to environmental demands. The quite different patterns of the defense-alarm reflex and of vasovagal syncope, i.e., the "playing dead" or fainting reaction, are two further types of such responses in the mammal.

Altitude Hypoxia

As the saturation of hemoglobin falls below 85% (which occurs at an altitude of 12,000–14,000 ft when breathing air), tachycardia and an increase in cardiac output develop. The hypoxia affects the brain, causing sympathetic arousal and a consequent stimulation of the pacemaker-conducting tissue, heart muscle, and most importantly, of the coronary vessels themselves, inducing vasodilation. In addition, there is increased cerebral blood flow. Both are probably due to local susceptibility to hypoxia. The muscle, renal, and skin vessels are not directly affected by the hypoxia, but the central control region does induce sharp vasoconstriction. In addition, the pulmonary vessels constrict in response to the hypoxia. This raises pulmonary arterial pressure. In persons suddenly exerting themselves at altitude without a period for acclimatization, as in weekend skiing, this reflex can occasionally lead to trouble. If the pressure in the pulmonary capillary bed exceeds the 25 mm Hg of the plasma osmotic pressure, there is danger of acute pulmonary edema. In general, hypoxia leads to an increase in the total peripheral resistance with an increased blood supply to the vital myocardium and brain, but a diminution of splanchnic and muscle blood flow.

The heart rate rise begins at 5,000 feet and progressively increases until, at altitudes above 20,000 feet, it is doubled. With acclimatization, the rate is reduced, but cardiac output remains elevated with an increase in stroke volume. Coronary flow increases in proportion to the increase in cardiac output. At altitudes of 18,000 feet and above, this output is doubled. There is no change in systemic arterial pressure. The electrocardiogram shows the same changes as those that occur due to local tissue hypoxia induced by coronary artery disease. The T-wave amplitude decreases; then later the S-T segment may be depressed. There are also disorders of conduction with depression of the SA node and ventricular escape, often with ventricular extra systoles.

The critical factor is the maintenance of an adequate cerebral oxygen supply; unlike the muscle cells, the brain has no anaerobic function to which it can revert. At arterial oxygen tensions above 50 mm Hg, vessel tone depends on CO_2 tension. This can have unfortunate effects since, if this is lowered by hyperventilation, there is reflex cerebral vasoconstriction, which can become serious in some people when alveolar CO_2 falls below 25 mm Hg. The varying degrees of mental impairment that are found in a group of persons at the same altitude may be due to differences in the sensitivity of this response. Vasovagal syncope becomes increasingly frequent. It is possible that its origin depends on a triggering of the syncope by afferent impulses from the stretch receptors in the ventricle. The impulses from these receptors increase in number with ventricular extra systoles and also, probably, with the increased mechanical stimulation that follows the lowering of end-systolic volume and intensive squeezing of the shortened ventricular muscle fibers.

A 50% rise in pulmonary arterial pressure will occur at altitudes in excess of 15,000 feet in a reflex that appears to be a local response of the vessels themselves. Its virtue is that it shifts blood flow from poorly- to better-ventilated areas. But at altitudes where there is general hypoxia, the reaction becomes deleterious, as in the previously mentioned occasional attacks of pulmonary edema in unsuspecting weekend skiers.

Circulatory Changes During Digestion

The resting man's splanchnic circulation receives 25% of the cardiac output. This implies a very high flow that, in fact, may attain 100 cc per 100 gm of tissue. It passes first through the gastrointestinal tract and then through the liver. After a meal has been taken, a slow wave of activity and consequent enhanced blood flow passes down the gut paralleling the passage of the food. Starting with a vigorous hyperemia in the secreting salivary glands, whose flow can attain 500–700 cc/100 gm tissue, an increase up to an average flow of 200 cc/100 gm tissue can be expected in the mucosa of the stomach and the duodenum. It is thought that the local release of vasodilator metabolites such as bradykinin are involved in this increase in gut blood flow. The total splanchnic blood flow in the postprandial state may be up from 1.5 liters to 3–4 liters. This is not an inconsiderable load, especially in a heart that has limited output capacity. When combined with the output requirements of the skin circulation, the approximately 10 liters needed for the two circuits would cut significantly into the reserves available for muscular exercise. Even with a normal vascular bed, a sweating man who has just eaten a heavy meal would find a considerable fraction of his potential output had been lost. In the man with coronary heart disease who has difficulty in putting out the 5 liters needed for resting metabolism, such an increase can precipitate angina and other symptoms of myocardial insufficiency.

Circulatory Changes During Heat Exposure

In a warm environment, heat is lost by the controlled opening of shunts in the skin, especially in the face, hands, and feet. This process of generalized dilation is called into play by the activation of "relay stations" in the anterior hypothalamus, under the combined influence of an increase of afferent impulse traffic from cutaneous thermal receptors, plus a local sensitivity in the hypothalamus to a temperature increase in the blood supplying it. The resulting adjustments of skin flow are accompanied by certain behavioral changes. Thus both dogs and men when hot lie stretched out, exposing a maximum relatively hair-deficient surface for cooling. By contrast, cold men and dogs curl up. The total blood flow to the skin of a hot man approximates 150 to 200 cc/100 gm. Since the 1.7 square meters of skin weigh some 2.5 to 3.5 kg, this implies that as much as 5–7 liters flow through the skin circuit when heat vasodilation and the effort to prevent a rise of core temperature is at a maximum.

The dog loses fluid by the tongue in the process of panting, and man has the generalized sweat mechanism of over 2 million individual glands to call on. However, both methods of control of body temperature use the latent heat of evaporation, and this is expensive in fluid. A man in the desert can lose as much as 1.5 liters an hour (Table 9-1). Replacement by drinking salt water is necessary when sweating is as profuse as this; if not available, collapse will soon ensue, for at these rates in four hours 10% of the body weight will be lost. Such losses are not uniformly distributed throughout the body fluids. There is a disproportionately high reduction of plasma vol-

TABLE 9-1.—ENVIRONMENT AND MEAN DAILY WATER EXCHANGES IN MAN

PLACE	MEAN TEMP. IN °F	WATER IN DRINK LITERS	WATER IN FOOD LITERS	URINE IN VOL. LITERS	SWEAT IN VOL. LITERS
Fairbanks, Alaska	17	1.20	1.13	1.20	—
Churchill, Canadian Arctic	−20	1.20	0.99	1.15	0.85
Ft. Knox, U.S.A. (temperate)	41	2.05	0.91	1.74	0.67
Desert	85	5.90	—	0.94	4.95
Tropics	80	3.26	—	0.92	2.33

The enormous difference in water requirements depends upon the environmental temperature. With vigorous activity in the desert, water requirements will exceed the given figures. (From Henry, J. P.: *Biomedical Aspects of Space Flight* [New York: Holt, Rinehart and Winston, Inc., 1966], p. 22.)

ume with a corresponding increase in blood viscosity. Even if fluid and salt are replaced, the great demands for skin blood flow encroach on the capacity of the heart to meet the needs for increased cardiac output with exercise. The result is that sympathetic vasoconstriction in the muscles may prevail, leading to a decreased work capacity.

The subject who is acclimatized to heat dilates his skin blood vessels earlier and sweats at a lower temperature than the nonacclimatized. His body temperature rises less, and he shows an increased production of sweat with a lower salt content. In all subjects, the rate of sweating is proportional to the difference between the actual hypothalamic temperature and a "set point" temperature at which the activities of anterior hypothalamic mechanisms, combating the rise of temperature, are balanced by those of the posterior hypothalamus, which are concerned with heat conservation. There is evidence that in states of intense physical exertion the "set point" may be raised so that the subject gains the advantage of the increased rate of chemical processes associated with a 2–3° F rise in temperature. This facilitation not only extends to skeletal muscle, but to the heart as well, increasing the stroke work and heart rate maxima feasible for any particular set of autonomic parameters.

Circulatory Changes During Exposure to Cold

If the preoptic area of the anterior hypothalamus is cooled below 37° C, thermoregulatory mechanisms are set in motion that induce vasoconstriction of skin vessels all over the body. The effects are due to the release of posterior hypothalamic sympathetic areas from inhibition by preoptic signals. The net result is to prevent

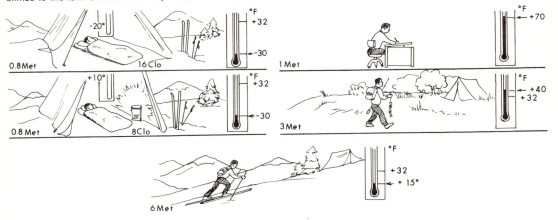

Fig. 9-6.—The importance of the metabolic rate (Met) in determining the clothing required in different environments. At the low metabolic rate and heat production of the sleeping state, a very thick layer of sleeping-bag insulation is needed, i.e., 16 clo. Even in a heated tent at +10° F, an 8-clo bag is required. But the skier working hard as he climbs to the tent is warm with only 1 clo; his heat production is over 7 times that of the sleeping man. A 1-clo unit, i.e., shirt, trousers, and coat, protects a man sitting at a desk only to 70° F, but the man skiing uphill with a pack will keep warm at +10° F in the same suit of clothing. (From Henry, J. P.: *Biomedical Aspects of Space Flight* [New York: Holt, Rinehart & Winston, Inc., 1966], p. 15, Fig. E.)

the radiator areas of the body from transferring heat from the core to the external environment. The blood flow may decrease in a finger to less than 1% of its value when warm. The layer of adipose tissue underneath the vasoconstricted skin protects the warm inner core from the direct conduction of heat. Because this layer is in general thicker in women than it is in men, they do better in tasks in which there is intense loss of heat from the skin. Thus it is the Ama women who dive for shellfish in the cold waters of Korea, while their menfolk, unable to endure such cold, must work in the boats.

There is a disadvantage to the intense vasoconstriction induced by cold. The reduction of the blood flow to the extremities such as the ears, fingers, and toes renders them susceptible to cold injury, even to freezing. If the threat posed by the cold is severe enough, the body temperature of the core is sustained even at the cost of peripheral damage. But the nature of the threat is important. If enough heat is lost to induce a fall in core temperature, then vaso-constriction proceeds at all costs. If, however, the fall is not severe, the exposure to cold is local (such as exposure of the hands to a strongly chilling activity like cleaning freshly caught fish in cold water), and the rest of the body is protected by adequate clothing, then vasoconstrictor activity in the chilled extremities may be far less marked. These regions have arteriovenous anastomotic shunts that stay open despite the local cold, especially in warmly clad and acclimated persons. This local protective vasodilation actually prevents cold injury at only a slight cost in extra heat loss.

A resource that is available to mammals other than man is the piloerection that raises the fur, trapping a thick layer of still, warm air within it. In the arctic fox, this will give as much as seven Clo units protection where one Clo is the protection given by a light suit of clothes (Fig. 9-6). In man, this is a residual function. The individual hair follicles respond to the autonomic impulses with the typical "goose pimples" of the person on the verge of

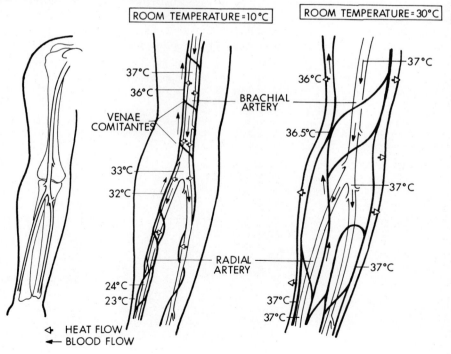

Fig. 9-7.—The countercurrent heat exchanger in the human arm. As cool venous blood moves toward the core and passes warmer arterial blood, heat passes through the vessel walls at a rate proportional to the arteriovenous temperature gradient and the area of contact. In the warm arm at 30° C the return flow is diverted to the superficial venous plexus facilitating loss of heat through the skin. (From Selkurt, E. E.: *Physiology*, 2d ed. [Boston: Little, Brown & Co., 1966], p. 624, Fig. 29-2.)

shivering. Shivering results from hypothalamic activation. There is a region of the posterior hypothalamus, near the third ventricle, that is the primary motor center for this activity. When the temperature of the preoptic center falls, the center for shivering is no longer inhibited, and impulses pass to the motor neurones in the spinal cord. At first, only muscle tone increases, and this alone is enough to lead to a 50% increase in heat production. With the onset of rhythmic shivering, which appears to be due to feedback oscillation of the muscle spindle stretch mechanism, heat production is readily doubled and may even rise four- or fivefold. Shivering automatically ceases when voluntary motor activity commences so that it does not affect the circulatory adjustments for physical work.

A basic mechanism of general physiological significance that is used in the kidney is found in the extremities of animals exposed to cold water immersion. It involves the countercurrent principle. The arteries and veins of the extremity are closely interwoven, forcing a heat exchange in which warm arterial blood from the central core of the body heats cold blood returning via the veins. The heat passes through the vessel walls at a rate proportional to the arteriovenous temperature gradient and the contact surface area. This is effective in wading birds that are exposed to cold water and in penguins that raise their young squatting on the ice. Rudiments of this mechanism can be demonstrated in man. On immersing the hand in ice water, arterial blood at the elbow is cooler than it is at the core (Fig. 9-7).

Circulatory Changes in Emotion

Defense-Alarm Response

In addition to changes in hormonal levels, obvious activities produced by laughing and crying, and glandular activity such as lachrymation, emotions are associated with discharges from the corticohypothalamic system that affect the cardiovascular system. In mammals, the responses to heat and cold and to the demand to fight or run away involve awareness of the event and often result in appropriate behavioral manipulation of the environment. Thus rodents increase the thickness of their nests in cold weather and make them shallower when it is hot. Most mammals use threatening or placatory symbolic gestures that are accompanied by the appropriate hormonal and cardiovascular adjustments. These responses to the animal's social and physical environment involve inputs that profoundly modify the ordinary reflex housekeeping control of blood pressure, blood volume, and blood flow distribution.

The exact mechanisms by which emotional cardiovascular changes are brought about are not worked out. This is a field for active research into methods of measuring pressure, flow, and volume in the various circuits in free animals whose reactions can then be measured in their normal social groupings. Nevertheless, there are clearly a number of different coordinated patterns with characteristic circulatory changes. Thus the cholinergic sympathetic vasodilator fibers of muscle are not affected by the stretch receptors of the high- and low-pressure system. They are triggered by hypothalamic stimulation of the "defense reaction" that simultaneously releases catecholamines from the adrenal glands and increases the stroke work potential of the heart. With lowered peripheral resistance as the muscles dilate, the cardiac output is increased without any rise of blood pressure. Found in men faced with emotional stress and in the alerted frightened animal who is not yet engaged in muscular activity, it appears to be an anticipatory response setting the stage for a hair-trigger explosion into the maximal effort of the charge of the predator and the flight of the victim. Where inches make the difference between survival and failure, the existence of this "cocking" mechanism becomes of potential evolutionary significance.

The defense-alarm reaction is more readily released in animals or men that have had certain types of training and experience in their early lives. On the other hand, its arousal can be made more difficult by the appropriate early social experience; that is, an isolated animal seems to be more readily aroused than normally socialized ones.

Another emotionally determined cardiovascular response is the cutaneous vasodilation of blushing that is accompanied by sweat gland reactions. This erythema may be induced by the bradykinin released by the glands in response to sympathetic stimulation. Lachrymation is accompanied by vasodilation in the gland and by the respiratory gasping and glottic spasm of crying and sobbing. Changes in blood flow in the stomach and intestinal mucosa accompany such emotions.

Vasodepressor Syncope

This condition is found in people who stand still for a prolonged period in hot weather, the classic example being the soldier drawn up at rigid attention on parade. A competitor who stands to talk with friends immediately after a marathon race is also liable to experience syncope, as the exertion leads to intense peripheral vasodilation. It is occasionally found after very severe coughing spells, as when there is a lesion obstructing the trachea. Vasovagal syncope also occurs following hyperventilation combined with the Valsalva maneuver and micturition when a person voids with great urgency immediately upon getting out of bed. These changes are all increased in persons having severe varicosities, which will pool extra amounts of blood in the legs. It is important in adolescence and critical for persons such as pilot candidates who cannot be accepted or kept on duty if subject to sudden loss of consciousness.

Vasodepressor syncope has a strong emotional component. It appears to be brought on by situations in which there is revulsion and fear, but escape is not feasible. Under these conditions, there is a strong vagal inhibition of the heart, giving intense bradycardia and evidence of marked vasodilation in the muscle bed due to inhibition of sympathetic vasoconstrictor tone, together with vasoconstriction in the skin and viscera and the release of large amounts of antidiuretic hormone.

This response may be bound up with sympathoinhibitory impulses, already described as running from the limbic cingulate paleocortex via the anterior hypothalamus to the thoracolumbar sympathetic outflow (Fig. 9-4). It is more frequent in adolescents, whom it serves as an escape from threat, as does the "freezing" of the young fawn and the "playing dead" of the opossum. It is not so easily elicited in elderly persons, although almost everyone can be made to faint given sufficient provocation.

Work on the pressure within the ventricular wall during systole, combined with studies of the factors affecting ventricular afferents, suggests that mechanical conditions causing a change in their firing pattern trigger the reflex. Fainting is uncommon in valvular heart disease, with the exception of aortic stenosis. Here, due to the obstruction in the outflow tract, tensions in the hypertrophied ventricular muscle wall rise to great heights during systole, especially when residual volume is deficient.

In studies of subjects exposed to lower-body negative pressure until they fainted, there was a severe vagal bradycardia, often with heart arrest for several seconds (Fig. 9-8). It is this bradycardia that causes the loss of consciousness; atropine will prevent the effect. In this work, limb plethysmography gave no evidence that dilation of the muscle bed was a significant factor in the collapse.

The prevention of episodes of vasodepressor syncope is directed primarily at organizing living habits so that the orthostatic loss of large volumes of blood, losses that can easily exceed 20% of the

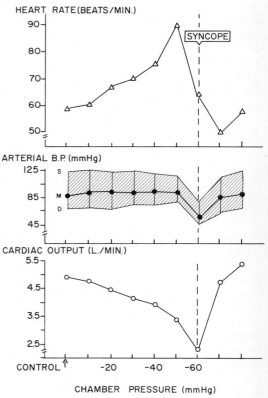

Fig. 9-8.—Hemodynamic effects of graded hypovolemia and vasodepressor syncope induced by lower-body negative pressure. Simulation of the effects of gravity in leading to the orthostatic pooling of blood by suction on the lower half of the body affects heart rate, arterial pressure, and cardiac output. The sharp fall in arterial pressure and cardiac output with the onset of bradycardia precipitates the syncope, which usually does not occur until more than 20% of the total blood volume has been removed. (Redrawn after Murray, R. H., et al.: Hemodynamic Effects of Graded Hypovolemia and Vasodepressor Syncope Induced by Lower Body Negative Pressure, Am. Heart J. 76:799–811, 1968.)

total blood volume, is avoided. It is possible that in orthostasis the addition of anxiety, leading to unduly vigorous heart beats, triggers the response. The onset of cerebral hypoxia can be so severe and sudden that acute hypoxic convulsions occur. This can lead to a snap diagnosis of epilepsy, a diagnosis that can be disproved by the history and by finding that the electroencephalogram is normal.

Summary

Various emotionally determined cardiovascular response patterns constitute a vitally important third order of control of the system. The first order consists of the local or autoregulatory processes, which proceed for the most part independently of the nervous system. The second order of control determines by mechanoreceptor feedback the maintenance of an adequate pressure and volume of the circulatory fluid, together with appropriate tonus of the vascular bed, in order to make best use of the volume available. These regulatory modes largely depend for their function upon the integration of the afferent and efferent autonomic nervous system in the spinal cord and medulla. Elements of this order of control exist at higher levels in the brain, as witness the antidiuretic hormone-release mechanism. For the most part, these regulatory responses to the mechanoreceptors proceed in the absence of conscious awareness. The third order of control, whose investigation so far has been sketchy at best, depends upon the interplay between the organism and its environment. It proceeds in response to emotional arousal and usually has a conscious behavioral component, but it also involves automatic adjustments of the cardiovascular system of which the organism is, for the most part, unaware.

REFERENCES

Adaptation to the Environment: Terrestrial Animals in Cold and Heat, in Dill, D. B. (ed.): *Handbook of Physiology: Adaptation to the Environment* (Washington: American Physiological Society, 1964), chaps. 20–39.

Andersen, H. T.: Cardiovascular Adaptations in Diving Mammals, editorial in Am. Heart J. 74:295–298, 1967.

Best, C. H., and Taylor, N. B.: *The Physiological Basis of Medical Practice,* 8th ed. (Baltimore: Williams & Wilkins Co., 1966).

Bevegard, B. S., and Shepherd, J. T.: Regulation of the Circulation During Exercise in Man, Physiol. Rev. 47:178, 1967.

Edholm, O. G.: On Being Lost on Mountains, in Deserts and at Sea, in Passmore, R., and Robson, J. S. (eds.): *A Companion to Medical Studies, Anatomy, Biochemistry, Physiology, and Related Subjects* (Oxford, England: Blackwell Scientific Publications, 1968), Vol. I, chap. 41.

Folkow, B., and Rubinstein, E. G.: Cardiovascular Effect of Acute and Chronic Stimulations of the Hypothalamus Defense Area in the Rat, Acta Physiol. Scandinav. 8:48, 1966.

Green, I. D.: The Circulation in Anoxia, in Gelles, J. A. (ed.): *A Textbook of Aviation Physiology* (Oxford: Pergamon Press, Inc., 1965), chap. 13, pp. 264–269.

Levi, L. (ed.): *Emotional Stress: Physiological and Psychological Reactions* (New York: American Elsevier Publishing Co., 1967).

Physiology of Muscular Exercise, in Chapman, C. B. (ed.): Circulation Res., Vol. 20, no. 3, Supp. 1, 1967.

Ruch, T. C., and Patton, H. D.: *Physiology and Biophysics,* 19th ed. (Philadelphia: W. B. Saunders Co., 1965).

Rushmer, R. F.: Cardiovascular Responses During Exertion, in *Cardiovascular Dynamics,* 2d ed. (Philadelphia: W. B. Saunders Co., 1961), chap. 8, pp. 193–210.

Sharpey-Schafer, E. P.: Effect of Respiratory Acts on the Circulation, in Hamilton, W. F. (ed.): *Handbook of Physiology: Circulation* (Washington: American Physiological Society, 1965), Vol. III, chap. 52, pp. 1,875–1,897.

10

Circulatory Failure: Shock and Syncope and Chronic Congestive Failure

Introduction

THE RATE at which circulatory failure develops will result in sharp differences in symptomatology. A sudden massive hemorrhage or a block to a major coronary vessel immediately compromises the brain blood perfusion; seconds after the arteriovenous pressure differential falls below 40 mm Hg, consciousness will be lost. This syncope, as it is called, occurs because the cerebral cells cannot maintain their coordinated activity without a constant exchange of metabolites. Some of the factors inducing such an abrupt failure are discussed in the first section of this chapter. A distinction is drawn between vasodepressor syncope with reflex bradycardia, orthostatic syncope with tachycardia due to blood pooling, and syncope due to a disturbance of heart action.

The next section is concerned with the factors responsible for an acute heart failure that takes only minutes to hours to develop. Various signs and symptoms appear as the nutrition of nonvital regions is progressively sacrificed in favor of the vital cerebral and coronary circuits. The consequence is the series of, first, reversible and, finally, irreversible changes that are characteristic of acute circulatory failure or shock.

A final section is concerned with the signs and symptoms of a heart failure that develops slowly over the days and weeks. At first, they appear and vanish in alternation as the fluctuation between the demands of exercise and rest successively exceeds and then falls below the heart's diminished capacity. The remarkable characteristic of chronic heart failure is the puzzling accompanying disturbance of fluid regulation with retention of water and sodium. This occurs so regularly that gradual cardiac decompensation usually takes the form of congestive heart failure, and any explanation of its mechanism must account for this expansion of the extracellular fluid space.

Syncope

INTRODUCTION

Syncope is characterized by a sudden and often unexpected loss of consciousness, with falling if the subject is upright. It is associated with an extremely acute circulatory failure, so severe that the brain circulation is grossly inadequate. Thus it results from an extreme fall in blood pressure that is often due to a slowing or temporary arrest of the heart. Vasodepressor syncope or simple fainting occurs most frequently in connection with the orthostatic pooling of blood. Since it is a reflex effect and not the direct result of the orthostatic blood loss, it has already been discussed under special responses of the cardiovascular system.

ORTHOSTATIC HYPOTENSION

Syncope associated with orthostatic hypotension differs from the vasodepressor response by virtue of the absence of heart slowing. It may occur due to surgical sympathectomy or to the use of drugs such as tranquilizers or ganglion- and adrenergic-blocking agents used in the treatment of essential hypertension.

In older patients with the so-called idiopathic, chronic, orthostatic hypotension, there is often a serious underlying disease of the nervous system with a clear deficiency of the peripheral sympathetic capability. This is betrayed by the loss of capacity to sweat and by impotence. Often there is an abnormal pupillary reaction, the so-called Horner's syndrome. These patients excrete little catecholamine and respond poorly to catechol administration. They fail to compensate by vasoconstriction, and there is no overshoot of pressure due to carotid sinus activation at the end of a Valsalva maneuver (Fig. 9-1). They do not pool excessive amounts of blood in the lower-extremity veins, but they do lack a normal vasoconstrictor response on the arterial side.

Treatment is difficult and may include the use of counterpressure elastic leotards if there is excessive pooling in the erect posture. Patients are cautioned to avoid sudden acts exposing themselves to gravity effects. They may sleep in a bed with the head elevated by 10–12 inches in the attempt to produce an increase of blood volume in response to the resulting prolonged minor blood pooling. The most effective step is to increase blood volume. An intake of sodium chloride as high as 30–40 gm/diem is combined with the use of long-acting fluorhydrocortisone acetate to retain sodium.

Cardiac Syncope

Cardiac syncope is yet another type of acute circulatory failure. It is due to cerebral anemia following ventricular asystole or to heart block (Adams-Stokes syndrome). Consciousness is lost when the circulation is arrested for more than approximately 5 seconds. The commonest cause is a disorder of the heart beat such as sinoatrial block, and a high degree of atrioventricular block. The treatment of Adams-Stokes attacks may include the use of a cardiac pacemaker. The condition is dangerous due to the risk of sudden, unexpected collapse at critical times when life would be endangered, as well as the possibility of sudden death due to an excessively long period of unconsciousness. The maximum period of cerebral anoxia that is tolerable is 4 minutes; the successful revival of persons who have suffered from heart arrest for periods longer than this becomes a questionable achievement because of the permanent cerebral damage that inevitably ensues.

Acute Circulatory Failure

Factors Inducing Failure

A sudden loss of blood or a sudden disruption of blood supply to a part of the heart can cause a deficiency of cardiac output within a few minutes. The symptoms and the compensatory changes that first occur in response to this failure differ from those characterizing a more gradually developing deficiency of the circulatory system. Most conspicuous is the absence of signs of congestion or excessive fluid accumulation in the vascular bed. In acute circulatory failure, the critical feature is the fact that flow through the microcirculation is impaired, with resulting damage to the organs involved. This impairment is exacerbated by the fact that compensatory mechanisms redistribute the already diminished output, so as to maintain as normal a flow as possible in some organs, while sacrificing less critical tissues. Thus the brain and heart receive the major share, while acute vasoconstriction shuts off the visceral blood flow.

The clinical signs of acute circulatory failure or shock are those of increased sympathetic activity. The skin is pale due to peripheral vasoconstriction. There may be some sweating of the hands and feet. Yet, they and the mucous membranes are cold and bluish due to an increased oxygen extraction from the blood. The face is haggard due to loss of interstitial fluid, as the changed pressure equilibrium at the venous end of the capillaries favors the withdrawal of fluid from the tissues. Urine flow always decreases and, in severe cases, will cease altogether. The pulse is fast and weak. The veins can be seen to be collapsed and are often in spasm so that injections are difficult to make. The arterial pressure is not necessarily reduced, although the pulse pressure is always decreased (Fig. 7-11).

A large number of conditions will bring about this type of failure. The blood volume may become deficient as a result of hemorrhage, crushing of muscle in trauma, or loss of plasma in burns. Another cause of blood volume deficiency can be the loss of water and sodium that occurs in acute vomiting and diarrhea, as in cholera, in the acute diarrhea of infancy, in acute obstruction of the intestines, or in a paralytic ileus. In adrenal insufficiency, there is sodium depletion; in heat exhaustion, there may be a loss of both water and sodium as a result of excessive sweating. There may be no absolute loss of blood volume, but only a relative one, as when the small vessels lose tone. This can occur after a severe stimulus to the autonomic system, as when there is damage to the abdominal viscera; in acute infections, such as peritonitis following rupture of an inflamed appendix; or in fevers and states of poisoning in the course of which peripheral vascular tone is disturbed.

Acute failure may result from the disturbance of the heart itself by a variety of causes. This may involve "paroxysmal" tachycardia due to a disorder of control, or a mechanical obstruction to filling such as pericardial tamponade by a blood or serous effusion. The heart itself may be mechanically damaged, as by myocardial infarction when the blood supply to a whole segment of the ventricular wall is impaired. Other conditions involve rupture of a valve cusp or the weakening of the muscle itself by virus disease, by rheumatic fever, or by diphtheria. Other events include massive embolism that obstructs the flow through the heart or major vessels, or the final extreme stages of contraction of the valve orifices such as mitral or aortic stenosis.

No matter whether it is hypovolemia, sepsis, or myocardial failure that leads to shock, there is a common, underlying mechanism that is responsible for the symptoms. This is a severe reduction of cardiac output with a failure of the pump to provide the blood needed by the body. The key factor responsible for the particular symptoms characterizing shock is the pattern of vasoconstriction that develops as a result of the sympathoadrenal arousal. This results in the most intense vasoconstriction in the skin, liver, and bowel, and later in the kidney and muscle. Emotion and pain appear to be especially effective in causing vasoconstriction in the kidney. In various individuals, the above organs probably respond to a differing extent to psychic stimuli. The same holds true to some extent for the heart and possibly the brain, and vasoconstrictor responses of the coronary circulation have recently been experimentally demonstrated.

A simple method of producing a controlled and steadily increasing degree of shock or circulatory failure is to remove blood volume progressively in 5% aliquots. If this is done, the sequence of compensatory changes can be closely followed, and it has been described in Chapter 6. For convenience, nonhypotensive hemorrhage can be distinguished from the later stages when the systemic arterial pressure falls significantly. The change-over occurs in the healthy animal at about 20–30% blood volume loss (Fig. 7-11). From this point onward, shock is likely to develop. The systemic arterial pressure can no longer be sustained by the full action of the compensatory mechanisms, and serious symptoms ensue. If the intense compensatory visceral vasoconstriction stays in full effect for several hours, irreversible changes may ensue. Consequently, this constitutes a convenient point of division for discussion of the mechanisms underlying reversible as opposed to irreversible acute circulatory failure. It is important to recognize that a hemorrhage that results in persistent hypotension and irreversible shock in a healthy animal usually means that an excess of 30% of the total blood volume has been lost (Fig. 7-11).

Mechanism for Compensatory Responses During Nonhypotensive Hemorrhage

The progressive removal of blood leads to a progressive fall in pressure throughout the low-pressure system. The resulting disparity between lowered atrial and constant sinoaortic receptor drives is probably responsible for the early cardiovascular and hormonal characteristics of moderate hemorrhage. These have already been described in Chapter 7. A few points may be raised in expansion and emphasis of this description. The work of Öberg and Folkow has shown that the ratio of resistance of precapillary vessels to the postcapillary venules actively changes in the early stages of blood volume loss as a result of nervous control. This increase in arteriolar resistance and the decreased tonus at the opposite end of the network decreases outward filtration and results in the transfer of fluid from the extravascular spaces into the circulation. It does much to compensate for the original loss of fluid volume and is an important volume regulatory mechanism in acute emergencies.

At a later stage, after the loss of about 20% of the blood volume, there is a constriction of the veins. This increases as the catechol levels rise progressively with further blood volume loss. The decrease in the size of the capacitance vessels helps to drive blood to the central regions. Over-all renal blood flow may or may not diminish during the loss of the first 30% of the blood volume (Fig. 7-11), and there is an early shift from a predominantly cortical to an outer-medullary pattern of blood flow. The sympathetic outflow to the kidney has a further important effect in the initiation of enhanced renin release, possibly by direct action on the juxtaglomerular apparatus. The increase in renin leads to enhanced levels of aldosterone, and this, in turn, to more reabsorption of sodium by the renal tubules. There is evidence that proximal tubular handling of sodium may be under the influence of factors that originate from the brain in response to decreased intravascular volume. An oxytocin-like polypeptide has been proposed, but the evidence is as yet slim. At the same time, assays of the blood for antidiuretic hormone show an early increase to very considerable heights in conscious animals submitted to progressive hemorrhage. This occurs even before there is any fall in systemic arterial pressure. The consequences of the combined redistribution of blood flow in the kidney and the activation of the renin angiotensin and antidiuretic hormone mechanisms are very complex. Initially, they serve to lead to a retention of the sodium and water needed by the hypovolemic organism that must conserve body fluid. In addition, high levels of these two hormones interacting with epinephrine and nor-epinephrine may enhance sympathetic effects upon the vascular bed and help to ensure the early contraction of the splanchnic circulation and of the skin.

Acute Circulatory Failure: Irreversible Shock

The disturbances induced by losses of blood volume insufficient to lower mean blood pressure include all the varied hormonal and vascular responses that are involved in diverting blood from the splanchnic, the muscle, and the skin bed and in facilitating flow through the heart and the brain. Throughout, the lungs remain passive and unaffected, the main focus for vasoconstriction being the skin and viscera, together with some reduction in muscle flow.

The catastrophic changes that accompany total blood volume losses of 30, 40, and 50% do not differ in kind; they are catastrophic because of the increased severity of the constriction in response to the baroreceptors of the now-failing high-pressure system. The flow through the gut decreases practically to zero. So, also, does that through the liver and, in later stages, through the kidneys. In these severe states of shock resulting from blood volume loss, or from a disturbance of cardiac function that results in lowered systemic arterial pressure, the return flow from the affected organs is a mere trickle and the great veins in the cold skin can actually be severed without bleeding.

In these circumstances, the normal functions of the affected regions can no longer be maintained. Little water is absorbed from the intestine. The production of bile and urine stops. Gluconeogenesis in the liver ceases and blood glucose levels fall, contributing to the weakness of the victim. On occasion in the so-called crush syndrome, the reduction in renal blood flow is so severe that renal tubular damage ensues. In such cases, despite a later recovery of blood pressure and general circulatory efficiency, death may result from renal failure.

A most dangerous disturbance is the loss of liver function, especially of its capacity to destroy bacteria and to break down endotoxin. This can occur after exposure to a couple of hours of hemorrhagic shock. In the intestine, an ominous simultaneous development is denudation of areas of mucosa, suggesting that the wall has lost its normal capacity to prevent the invasion of the blood stream by bacteria. It appears probable that the final fatal outcome of prolonged hypotensive shock arises because of this combination of loss of the normal defenses against bacterial invasion from the gut and weakening of the endotoxin-detoxifying capacity of the reticuloendothelial system, especially in the liver. The result is that bacterial toxins build up in the blood stream and are circulated to the brain where they further stimulate the already excessive sympathetic activity. Thus there is a vicious circle, with steadily increasing catecholamine levels in the tissues that can result in irreversible damage to the tissues and particularly to those of the splanchnic area.

Treatment of Acute Circulatory Failure

Treatment centers around the prevention and, finally, the alleviation of the vasoconstriction that perpetuates the shock. The first step is to monitor the filling of the low-pressure system, if possible, by a catheter introduced through the brachial vein into the right atrium. The monitoring of this pressure and provision of adequate fluid or blood to raise the central venous pressure to some 3 mm Hg or 4 cm H_2O is vital when the prime cause of the shock is deficiency of circulating blood volume. However, when the heart itself is responsible for the circulatory failure, the blood volume may be normal and the tonus of the vascular bed may not be deficient. In such circumstances, extra fluid must be added with great caution to avoid excessive elevation of central venous pressure. Survival rates can be greatly improved, despite the lowered systemic arterial pressure, if the excessive tonus in the peripheral vascular bed is reduced. Experimentally, this can be done by prior repeated exposure to epinephrine injections, thus creating some habituation and an increased rate of catecholamine removal. Clinically, a vasodilator agent such as phenoxybenzamine can be used to block the α-adrenergic activity. The reason for the success of these maneuvers appears to be that the vicious circle of excessive vasoconstriction with progressive loss of the vital function of the visceral circulation is broken. Cardiac output measurements can be deceptive in certain types of shock. Thus, in peritonitis, there may be a normal cardiac output, yet most is wasted in a shunt through the hyperemic peritoneum, and death may occur due to the accompanying excessive vasoconstriction in the viscera.

The treatment of shock requires the earliest possible elimination of sources of afferent stimuli that precipitate an excessive sympathetic outflow. These include the control of pain, the allaying of fear, the setting of broken bones, the use of antibiotics whenever there is infection, and the control of excessive body temperature. Where there is anaerobic infection, treatment may include use of hyperbaric oxygen, and when anaphylactic responses are involved, epinephrine and glucocorticoids are indicated. Appropriate fluids must be administered to replace the lost blood component. Hemorrhage requires blood replacement. In burns, plasma is indicated; in diarrhea, when there has been no loss of blood, sodium chloride in normal solution may be given in large amounts. In all cases, the central venous pressure must be watched to ensure that it does not exceed an upper limit of some 10–15 cm H_2O, for to do so is to run into the danger of pulmonary edema and heart failure.

In cases in which the arterial pressure has fallen to critical values, below 70 mm Hg, drugs that have a beta-adrenergic and inotrophic effect like isoprotenerol may be infused until the pressure rises to acceptable levels. This must be done because in hypotension a brain or a heart exposed to arteriovenous pressure differences of less than 50–70 mm Hg may be permanently damaged. However, the moment the hypotensive crisis is over, attention has to be paid to the improvement of peripheral blood flow if the ever-present danger of tissue damage due to persistent vasoconstriction is not to be exacerbated. In summary: the handling of acute circulatory failure is rendered easier by the monitoring of the state of filling of the low-pressure system. Reliance upon systemic arterial pressure alone is contraindicated because states of irreversible damage can develop in subjects who have not lost more than 30% of their blood volume and show no gross fall of mean arterial pressure. By watching right atrial pressure, the amount of fluid replacement required can be determined and therapy pushed without fear of slipping into the equally serious difficulty of excessive filling of the low-pressure system.

Congestive Heart Failure: A Disorder of Regulation of the Low-Pressure System

Symptoms

Many of the signs of chronic circulatory failure are due not to the inadequate heart output itself, but to changes in fluid volume that lead to venocapillary engorgement, to elevation of capillary pressure, and to increased circulatory and extracellular blood volume. It is because these symptoms are so prominent that emphasis is laid on these "congestive" features. Instead of speaking of chronic circulatory failure, it is customary to refer to congestive heart failure. In acute failure, the compensatory mechanisms redistribute the diminished available output so that a normal blood flow will be maintained to the heart and brain. This persistent redistribution of flow in the chronically failing circulatory system induces disturbances of function that gradually result in a grossly abnormal and functionally disturbing accumulation of sodium and water. It will be the purpose of this section to describe these symptoms and to propose the mechanisms that cause the organism with a deficient cardiac output to act as though its blood volume is inadequate.

Stead describes the typical case of commencing congestive heart failure as follows: "He may complain that he becomes increasingly tired and dyspneic during the week's work but that after a weekend of rest he can go back with renewed vigor. He notices a lag between drinking and urinating. The normal man drinks, eats and voids during the day and sleeps soundly at night. As failure begins he notices that during the week while he is working his urine output during the day is low and yet at night it is large enough to disturb his sleep. There is a slight increase in body weight as subclinical edema collects. He notes that when he is off work from Friday afternoon to Monday morning he loses weight and is not aroused on Sunday night to void. If he restricts salt he finds that his weight gain is less and nocturia less bothersome."

As the condition becomes more severe, edema fluid begins to form and accumulate in the lungs, especially in the alveoli, impairing respiratory function. The engorgement of the lungs with blood and the accumulation of edema fluid impairs the mechanism of ventilation and increases the work of breathing; this leads to breathlessness. Secretions may accumulate, and alveolar membranes thicken and become edematous. Finally, the patient develops dyspnea, rapid shallow breathing of which he is conscious, together with orthopnea or difficulty in breathing when recumbent. Paroxysmal nocturnal dyspnea develops. The patient who goes to bed lying flat, wakes feeling suffocated. He sits up coughing and wheezing, but, as the blood and tissue fluids are transferred back to the legs, his symptoms lessen. This dyspnea is not so much due to lowered oxygen and increased carbon dioxide tension in the blood as it is to stimulation of vagus nerve stretch receptors in the lung.

Another set of symptoms of chronic heart failure is connected with the increase in systemic venous pressure. This may reach 25 cm H_2O, and the jugular veins can be seen to be filled to the angle of the jaw even when the patient is upright. This increase of central venous pressure is a direct expression of the gross increase in the blood volume with, perhaps, some venoconstriction as a result of adrenergic activity. The increase of blood volume is demonstrated by the fact that, even after death, the venous pressure of a man with congestive failure greatly exceeds that of a normal person. Evidence that venoconstriction can play a part is the fact that ganglionic-blocking agents such as dibenamine will decrease the venous pressure in congestive failure.

After an irreversible weight gain of some 5 to 10 pounds, the ankles begin to swell. Pitting edema develops. This can be detected at the ankles of the ambulatory and over the sacrum of the bedridden by firm pressure with a finger. It not only accumulates in the swollen legs, but also in the abdomen as ascites, and even in the thorax as hydrothorax. Since the intake of fluid is normal, it is the abnormal accumulation of water and salt that appears to be the key to the peculiar "congestive" aspects of chronic heart failure.

Exercise, Adrenergic Activity and Heart Failure

As Stead's "typical history" points out, the early heart failure patient only complains of fluid accumulation during the period he is up and about and working. Thus there is a connection with exercise, and indeed by far the greatest demand on the heart is that of the skeletal muscles. Standing, washing, shaving, and driving a car demand up to twice the cardiac output needed to maintain the organism at rest in bed. In heavy exercise, such as walking upstairs, the demand increases fivefold or more. The requirements of digestion and temperature regulation are smaller. The cardiac output is doubled in a sweating man; the relief afforded by air conditioning, which removes the need for sweating and peripheral vasodilation, can make this a lifesaving provision for those with failing hearts.

Braunwald has made comprehensive studies of the effects of exercise on both normal and damaged hearts. In normal persons when left-ventricular end-diastolic pressure increases slightly, there is a considerable increase in stroke work, where stroke work is the force exerted by the ventricular muscle in overcoming the aortic pressure times the volume ejected, i.e., a measure of the distance traveled by the contractile elements or muscle shortening (see Chap. 3). However, in left-ventricular disease, large increases in left-ventricular diastolic pressure lead only to a small increase in stroke work (Fig. 10-1). Hence cardiac patients cannot rely on the simple law of the heart, with increased response to increased diastolic lengthening to increase the performance of the organ. Instead, they must resort to inotropic stimulation with increase of heart rate and contractility to force the ventricle to a better performance. There was evidence of marked sympathetic stimulation in his patients. By using guanethidine to inhibit the sympathetic resources, he caused an exacerbation of the symptoms of persons with moderate heart failure. When this blocking agent was used, the patient's dyspnea and orthopnea were more severe, probably as a consequence of the stimulation of Paintal's juxtacapillary receptors by early edema in the lung parenchyma. Sodium output decreased, and the patient's weight and central venous pressure increased, i.e., extracellular fluid accumulated (Fig. 10-2). Braunwald also

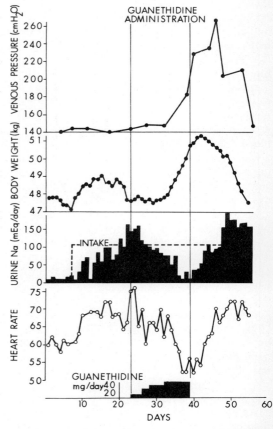

Fig. 10-1.—Diagrammatic representation of the ranges of left-ventricular function curves produced by angiotensin infusion in three groups of subjects. **(1)** in normal subjects, angiotensin produces large increases in stroke work. **(2)** In left ventricular disease without heart failure, end-diastolic pressure increases more for less increase in stroke work. **(3)** In heart failure, despite great increase in left-ventricular diastolic pressure, stroke work remains constant or even declines. (From Braunwald, E.: Control of Ventricular Function in Man, Brit. Heart J. 27:1–16, 1965.)

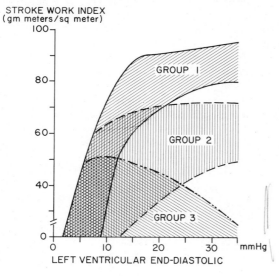

Fig. 10-2.—Changes in venous pressure, body weight, sodium balance, and heart rate—before, during, and after the administration of guanethidine. The drug causes adrenergic blockade and prevents the action of the sympathetic system in maintaining ventricular contractility, in spite of depression of myocardial function. With the blockade, sodium is retained, body weight and venous pressure rise, and the orthopnea of congestive failure worsens. (From Braunwald, E.: Control of Ventricular Function in Man, Brit. Heart J. 27:1–16, 1965.)

found that if a normal man is required to exercise, his catechol levels rise little in the blood. However, a man suffering from heart failure will show up to a fourfold increase. In addition, the heart muscle in congestive failure is depleted in catechol content. He suggests exhaustion due to sustained and intense adrenergic stimulation (Fig. 10-3).

His conclusion is that the normal moderate exercise of walking, driving, climbing stairs, standing, conversing, etc., that the healthy man takes in his stride forces the man with a chronic heart impairment to use the adrenergic nervous system to make up the imbalance between his restricted cardiac output and the perfusion requirements of the peripheral tissues. These observations support older studies that have shown that the patient in heart failure cannot meet the stress of exercise with an increase in cardiac output, and that renal blood flow may be normal when at rest, but inadequate with exercise.

The concept of persisting adrenergic activity in chronic circulatory failure is supported by Barger's now-classic observation on dogs in which congestive failure was induced by the combined lesions of tricuspid insufficiency and pulmonary stenosis. Not only did they retain sodium and water, but when the adrenergic-blocking agent, dibenzlyine, was introduced via the renal artery, the kidney started to increase its excretion of salt (Fig. 10-4). In normal animals, this does not occur. Thus Barger's data showed that there is an increased sympathetic activity in the kidney nerves of animals in congestive heart failure.

It is not necessary to postulate a gross decrease in glomerular filtration to account for sodium retention in such animals, although this, too, does occur in severe heart failure. There is evidence that an increase in renal sympathetic activity, such as that observed by Barger, may redistribute blood from cortex to outer medulla and that this redistribution is associated with sodium retention. In addition, Vander has directly related the increase in renal sympathetic nerve activity to renin release. Since these nerves supply the juxtaglomerular apparatus, the effects may well include a direct stimulation of the renin-containing cells.

Thus the question of the mechanism of sodium retention in congestive heart failure appears to be reduced to the question of why the adrenergic sympathetic activity is so high. The fact that exercise increases the level of adrenergic activity focuses attention on the mechanism of this effect. The response to exercise of the man with chronic circulatory deficiency does not differ in kind but in intensity from that of the normal man. In both, the adjustments that occur are determined in the higher levels of the reticular formation including the hypothalamus. Asmussen has pointed out that in exercise there is an unknown "work factor" that adds to the effect of CO_2 on the respiration and interacts with the effect of hypoxia on ventilation (Fig. 9-3). This "work factor" increases pulse rate and stroke volume, and adjusts heat dissipation so precisely that body temperature increases only to the level corresponding to the metabolic rate of the exercise and then remains constant. The

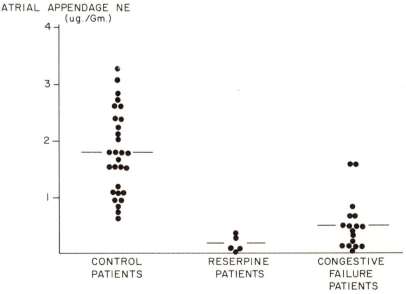

Fig. 10-3.—Concentration of nor-epinephrine in the atrial appendages of patients who had been in congestive failure is greatly diminished, suggesting intense and prolonged activity of the sympathetic nervous system. (From Braunwald, E.: Control of Ventricular Function in Man, Brit. Heart J. 27:1–16, 1965.)

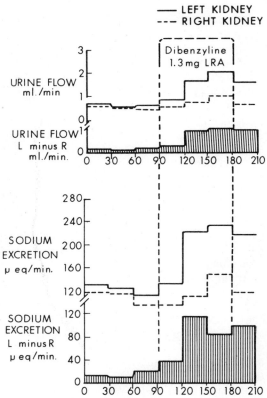

Fig. 10-4.—Effect of left renal artery *(LRA)* infusion of the adrenergic-blocking agent, dibenzyline, on sodium and water excretion in a dog with tricuspid insufficiency. The sharp increase of these parameters suggests that the kidneys are under strong adrenergic influence in congestive failure. (From Barger, A. C., Liebowitz, M. R., and Muldowney, F. P.: The Role of the Kidney in the Homeostatic Adjustments of Congestive Heart Failure, J. Chron. Dis. 9:571–582, 1959. Reprinted with permission from Pergamon Press.)

remarkable adjustment of ventilation and heart output to levels manyfold the resting values, without any gross changes in readily measured parameters such as CO_2, O_2, and pH levels, can only be explained on the grounds of a highly sensitive integration in the central nervous system. This probably demands the alert, conscious organism for its effective operation.

Asmussen proposes that muscle spindle and articular receptors may be involved in the reflex control of ventilation during muscular exercise. He suggests that the stream of sensory impulses that run up from the muscles to the coordinating centers in the brain may actually interplay with nonrespiratory parts of the reticular formation. Hence his "work factor" represents the integrated response of higher centers in the brain to the total information flow associated with the exercise.

A Suggested Role for Receptors in Heart Failure

Extending the above concept, we would add to the list of inputs that may prove to be important during exercise. The temperature sensors in the hypothalamus are capable of very accurate assessment of the work being done by the organism. They may do this by comparing the rate of change of blood temperature with an established regulatory "set point," by reference to which the body temperature is kept in balance. For any given work load imposed on the muscle mass, a certain amount of extra heat is generated and must be dissipated. The adjustments required for this dissipation, as Asmussen points out, are very accurate and sensitive. Indeed, it is theoretically possible that heat production is used as an indirect measure of the work output by the muscles and, hence, a measure of the increased cardiac output that is being required of the organism.

In order to assess the difficulty of the failing heart, the organism needs a measure of the cardiac output requirement against the actual output. In the foregoing, it has been proposed that some measure of the requirement can be made in terms of heat production and activity levels of afferents from muscles and joints. Various receptors could give valuable information as to the actual output of the heart. Thus the atrial receptors would tell the level of end-diastolic pressure, whereas the sinoaortic receptors tell the level of force needed for ejection. Hence a measure of stroke work is available by which this aspect of the effectiveness of muscle could be gauged by the central mechanism. In the disabled heart, stroke work does not match this level appropriately.

The end nets in the ventricular endocardium and on the atrioventricular valve leaflets will fire during the isometric phase of contraction as closure occurs and pressure rises, but the baroreceptors in the aortic arch reach a peak with the ejection phase. The time lag between these two bursts of impulses will give the organism the second critical piece of information—that is, ventricular contractility or the rate of rise of intraventricular pressure. Thus the cardiovascular receptors may supply the information needed to gauge both stroke work and contractility.

It is suggested that the combination of conscious awareness of the environmental conditions, proprioceptive inputs from the active muscles and joints, information as to the rate of heat production and, hence, of work by the muscles involved, together with measures of contractility, stroke work, and other aspects of the actual mechanical performance of both high- and low-pressure portions of the heart furnished by the built-in receptors, are all smoothly integrated in normal animals in order to produce the appropriate performance of the cardiovascular system for various outputs ranging from modest activity to sustained violent exertion. It is postulated that the information derived from the failing ventricle with its slowed rate of rise of intraventricular pressure (Fig. 10-2) may create a disparity when contrasted in the central regions with the normally anticipated and programmed pattern of afferent impulses.

In this way, the failure of the heart muscle to handle the demands being made on it may well lead to central nervous responses that trigger the increased sympathetic drive characteristic of the individual with chronic circulatory failure. Given this increase in over-all adrenergic activity, which is primarily aimed at raising the contractility of the flagging ventricle, there will follow as an unwanted side effect the retention of sodium, leading to the classic congestive features of chronic heart failure.

The role of the CUE Nonidez receptors in the low-pressure system that control the release of antidiuretic hormone has not been determined during heart failure, nor do we know the role of the end nets. However, observations

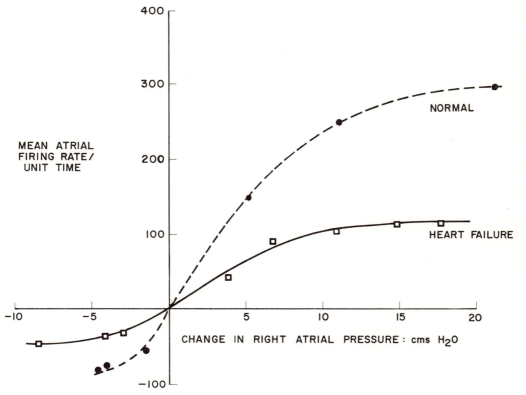

Fig. 10-5.—The broken line represents the change in the mean atrial firing rate (CUE) per unit time when the right atrial pressure is varied in normal animals. The response is contrasted with the change in rate in dogs in experimental heart failure induced by combined tricuspid avulsion and pulmonary artery stenosis *(solid line)*. The slope of the curve is steeper in the normal animals, both when venous pressure is increased by transfusion and when it is reduced by hemorrhage. See also Zehr *et al.* for similar observations of ADH levels in heart failure.

suggest that this part of the cardiovascular system may be involved. Progressive distension of the low-pressure system with dextran leads to an increasing pulsation of the atria and hence to an increase in mean atrial firing rate (Fig. 10-5). This increase tapers off at pressures above the 20 cm H_2O range; further distension leads to no further increment in impulse traffic. Animals in spontaneous or experimental heart failure, due to an induced tricuspid regurgitation together with pulmonary stenosis, have been studied to determine the response of atrial receptors to transfusion. The solid curve in Figure 10-5 shows that small changes of right atrial pressure, such as might occur with exercise, do not lead to the same rise in mean atrial firing rate in heart failure as in the normal heart. It remains to be seen whether the paradoxic retention of sodium and water, despite the great atrial distension of congestive failure, can be explained by this failure of the firing rate of the CUE and/or end-net receptors to increase. These firing rate anomalies may contribute to the fluid retention by giving information suggestive that heart filling is inadequate despite the gross mechanical overdistension of the atria. An additional factor contributing to the sodium retention of the man with chronic heart failure is that the distress that he experiences may contribute to the strong adrenergic activity with its consequent elevation of ADH levels, renin release, and renal blood flow redistribution.

The theme of the foregoing is that, in man, much of the burden for the complex autoregulation of the circulation is carried by the central nervous system. The various networks of receptors, demonstrated in the atria, the ventricles, and the great arteries, supply vital information concerning the status of the low- as well as the high-pressure systems.

Difficulties with congestive failure have followed the orthotopic autotransplantation of the heart by those using operative techniques that did not preserve the afferent CUE and end net receptors in the posterior atrial wall. Lower has suggested that the excellent results that have been obtained with recent heart transplants from the viewpoint of fluid balance may have been because the new technique leaves portions of the posterior atrial wall of the recipient intact and retains the afferent nerves from the low-pressure system (Fig. 10-6). This hypothesis could be evaluated experimentally. Not only may the cardiac transplant carried out in this way enjoy an advantage from the viewpoint of cardiovascular regulation, but, if confirmed, the result would point to the importance of the complex afferent information carried from both the high- and the low-pressure systems in the regulation of the normal circulation and in the genesis of the fluid retention that characterizes chronic circulatory failure.

Treatment of Chronic (Congestive) Heart Failure

Prime effort is directed toward removing the cause of heart failure by treating the underlying condition, if at all possible. Replacing or repairing defective heart valves, the use of a pacemaker to correct unfavorable cardiac rhythms, the

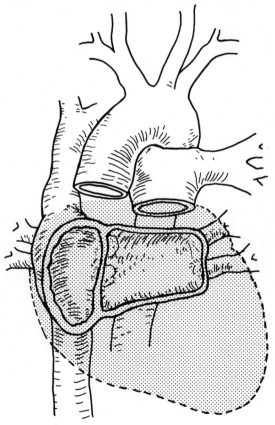

Fig. 10-6.—Showing the extent of posterior atrial wall left in situ with recent techniques for heart transplantation. Compare with Figure 7-1 for distribution of receptors in the region left behind. (From Cooley, D. A., et al.: Transplantation of the Human Heart, J.A.M.A. 205(7):480, 1968.)

management of metabolic problems such as thyrotoxicosis, etc., are some of the measures that may be effective. The general principles that are followed involve two approaches. The first sharply limits physical activity, often by strict bed rest, thereby reducing the work load of the heart. Digitalis is frequently used. It has remarkable effects on contractility and often dramatically improves cardiac function; there is evidence that it increases the utilization of the energy provided by the cell's phosphate mechanism. The second approach involves the direct control of sodium and water retention. This may be accomplished by limiting sodium and water intake and also by using pharmacologic agents that enhance the excretion of sodium and water by the kidney.

Postmitral Commissurotomy Dilutional Syndrome

The evidence available concerning the mechanism of sodium and water retention in chronic circulatory failure points to a breakdown of the normal regulation of fluid volume. It has been suggested that the receptors in the cardiovascular system produce a pattern of responses that leads to an overwhelming adrenergic sympathetic arousal, resulting not only in activation of the renin, angiotensin, and aldosterone mechanisms, but also in intrarenal changes in blood flow increasing the relative perfusion of juxtamedullary nephrons. As a result, there is progressive distension of the blood volume. This may lead to a direct failure of the mechanical stimulation of the atrial receptors themselves, as impaired pulsation in the overstretched, thin-walled chambers fails to excite an adequate train of impulses. This failure of regulation of the low-pressure system in chronic disease may be contrasted with two conditions in which there is radical alteration of fluid output in association with an acute change of state of the region carrying the atrial receptors.

Surgical intervention with the mitral valve in stenosis, when the orifice is greatly restricted, is now a common practice. Moran and Zimmerman have described the sharp reduction in ADH in the blood with distension of an atrial balloon and the interesting rebound that follows it (Fig. 10-7). They have also described a moderate diuresis and an accompanying reduction of ADH levels when a ligature acutely constricts the mitral ring; this is followed by a rebound of the ADH

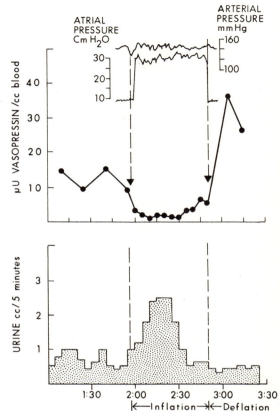

Fig. 10-7.—An experiment in which a balloon in the left atrium is inflated, causing an increase of left atrial pressure to 30 cm H_2O, a sharp fall in vasopressin levels to less than 2 μU/cc, with consequent development of a diuresis. (From Shu'ayb, W. A., Moran, W. H., and Zimmerman, B.: Studies of the Mechanism of Antidiuretic Hormone Secretion and the Post Commissurotomy Dilutional Syndrome, Ann. Surg. 162:690–701, 1965.)

levels on its release. They showed that when the chronic obstruction and atrial distension is released by mitral commissurotomy, there is a sharp rise in ADH blood levels that persists for days and is accompanied by a retention of water and a fall in serum sodium levels because of blood dilution. The condition is controlled by giving alcohol, suggesting that antidiuretic hormone is involved. The water balance can also be restored by overtransfusing the patient and so sustaining high levels of central venous pressure. This suggests that the changes that occur in the atrial walls in these long-standing cases may have impaired the delicate receptor networks, and time may be required before the atria slowly return to normal.

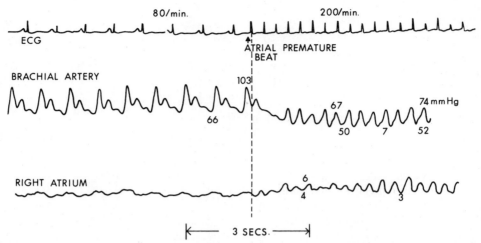

Fig. 10-8.—Brachial arterial and right atrial pressures before and at the onset of paroxysmal tachycardia at a rate of 200 per minute. The brachial arterial blood pressure fell from 103/66 to between 67/50 and 74/52 mm Hg; the right atrial pressure rose from 2 mm Hg (mean) to between 6/4 and 9/3 mm Hg (mean, 5 mm). (From Wood, P.: Polyuria in Paroxysmal Tachycardia and Paroxysmal Atrial Flutter and Fibrillation, Brit. Heart J. 25:273–282, 1963.)

Fig. 10-9.—The renal response to paroxysmal tachycardia is variable. It may involve a simple increase in free water excretion, though there is also often an increase in salt output. (From Wood, P.: Polyuria in Paroxysmal Tachycardia and Paroxysmal Atrial Flutter and Fibrillation, Brit. Heart J. 25:273–282, 1963.)

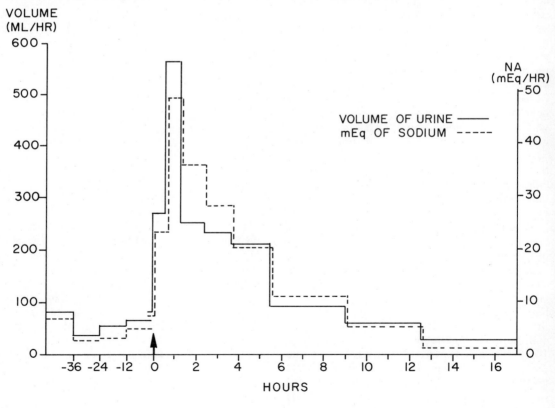

Paroxysmal Atrial Tachycardia

Paroxysmal atrial tachycardia, which results from the rapid succession of rhythmic impulses arising in an irritable ectopic focus in the atrium, is characterized by pulse rates in the order of 170–200/min, which may last for hours in an otherwise normal heart. Attacks occur suddenly, without warning, with a sense of fluttering in the chest and may proceed with few symptoms in persons with healthy hearts, as long as the rate is not in excess of 200. However, patients often complain of fullness and throbbing in the neck. A progressive rise in left-atrial mean pressure and pulse pressure until they are approximately doubled has been demonstrated in the course of an attack (Fig. 10-8). At the lower heart rates, there are usually no overt signs of heart failure, but a water or salt diuresis occurs in a majority. This diuresis has been attributed to the extreme increase in afferent impulses from the atria as a result of the combined effect of violent pulsation together with the very high frequency (Fig. 10-9). The Londoner, Adams, presents a vivid "typical" history, saying that the diuresis usually develops in 20 to 30 minutes, the time interval being very constant for each case. He wryly comments that "another woman learned something of the occupants of houses near the bus stops on her route between her home and work. Her diuresis began rather soon after the onset of an attack and she was not infrequently caught out on the bus. She had made it her practice to get out at the next stop and to knock on the door of the most hospitable house."

However, the increase of water and salt excretion is not always observed. This may be because, if the condition progresses to circulatory failure and discomfort, anxiety, and a deficiency in cardiac output despite adrenergic sympathetic stimulation, then antidiuretic hormone levels can be expected to rise above the critical 4–6 μ units/ml level. Under these circumstances, the condition will change from one of increased fluid elimination to the pattern of sodium and water retention familiar in congestive failure. Thus paroxysmal tachycardia appears to constitute an intermediate state between acute circulatory failure and the chronic, slowly developing disturbance of congestive failure with increased venous pressure and atrial overdistension.

REFERENCES

Braunwald, E.: The Control of Ventricular Function in Man, Brit. Heart J. 27:1–16, 1965.

Davis, J. O.: The Physiology of Congestive Heart Failure, in Hamilton, W. F. (ed.): *Handbook of Physiology: Circulation* (Washington: American Physiological Society, 1965), Vol. III, chap. 59, pp. 2071–2122.

Fine, J.: Shock and Peripheral Circulatory Insufficiency, in Hamilton, W. F. (ed.): *Handbook of Physiology: Circulation* (Washington: American Physiological Society, 1965), Vol. III, chap. 58, pp. 2037–2070.

Friedberg, C. K.: Circulatory Failure, Part II, in *Diseases of the Heart,* 3d ed. (Philadelphia: W. B. Saunders Co., 1966), pp. 137–474.

Gauer, O. H., and Henry, J. P.: Negative Acceleration in Relation to Arterial Oxygen Saturation, Subendocardial Hemorrhage and Venous Pressure in the Forehead, Aerospace Med. 35:533–545, 1964.

Gauer, O. H., Henry, J. P., and Behn, C.: The Regulation of Extracellular Fluid Volume, Ann. Rev. Physiol. 32:547–595, 1970.

Guyton, A. C.: *Textbook of Medical Physiology,* 3d ed. (Philadelphia: W. B. Saunders Co., 1966).

Guyton, A. C.: Cardiac Output, Venous Pressure, Cardiac Failure, and Shock, in *Function of the Human Body* (Philadelphia: W. B. Saunders Co., 1969), chap. 13.

Keele, C. A., and Neil, E.: in Wright, S.: *Applied Physiology,* 11th ed. (New York: Oxford University Press, 1965).

Paintal, A. S.: Mechanisms of Stimulation of Type J Pulmonary Receptors, J. Physiol. 203:511–532, 1969.

Rushmer, R. F.: *Cardiovascular Dynamics,* 2d ed. (Philadelphia: W. B. Saunders Co., 1961).

Shu'ayb, W. A., Moran, W. H., and Zimmerman, B.: Studies of the Mechanism of Antidiuretic Hormone Secretion and the Post Commissurotomy Dilutional Syndrome, Ann. Surg. 162:690–701, 1965.

Wood, P.: Polyurea in Paroxysmal Tachycardia and Paroxysmal Atrial Flutter and Fibrillation, Brit. Heart J. 25:273–282, 1963.

Zehr, J. E., Harve, A., Tsakiris, A., McGoon, D. C., and Segar, W. E.: Effects of Chronic Mitral Stenosis on ADH Release in Dogs, Physiologist 13:354, 1970.

11

High Blood Pressure

Introduction

THE EXPLANATION for the gradual increase in arterial blood pressure characteristic of essential hypertension has been elusive because of the numerous interacting mechanisms involved in the development of this phenomenon. Early experiments implicated the kidney as having a primary role. More recent evidence indicates that the renal involvement may be secondary, and an excessive response to environmental stimuli may be the initiating factor.

Various influences work through the mechanisms that extend from the hypothalamus via sympathetic system and the adrenal gland to the peripheral vascular bed. Others can be postulated that extend upward from the hypothalamus to the higher centers of the brain, namely the cortex and the limbic system. These structures serve in the evaluation of the environment and appear to be associated with the determination of the magnitude of emotional responses. The various factors working from the hypothalamus downward via the sympathetic system are discussed first in order to show how their persistent arousal can eventually lead to renal hypertension.

High Blood Pressure and Mechanisms Distal to the Hypothalamus

In the healthy organism, a systolic blood pressure as low as 80–100 mm Hg is quite compatible with tissue needs. Yet a hypertensive individual may have a resting systolic pressure of 200 mm Hg. The consequences to the tissues of high blood pressure are determined by the level at which it is sustained. The increased stroke work imposed on the heart will not, by itself, lead to heart failure. The healthy ventricular muscle can hypertrophy until it is as much as 20% larger than normal. The real problem is that at high systemic pressures the walls of the small arteries become sclerotic, and tissue nutrition fails due to a developing obstruction to the blood supply. This initiates responses that call for still-greater increases of blood pressure. In the heart, the vascular damage of arteriosclerosis impairs the muscle blood supply, making the increased work load imposed by an elevated pressure less tolerable. In the brain, the progressive deterioration of the arteries results in an ever-increasing risk of rupture and death or disablement from brain hemorrhage.

The fact that excessive pressure pulses in the arterial tree can by themselves lead to damage is clearly illustrated by the results of overly rapid surgical release of coarctation of the aorta. This congenital restrictive lesion results in a grossly impaired blood supply to the trunk. The response to the ensuing inadequacy of blood flow to the kidneys and other regions is a marked elevation of blood pressure. Sudden and complete relief of the obstruction by an operation substituting a normal-sized channel for the restricted portion results in the impact of the very high pressures on a vascular bed in the rest of the body hitherto adapted to far-lower values. A variety of clinical symptoms ensue. All appear to be due to swelling and necrosis of the arterial wall that obstruct blood flow. If the relief is deliberately made less dramatic, and the blood pressure is kept down after surgery by antihypertensive drugs, the arteriolar lesions do not develop.

This acute condition draws attention to the

possible role of mechanical pressure effects in inducing the more slowly progressive lesions that accompany chronic high blood pressure. Certainly, necrotic arterial lesions will develop rapidly with consequent intense impairment of the blood supply if the pressure exceeds the 180–200 mm Hg range for long periods.

The clinical conditions affecting the viscera that lead to high blood pressure include, first of all, infective and other disorders of the kidney that result in progressive vascular derangement and impairment of its function, i.e., glomerulonephritis and, less frequently, pyelonephritis. This impairment may stem from fibrosis and damage to the small vessels within the organ, including the glomeruli themselves. But the lesion does not have to be confined to the intrarenal vessels. The main artery leading to the kidney can be obstructed by embolism or by an arteriosclerotic plaque. The organ beyond is affected to a degree that is dependent on the severity of the lesion. With progressive obstruction, there is a progressive elevation of blood pressure. If rapid and severe, it will be associated with an increased release of renin from the juxtaglomerular apparatus, and the blood pressure can proceed to levels in excess of 200 mm Hg in a matter of weeks. Such "malignant" hypertension will be fatal within a few months if unchecked by the use of drugs. Renovascular disease obstructing the large vessels of the kidney does not occur in more than 1 patient out of 20 with high blood pressure. Approximately one half of these can be treated by surgery with success.

There are a number of uncommon conditions associated with sustained high blood pressure. These include Cushing's disease, which usually affects women and is associated with a "moon face," obesity, acne, and polycythemia. It is due to the excessive production of cortisone and other glucocorticoids by an adrenal tumor or hyperplasia. If large amounts of cortical hormones are given to a normal person or a person having adrenal deficiency, a similar excessive weight development and blood-pressure increase can also be observed. Hyperaldosteronism or Conn's syndrome results when a benign adrenocortical adenoma pours out an excess of aldosterone, causing high blood-pressure levels and suppressing the blood renin and angiotensin. There is polyuria, weakness, increased serum sodium, and an increased circulating blood volume. It has been suggested that such tumors may represent malfunctions of the zona glomerulosa of the adrenals in response to sustained stimulation. Indeed, Gifford and Gunderson have recently presented the case for considering Cushing's disease to be a psychosomatic disorder. Certainly, Selye long ago described adenoma formation in the adrenal cortex of the chronically stimulated rodent.

A high salt intake may contribute to the development of severe hypertension. This mechanism may play a part in the great incidence of extremely high blood pressure in areas such as northern Japan, where the salt intake is high and high blood pressure in the older segment of the population is the rule. Such populations can have considerable kidney disease. As Shapiro has shown, hypertension from any cause that persists for long periods leads to an increased susceptibility of the kidneys to bacterial infection and eventual damage. Once such damage has developed, a high-salt diet will increase the severity of the high blood pressure, so completing the cycle.

Experimental Observations Demonstrating the Role of Subhypothalamic Mechanisms in the Development of High Blood Pressure

Hypertension can be produced in animals by methods that throw light on the mechanisms underlying the foregoing naturally occurring conditions. If the renal artery is constricted by means of a clamp that does not cut off the entire blood supply, then, as Goldblatt first showed, there will be a progressive elevation of blood pressure. This is made worse by giving salt and/or corticosteroid, which enhances salt retention. Indeed, desoxycorticosterone given with sufficient salt will cause hypertension in normal animals. The genetic constitution of the animal is important; Dahl has shown that in certain inbred strains of rat, the susceptibility can be increased to the point at which salt alone will induce hypertension. Finally, Okamoto in Japan has bred strains of rats that develop high blood pressure without either the added influence of salt or adrenal cortical hormone.

The resemblance of the foregoing disturbances to cases with deficient renal arterial supply or with an adrenal tumor is suggestive, but the mechanism of the increase in pressure is not yet clear. In the early stages, it may be related to an increase in cardiac output, which, in turn, is believed related to an increase in plasma volume, venoconstriction, and increased myocardial contractility. Later, a role is attributed to an increased resistance to flow through arteries whose distensibility has changed due to an altered sodium-and-water content of the walls.

Underlying the above changes may be an increase in the sympathetic nervous outflow due to exaggerated subcortical responses to environmental stimuli. The possible stimuli originating these changed levels of response are the subject of the ensuing sections of this chapter.

The development of extremely rapidly mounting so-called "malignant" hypertension is associated with demonstrably elevated levels of renin and gross retinal changes including exudates, hemorrhage, and optic nerve swelling or papilloedema. At autopsy, there is a renal arteriolar necrosis. Such cases throw light on the very common condition of essential hypertension. In this case, the vascular damage is far less. There is thickening of the media without necrosis and swelling; the pressures are lower, and renin levels are not measurably elevated. It is suggestive that the pressure level itself is the damaging agent that sets various vicious cycles into motion. Thus hypertrophy of the smooth muscle of the arterioles will result for purely mechanical reasons in an excessive response to a normal flow of sympathetic stimuli. This process may be reversible. Evidence is accumulating that, by using antihypertensive agents on a large scale, it is possible to reduce the incidence of the dangerous complications of high blood pressure. Thus, in Sweden, the mortality and morbidity rates from cerebral hemorrhage have fallen significantly, and it has been concluded that "patients under good control of their blood pressure are less at risk."

The functional disturbance in the later stages of experimental renal hypertension involves a return of the cardiac output to normal and an increase in peripheral resistance, with no change in heart rate or of blood volume. Because neither renal nor heart denervation nor even destruction of the spinal cord will affect severe renal hypertension, a humoral agent has been suspected. The theory is supported by various facts. For example, transplantation of a graft of ischemic kidney to the neck of a nephrectomized dog leads to hypertension, and renin can be demonstrated in the perfusate from the ischemic kidney.

The recent comprehensive review edited by Page and McCubbin epitomizes the successful effort to work out the complex reactions by which renin leads to the release of the polypeptide angiotensin from plasma globulin. Angiotensin is a potent pressor agent that, when continuously infused in subpressor amounts for several weeks, will lead to a labile hypertension in animals. This is most marked when they are alert, for the pressures are near normal when sleeping. There is some evidence that angiotensin intensifies the effects of sympathetic nerve activity and increases sensitivity to the catecholamines normally present in the organism. Although renin is not found in large amounts in the blood except in severe kidney damage, these results suggest that some clinical effects may be due to small, as yet nonmeasurable amounts of renin at work over long periods.

The release of renin may well be a response to direct stimulation of the sympathetic nerve supply to the juxtaglomerular complex, that, in turn, determines aldosterone production, so influencing sodium and, therefore, fluid retention. It is also possible that the increased sympathetic discharge has some direct effect upon sodium retention by the tubules. Since the release of renin in the intact animal appears to be related to sympathetic activity, this constitutes a positive feedback system with a probability of high blood pressure if any link in the chain is overactive. The factors controlling the reactions of the renin-angiotensin-aldosterone mechanism are still incompletely understood. However, Page and McCubbin suggest that the internal distribution of sodium may be important. It is already clear that hypertension can occur without high plasma renin levels and that the hypertensive effect of aldosterone does not parallel sodium-retaining activity.

In malignant hypertension, kidney function is significantly impaired, and there is an excess of aldosterone, probably because of the high renin-angiotensin production. However, it is also true that aldosterone levels can be very high in other conditions without any change in arterial pressure. It is known that even nonpressor doses of angiotensin will lead to an elevated aldosterone level, if given for several days, and aldosterone levels can be elevated in men and animals suffering from decreased blood volume. This may occur because decreased filling of the low-pressure system can change afferent impulses leading to sympathetic arousal and hence to increased renin levels in the blood. It is significant that the blood pressure is not necessarily elevated in such cases, despite the enhanced renin secretion. Here again, the presence of salt and its internal distribution appear to be critical factors whose underlying mechanism is not yet understood.

If a gross excess of salt is given, even normal animals will develop hypertension. In the rat, this occurs after drinking 1% salt solution for a year. The strains of animals that are susceptible to salt hypertension show an abnormally intense reactivity to angiotensin and nor-epinephrine. They are also more prone to develop renal hypertension if the renal artery is clamped.

The condition of animals suffering from experimental hypertension appears to be due to the release of renin by the kidney, but, as the preceding has indicated, this may be only the second stage of essential hypertension. In this common, naturally occurring condition, the first step may be an increased vascular response and sympathetic activity that, in turn, induces the kidney malfunction and renin release.

Such conclusions turn attention to the role of the nervous system and the possible effects of denervating the zones in the aorta and carotids carrying the baroreceptors. If this is done, chronic high blood pressure does indeed ensue. But it can be shown that, after the hypertension has persisted for some time, there is an adaptation of the responses so that the reflex is reset to operate at higher pressure levels. The mechanism underlying this change of sensitivity is not known, but the fact that it occurs suggests that the end organs in the adventitia of the great arteries are not the critical "barostat" controlling blood pressure that is set to higher levels in the essential hypertensive. Recent observations suggest that the olivary nuclei control the development of hypertension by permitting escape from control by the baroreceptors. Impulses coming down to the hind brain from the hypothalamus will prevent the fall in blood pressure that would otherwise occur on stimulating the carotid sinus region. This work provides a link between the physiological mechanisms controlling the cardiovascular system and the psychologically significant defense-alarm response, which Charvat, Dell, and Folkow have proposed as playing a central role in essential hypertension.

High Blood Pressure and Mechanisms From the Hypothalamus Upward Involving Higher Centers in Inducing High Blood Pressure

Only systolic arterial pressures will be discussed, not only because the data on this parameter are less subject to error than the data on diastolic pressure, but also because it is the height and duration of the systolic pressure in the vascular bed that are critical for the development of pathological changes. Indeed, even when a systolic pressure elevation occurs without any elevation of diastolic pressure, it is associated with a significant increase in the mortality from cardiovascular and renal disease. Recent work has established that the increased pressures found so commonly in the peripheral pulses of the aged are also present at the arch of the aorta. Only in those—like young children—whose elastic arterial tree is free from arteriosclerosis does a reflection in the elastic terminal arterioles lead to a building-up of the pressure wave as it is reflected from the periphery. Contrary to the generally accepted opinion, the rigid vessels of arteriosclerotic persons actually transmit a pulse wave of unchanged systolic pressure from the root of the aorta right out to the periphery, where the capacity of the small vessels to reflect the wave is impaired.

More than 90% of cases of high blood pressure start off without showing any signs of organ damage. The subject is "healthy." There are no symptoms, and the bodily functions are all normal; only the arterial pressure is elevated. But it has been indicated that, if the systolic pressure remains in the 180–200 mm Hg range for any significant period, there will be progressive damage of the blood vessels, including those of the kidney, heart, and brain. It appears that, regardless of the mechanism causing them, episodes of elevated vascular pressure that are repeated many times over a period of 10–30 years will result in generalized disease of the vascular bed and eventually lead to organ dysfunction.

As Smirk points out, it is rare that the young adult with essential hypertension has a high enough resting or basal blood pressure to cause symptoms. If, however, the physiologically determined pressure rises that occur with emotional and other stimuli are, as he says, "perched on top of high basal physiological levels," they may carry the final height of the blood pressure to degrees that are associated frequently with hypertensive disease. Perhaps as age advances, various organs gradually deteriorate under the influence of these repeated pressure elevations. One problem is that repeated periods of vasoconstriction enhance the kidney's susceptibility to infection. Another is a purely mechanical arteriolar hypersensitivity due to hypertrophy of the smooth muscle; yet another is arteriolar deterioration as a consequence of high local pressures. Once these processes have gone far enough in the kidney, there is set in motion the sequence of events that has been described briefly in the first part of this chapter and that is discussed in detail in the monographs by Page and McCubbin cited earlier. The sequence starts with renin release, which, in turn, leads to an exacerbation and perpetuation of the hypertension. Thus what commenced decades before as transient, innocuous elevations of blood pressure due to physiological causes can end as self-perpetuating hypertensive disease with eventual severe lesions in vital organs.

It becomes important to look above the hypothalamus for causes of often-repeated elevations of blood pressure. The brain is constantly receiving information from receptors both in the viscera and in the sense organs telling of the threat or the promise of support presented by the environment. The higher centers integrate this input so that a given stimulus has an effect upon a certain sensory projection area and gives rise to the appropriate motor response. In addition, there are cardiovascular response patterns due to inborn schemata that are set in motion by the activation of the brain stem reticular formation. As Folkow has emphasized, one of the most important of these is the defense-alarm reaction, which can be induced by stimulation of the anterior hypothalamus (Fig. 11-1). It puts the animal into a state appropriate for either attack or flight. It can be excited from the cortex and can be activated by situations that are not directly threatening but involve the need for alertness. It can be induced by conditioning an animal to anticipate stress by the repetitive association of some event with a painful stimulus. This is presumed to be due to stimulation of corticoreticular pathways. In addition, reticular deactivation or inhibition of the same defense-alarm reaction can also be induced from the cortex, if the organism perceives the environment as supportive and nurturant.

Folkow and Rubinstein have shown that, if an electrode implanted in the defense-alarm area in the lateral hypothalamus is mildly stimulated, signs of alertness without violent symptoms of attack or flight will appear. If these alerting stimuli are repeated again and again for days and weeks, a moderate, sustained hypertension ensues. This occurs despite the fact that the individual stimuli are set to last for no more than 10 seconds; nor do the stimuli cause the animal to show signs of fear or upset his eating and drinking patterns.

This "alerting" response can also be induced by symbolic stimuli. Thus Brod, *et al.*, have shown that mental arithmetic performed under the harassment of a time stress caused by a ticking metronome with which the subject is heckled to keep pace, will lead to a syndrome of hormonal and neurogenic cardiovascular changes that are typical of the defense-alarm state. They include an elevation of arterial pressure, increased heart rate and, often, cardiac output, and increased blood flow to the muscles, while the flow through the gastrointestinal tract and kidneys is radically reduced (Fig. 11-2).

In addition to the above pattern typical of autonomic nervous system arousal, a number of studies have shown an increase in the output of 17-hydroxycorticosteroids in persons who are experiencing a stimulation of the defense-alarm

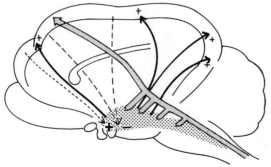

Fig. 11-1.—Schematic drawing of a mammalian brain, illustrating the location of the diencephalic defense-alarm center in the hypothalamus. The reticular formation *(coarse dotted shading)*, which is strongly influenced by the specific afferents running to the cortex *(heavy line with offshoots)*, sends stimuli to the cortex *(solid lines)*. The cortex, in turn, has both an activating and deactivating influence *(two types of broken lines)* on the defense-alarm reaction area in the hypothalamus, i.e., + and −. (Modified from Charvat, J., Dell, P., and Folkow, B.: Mental Factors and Cardiovascular Diseases, Cardiologia 44:124-141, Fig. 2, 1964.)

reaction. A fall in level occurs in response to soothing, relaxing inputs.

There is also an increase in catecholamine discharge. Furthermore, studies of adrenal enzymes show an increase in tyrosine hydroxylase, which is rate limiting in catecholamine synthesis, and in the phenylethanolamine transferase that converts nor-adrenalin to adrenalin. This increase occurs both in animals made hypertensive by sectioning of the buffer nerves and in hypertension following months of psychosocial stimulation. Since these enzyme changes take a significant length of time to develop, these results imply that the biochemical consequences of the increased sympathoadrenal drive do not merely involve a brief discharge of hormone, but prolonged readjustments of enzyme production as well.

The result of all these combined changes is, on the one hand, to sustain blood volume, mobilize glucose, and, in general, to prepare the organism for action, or, on the other hand, to turn the organism towards nurturance. Thus the three major efferent channels for the mobilization of the organism are all engaged by the alarm situation, which is as fully developed in man as in the most primitive mammals.

In the 1950's, Russian workers experienced with dogs that had been exposed to prolonged Pavlovian training reported a number of unequivocal cases of sustained high blood pressure. Special studies were initiated with monkeys and baboons that led to the conclusion that development of high blood pressure seemed to depend on interference with basic responses, such as the "sexual or the self-protective reflexes."

In a recent follow-up of the observation of the development of high blood pressure in chimpan-

Fig. 11-2.—The hemodynamic effects of emotional stress induced by doing mental arithmetic under the duress of a metronome. Cardiac output increases together with systemic arterial pressure. Despite the increase in renal vascular resistance, the resistance to blood flow through the muscles of the forearm decreases. (From Brod, J., et al.: Clin. Sc. 18:269, 1959.)

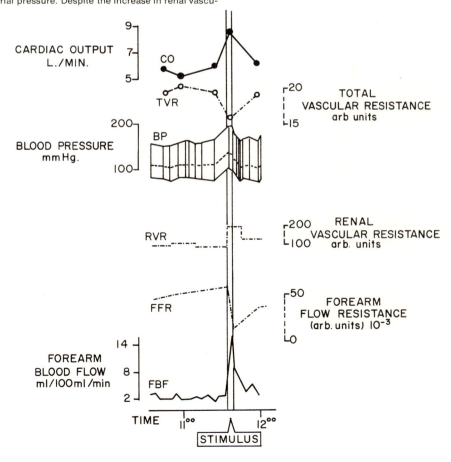

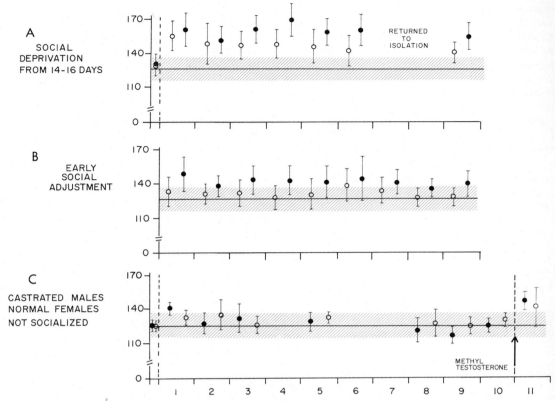

Fig. 11-3.—Observations of systolic arterial pressure of groups of 34 CBA mice in interconnected box systems. Equal numbers of males and females were placed in the system when 4 months old. Pressures were measured weekly in most cases. Open circles: females; solid circles: males. Horizontal band represents one standard deviation above and below the pressures of the normally boxed sibling CBA's. The first set of readings before the first month were obtained before placement in the box system.

A, thirty-four males and females were maintained in isolation in pint jars until 4 months old. They were then placed in a 6-box system where fighting and tail biting were persistent and severe, resulting in epilation of tail and rump. There were only a limited number of pregnancies and no infant survival beyond 24 hours due to cannibalism. Hypertension persisted for months despite return to the minimal psychosocial stimulation of isolation.

B, thirty-four males and females in equal numbers had lived together in this 6-box system from birth. There was vigorous fighting, but it stopped short of tail biting. There was no scarring or epilation. Pregnancies occurred and many litters survived to weaning age.

C, seventeen males were castrated at 12 weeks and, when 10 months old, were put with an equal number of intact females of the same age into a 6-box intercommunicating system. There was no fighting or other evidence of antagonistic behavior. When given methyltestosterone, the fur became disarrayed and the arterial pressure of both males and females increased. Some tail scarring—but no rump epilation—suggested moderate fighting. No sexual behavior was observed. (From Henry, J. P., and Cassel, J. C.: Am. J. Epidemiol. 90(No. 3):181, Fig. 4, 1969.)

zees undergoing intensive training in preparation for space flight, mice were placed in an intercommunicating box system. This was done both with normal mature siblings that had been raised together and with animals that had been isolated from weaning until maturity to deliberately stunt the development of their social responses. Weight loss, failure to breed, cannibalism of the newborn, adrenal hypertrophy, thymus atrophy, and chronic blood pressure elevation to a mean of some 160 mm Hg developed in the previously isolated animals as a result of intense mutual stimulation. There was a conspicuous failure of the male animals in this group to respect each other's need for territory and to control their aggressive responses (Fig. 11-3-A). The contrast with animals in a similar box system that had lived together from birth was clear-cut (Fig. 11-3-B). The "socialized" animals raised with each other wrestled and "boxed" with energy, but they did not attack and bite each other in the perineum and base of the tail as did the socially deprived animals. Unlike the deprivates, which killed their young, they raised healthy litters. The hypertension of the socially deprived animals was sustained, and it did not subside on returning them for several months to isolation.

If the males were castrated, they lost their drive to develop territory, and they lived even more peaceably with each other than did previously socialized normal males. Pressures of the members of a mixed colony of 17 normal females and the same number of castrates remained well within normal limits in an intercommunicating box system for a period of nine months. However, on giving testosterone to these males, blood pressures rose in both sexes, and there was evidence of fighting (Fig. 11-3-C).

Fig. 11-4.—Blood pressure elevation of male CBA mice with coffee brewed for human use as their only fluid.
Upper diagram: Males mixed together from separate boxes at 4 months fight and show significant pressure elevation when caged 8 to a standard box. Their pressure is greater when on coffee than when on water.
Middle diagram: Siblings caged 8 to a standard 23 × 11 × 11 cm box and drinking coffee show a significant pressure elevation. On water, they remain normotensive. Siblings similarly boxed and on decaffeinated coffee show no significant rise in pressure.
Lower diagram: Animals isolated in pint fruit jars show a modest pressure elevation in the later months on coffee. (From Henry, J. P., and Cassel, J. C.: Am. J. Epidemiol. 90(No. 3):182, Fig. 5, 1969.)

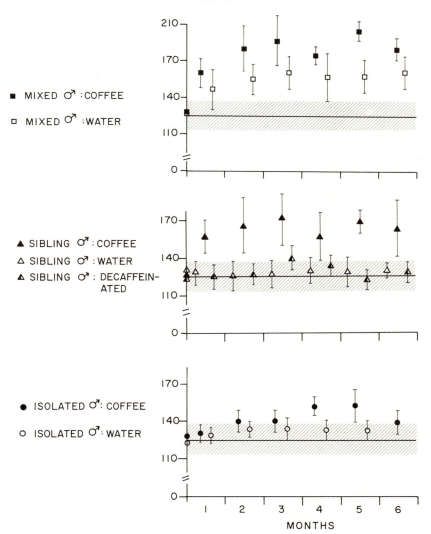

Further, if animals are put in circumstances that stimulate cortical activity, then the interaction of both socially adjusted and deprived animals becomes more violent. Animals raised from birth with each other and separated as to sex retain low systemic arterial pressures of the order of 120 mm Hg all of their lives. But if the beverage "coffee" containing the usual 70 mg of caffeine per 100 cc is substituted for their drinking water (Fig. 11-4), their pressure will rise to the 150–160 mm Hg level; whereas that of socially deprived animals that were already fighting will rise still further to the 180 mm Hg range.

These various animal observations suggest that, in a constant physical environment, the systemic arterial pressure of a group is a measure of the symbolic and the direct physical stimuli received during social interaction, and that early experience plays a role in determining the arousal value of the stimuli perceived. There is also evidence of such effects in the epidemiology of human hypertension.

Role of Various Environmental Factors in the Development of High Blood Pressure

Introduction

A number of factors that have long been suspected of playing a role in the development of essential hypertension should be discussed in the light of recent work, much of which is summarized in the text entitled *The Epidemiology of Hypertension*. They include exercise, the intake of salt, the amount of fat and protein in the diet, malnutrition, disease, obesity, the influence of heredity, and smoking. It appears that some of these factors protect against and some may contribute to essential hypertension in its later stages, but none is dominant or necessary for its initial development.

Exercise

Exercise, in itself, does not appear to play a determinant role in the development of high blood pressure. For if it were critical, it might be expected that older people living in communities in which there is much physical exertion might show lower or higher pressures than those in communities in which there were fewer physical demands. In practice, at the age of 60, there are groups that fit into all 4 categories.

HIGH EXERCISE WITH HIGH BLOOD PRESSURE.—The Indians working in the hilly Assamese tea plantations are exposed to a lifetime of considerable exertion; nevertheless, their blood pressure at 60 years is approximately 150 mm Hg for both sexes.

In the sugar cane plantations of the Caribbean island of St. Kitts, the male workers average 150 mm Hg and the females, 160 mm Hg. The same is true for Jamaican hill farmers in which the male pressure is 150 mm Hg and the female, 172 mm Hg.

LOW EXERCISE WITH HIGH BLOOD PRESSURE.—There are relatively sedentary groups that can be compared with the above. Czechoslovakian clerks, doctors, lawyers, technicians, and teachers at 60 years have a mean pressure of 160 mm Hg, in contrast with Czech farmers and industrial workers whose mean is 148 mm Hg. The women in the United States general population at 60 years are on the whole not exposed to heavy exercise demands. Their mean pressure is 150 mm Hg. Professional workers in India—doctors, lawyers, and managers—average 140 mm Hg, as contrasted with the peasant blood pressure of 120 mm Hg. Not only can high blood pressure be found in both the high and low physical activity groups, but the same picture can be presented in reverse.

HIGH EXERCISE WITH LOW BLOOD PRESSURE.—The Mayan Indians of the mountain country near Lake Atitlan in Guatemala have recently been studied. They work on steep farms and carry large burdens long distances on hilly paths. The mean systolic blood pressure of the 60-year-old males is 120 mm Hg. The same 120 mm Hg was found in the 60- to 70-year-old males in the Indian mountain village of Macusani in the Andes.

The vigorous, canoe-loving Polynesian males of the Cook Islands atoll, Puka Puka, in the Pacific have a blood pressure of 105 mm Hg at 60 years.

So, too, have aged African bushmen hunters.

LOW EXERCISE WITH LOW BLOOD PRESSURE.—Examples can be found in more sedentary groups, such as members of the Indian Statistical Institute in Calcutta whose mean pressure at 60 years is 130 mm Hg. Female, rural northern Indians by reason of the practice of purdah are largely confined to a small house and courtyard, yet their pressures are 120 mm Hg at 60 years. The staffs of the American hospitals in China in the 1920's, both doctors and nurses, did not have strenuous physical duties. However, at 50 years their systolic pressures averaged 110 mm Hg. Of the group of German contemplative monks studied in the 1930's, the Trappists took moderate and Carthusians very little exercise; yet at 60 years, both had an average systolic pressure of 120 mm Hg. The relatively inactive ruling elders of the Kenyan nomadic Samburu tribe have a mean systolic pressure of 112 mm Hg at 60 years.

These examples are sufficient to indicate that variations in exercise alone are not adequate explanations for variations in blood pressure levels in different populations.

Salt

Salt is eaten in large amounts by rice-growing Buddhist farmers of Thailand (20 gm/diem); yet, a recent nutritional survey found them to have uniformly low blood pressure, i.e., 120 mm Hg at 60 years. By contrast, there is much high blood pressure among the peasantry of the crowded sugar plantations of St. Kitts (Fig. 11-5). They are descendants of former slaves, and their economic and social position has changed little in the last 100 years. The salt intake of these people has been recently evaluated. They drink stored rainwater, and their total salt consumption is one half that of the Thai farmers.

Salt intake may well play a role in the very high blood pressure of the older farm population of Akita on Japan's northern island. However, it can hardly be the initiating cause, for the 18 gms taken per diem is not as much as in the diet of the low-pressured Thai farmers; it is, in fact, only 3–4 gms higher than the intake in Japanese provinces with a far lower incidence of high blood pressure. Further, the freely salt-using coastal natives of New Guinea have the same blood pressure as the salt-hungry natives of the high country of the interior.

It is added evidence that the detailed evaluation during the Framingham study of the various factors concerned with the development of cardiovascular disease in a population of a Massachusetts town has shown no relationship between urinary sodium excretion and blood pressure level. While a high-salt diet probably plays an important role in the deterioration of those suffering from high blood pressure, it does not appear to commonly determine the onset of the condition.

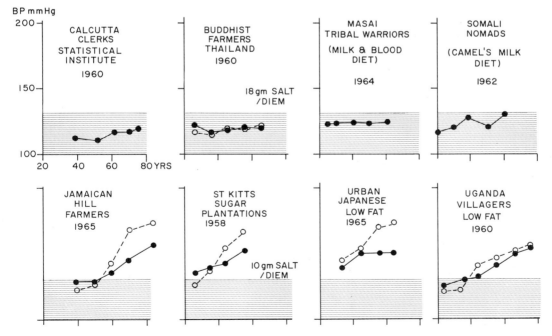

Fig. 11-5.—Current evidence points away from a dominant role for exercise, salt, or fat in the determination of the asymptomatic rate of rise of blood pressure with age. Thus the four pairs of curves contrast groups without significant pressure elevation that perform little exercise at work or have a high salt or a high fat intake with groups with higher pressures that engage in heavy physical labor or have a low salt or fat intake. (From Henry, J. P., and Cassel, J. C.: Am. J. Epidemiol. 90(No. 3):184, Fig. 6, 1969.)

Fat and Protein

The last two pairs of diagrams in Figure 11-5 refer to two groups of Africans who still live in their ancient and traditional style. The Masai warriors eat a high-animal-fat diet of milk and meat, as do the Somali nomads in the desert country to the north. On occasion, as much as 65% of their caloric intake is in animal fat.

The Masai diet is stated to contain 300 gm protein and 160 gm fat per diem. These figures apply during the season when food supplies are adequate. In the "famine months," they fall sharply. Both groups of men had been little disturbed at the time of measurement by Western technology or social patterns, but continued to follow their old patterns of living and to hold to their ancient beliefs. Their freedom from high blood pressure is not shared by the urban Japanese living on a low-fat diet, nor is it shared by socially and economically moderately advanced Ugandan villagers living a few miles from the modern medical school and other facilities of the town of Kampala. These people live on a largely carbohydrate diet with plantain (green banana) as the staple food; protein and fat contribute relatively small proportions to the total caloric intake (Fig. 11-5).

Protein was very high in the traditional meat-eating diet of the Eskimo, for they used much of the fat from their catch for heating and lighting. This does not hold for the pastoral nomadic tribes, such as the Samburu, who, like the Masai and Somali groups, live on meat and milk. The animal fat intake of the warriors reaches some 200–400 gm a day for two thirds of the year, for they drink up to 7 liters of milk with a 5% fat content per day. Only during the dry season, as milk production fails, does the intake drop; then they subsist on a low-calorie intake of meat only. The uniformly low pressures of all these people, when living in their traditional style, speak against animal fat having a controlling influence on blood pressure. This is not to deny that its potential role in the development of renal vascular atherosclerosis could, however, determine the eventual development of renoprival hypertension.

Malnutrition

As for nutritional levels in general, it has been reported that in starvation the blood pressure will fall. However, the changes are moderate even in severe famine. A group of starving Europeans showed a fall from 132 to 125 mm Hg systolic in 20- to 29-year-olds, and, at the age of 60 to 75, the fall was from 164 to 144 mm Hg. The rise of blood pressure with age was thus still apparent. Studies in malnourished Javanese villagers have shown a moderate increase in blood pressure with age.

It has indeed been claimed that the low blood pressure of various native groups was an expression of chronic or periodic malnutrition and disease. With regard to the former, the nutritional state of young adult Masai has been evaluated, and they have been shown, despite their slender build, to have the same body weight as British men and women of the same age. Two thirds of the Masai children of both sexes were described as in excellent physical condition and the majority of the rest as satisfactory. The Pacific atoll-living Gilbertese have been examined from the viewpoint of body build. At 20–30 years, both these and the New Guinea highlanders averaged an ideal weight for their height.

Indeed, when arm circumference is taken as an index of bulk, the Gilbert Islanders are found to be somewhat larger than Welsh coal miners. However, there is no change in this dimension either in the islanders or the New Guinea natives with age. When there is an increase of blood pressure with age, it is not due solely to the effect of using a cuff of constant size on arms of varying girth. Only when the arm is very large and flabby, as in gross obesity, is there a significant effect of arm girth on the blood-pressure readings. According to an extensive, recent survey of the United States population, the same conclusion was reached that larger arm girth is not alone responsible for the high blood pressure of the obese.

The idea that certain groups were suffering from malnutrition may have crept in because, unlike the Europeans and Americans, many of whom become obese as they age, these people's body weight stays unchanged throughout their lives, as does their systolic blood pressure. The facts are that the nutrition of the average Masai and Samburu, Ponapean and Gilbert Islander is not inadequate, and the failure of their blood pressure to rise with age is not an expression of physiological inadequacy.

Disease

The suggestion that the lower blood pressure of these peoples might be due to tuberculosis was dismissed by the clinician studying the lean and active Samburu with the statement that clinical examination had excluded any cases with pulmonary disease. He further dryly commented that "if you had seen these people herding camels you would know this is not a community universally afflicted with pulmonary tuberculosis."

The same applies to the Gilbertese and Ponapean Pacific islanders who for decades have had medical services adequate to pick up and report on the prevalence of such conditions. It is this relative adequacy of contemporary medical services that permits dismissal of the suggestion that the rarity of high pressures among older Fijians and Gilbertese might be due to an early selective mortality among those who might develop high pressures. It appears that what hypertension is seen coming from nomadic tribal groups is usually of renal origin; when essential hypertension does develop, it runs a normal and not an accelerated course.

The idea that the low blood pressure and failure of the pressure to rise with age in a population might be due to anemia secondary to hookworm infestation was raised following a 1947 study showing uniformly low blood pressure of the Ponapean islanders living in the Eastern Carolines in the Pacific. More recent medical surveys that have accompanied the blood pressure surveys have eliminated this possibility in a number of groups. Thus the infestation rate with parasites was less than 20% in Masai women, while New Guinean highlanders have, together with their good nutrition, the high hemoglobin levels to be expected of the residents of a country at 6,000 to 9,000 feet.

Indeed clinical experience shows that anemia and chronic infections, such as tuberculosis, are not associated with uniformly low pressures in ambulatory subjects. In keeping with the above, a moderate reduction in food intake has been shown in the Framingham study to have no direct association with blood pressure.

Obesity

The question of the role of obesity in inducing high blood pressure has been thoroughly reviewed in a study of the difference between the Australians, who show the same increasing weight and incidence of high blood pressure with age as the Western Europeans, and the New Guinea tribesmen, who do not. The heavier Australians do have, on the average, higher blood pressure; but to increase the blood pressure by 10 mm Hg, would require some 40 pounds of overweight. Further, in dockside stevedores of European extraction, it was found that by the critical sixth decade there was no further correlation between blood pressure and obesity, so that at least at this age, the blood pressure is predominantly controlled by other factors. Recently the population of women in a city near Warsaw was divided into underweight, normal, and overweight persons. Figure 11-6 shows that, although the systolic pressure of the obese averages some

Fig. 11-6.—Comparison of mean systolic pressures of normal, overweight, and underweight women. (From Alexsandrow, D.: Studies on the Epidemiology of Hypertension in Poland, in Stamler, J., Stamler, R., and Pullman, T. N. (eds.): *The Epidemiology of Hypertension* [New York: Grune & Stratton, Inc., 1967].)

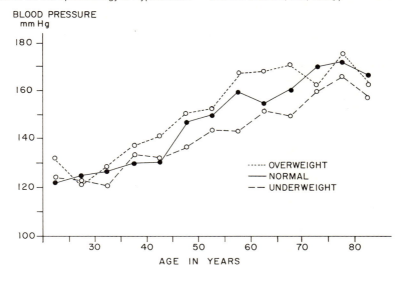

10–15 mm Hg higher than that of the underweight, this does not account for the change in blood pressure with age, but rather represents an added factor.

HEREDITY

In a continuation of their long-standing friendly controversy, the problem of the influence of heredity in the etiology of essential hypertension has recently been reviewed by both Platt and Pickering. Platt, today, considers that the mechanisms underlying that complex known as essential hypertension must be too various to be accounted for by a single gene. However, he thinks that single, unique conditions such as pheochromocytoma might be determined by a simpler genetic mechanism. Pickering considers that arterial pressure is inherited polygenically as a tendency to high or low pressures at all ages. He does not regard the rate of rise of pressure with age to be inherited and considers that the environment determines pressures in middle age and beyond. He urges effort to identify those factors in the environment that affect this rise, citing those that operate through the mind as being perhaps the most important.

Recently, a set of prospective observations of blood pressures of 500 insurance company employees for periods ranging up to 30 years has been published. It presents varying rates of rise with age, ranging from zero to the most extreme cases in a continuously graded distribution. These results accord with Pickering's hypothesis; for the opposing viewpoint would predict that, in such longitudinally collected data, most slopes would be close to zero, with a minority having distinctly faster rates of rise.

Discussing Platt's remarkable cases of hypertension in identical twins, Pickering points out that one can argue that, just because they are so alike, they tend to share their lives much more than nonidentical twins. Thus their identity of blood pressure may merely be an expression of identity of response to the environment. It is for this reason that the role of heredity in determining family pressures is very hard to ascertain because the child shares his early environment with the family, as well as his genes.

It is known that the variance of blood pressure is considerably less within families than between families; i.e., elevated blood pressures tend to run in families. None of the children investigated were younger than two years; the question was raised whether there was a specific age range at which this effect first appears. The answer would appear to be very early, in view of another recent study of the effects of the parental environment upon the blood pressure of infants sleeping in their beds at home. By the use of a pretested, semistructured interview schedule, relative stress ratings were assigned to different families. The data plot of this preliminary study in 43 infants, the majority of whom were less than 1 year of age, fitted a linear regression with the most stressful environments rating an excess of some 10 mm Hg.

Nevertheless, animal studies using inbred rats and others using various inbred strains of mice demonstrate that heredity is most important as one of the determinants of blood-pressure level. However, the phenomenon of the influence of psychosocial stress upon blood pressure is a general one, having been demonstrated in rodents, carnivores, and the lower primates. In man, both a rise and a lack of rise with age can be found in every racial group in which it has been studied. It is probable that the extent of the rise is determined by the individual's genetic predisposition to respond to environmental insults by vasoconstrictive reactions. However, people similarly predisposed (at least as measured by belonging to the same race) who are not exposed to these environmental insults (as measured by belonging to insulated cohesive cultures) do not show a rise with age.

It must further be noted that, in addition to the influence of heredity, studies with animals suggest very early experience may determine the later arousal value of environmental stimuli.

SMOKING

The Framingham study confirms the already well-known fact that smoking does not lead to high blood pressure; if anything, smoking is found to be associated with lower-than-average values.

Role of Psychosocial Stimuli and the Increase of Blood Pressure of Human Populations

PRESSURE CHANGES WITH AGE IN DIFFERENT COMMUNITIES

Impressive evidence of the role of environmental stimuli was the finding by Graham in 1943 of high blood pressure (i.e., 180 mm Hg or more) in over 30% of a victorious battalion resting on the beaches after 2 years of continuous mobile warfare in the Libyan Desert. In the course of a few weeks, their pressures started to return to normal. Miasnikov observed a similar epidemic of high blood pressure during the siege and bombardment of Leningrad. Figure 11-7 presents an example of the opposite effect. It is based on work published in the 1920's showing that the blood pressure of two groups of American nurses and doctors, all of whom had worked for years in mission hospitals in China, had fallen significantly on moving from America to China. That this was not a result merely of "regression to the mean" can be seen from the fact that, at all levels of initial blood pressure, a greater proportion of individuals showed a drop rather than a rise in pressure on moving to China. It was the opinion of the American physicians reporting on the case that the fall had something to do with the culture of the Chinese during the 1920's. At that time, the Chinese populace regarded their culture and their environment as "the natural order of things." Possibly the favorable "ambiance" in China, including the role in which they saw themselves as missionary hospital staff, decreased the anxiety level of these American men and women and increased their sense of self-esteem.

In Figure 11-8, a series of observations made on a number of social groups is arrayed to show the variations in the rate of rise of blood pressure with age.

During the past 20 years, a large number of such cross-sectional blood pressure surveys has been made at single points in time for different populations all over the world. The measurements have involved either a sampling or, in the case of small groups, the entire population. Everyone is measured at one session; the method has the advantage of applying the same technique to all subjects. The disadvantage of such cross-sectional studies is that they ignore the fact that the experience of the older members will stretch back through 50 more years of the group's history than that of the younger members.

A theoretical drawback to making inferences concerning the relationship of age to blood pressure levels from cross-sectional data is that the failure of blood pressure to rise with age might

Fig. 11-7.—A majority of American nurses and doctors working in two Chinese mission hospitals in the 1920's showed a decrease of casual systolic blood pressure below stateside values. Possible reasons for this in terms of changes in psychosocial stimulation are presented in the text. (From Henry, J. P., and Cassel, J. C.: Am. J. Epidemiol. 90(No. 3):188, Fig. 8, 1969.)

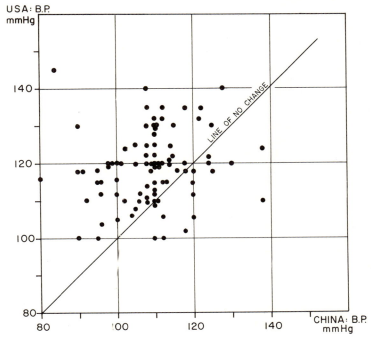

188 THE CIRCULATION: AN INTEGRATIVE PHYSIOLOGIC STUDY

simply be a reflection of selective survival. It could be argued that the lack of rise of blood pressure with age in some of the societies illustrated in Figure 11-8 can be explained on this basis, especially as the level of medical care in these particular societies is likely to be low. As already stated, such an argument does not hold where medical observations would be sufficient to exclude this factor. It does not apply where there is a rise in blood pressure with age in groups that presumably have equally poor medical care facilities, e.g., hypertensive farm populations in Japan; it does not apply where there is no pressure increase with age and medical care is good, e.g., U.S. Naval aviators and arctic industrial city inhabitants.

Despite the nonrepresentative nature of many of the groups studied, the differences in the rate of rise of blood pressure can often be linked sufficiently meaningfully to the social history of the group to give credence to the hypotheses of Scotch and Geiger, who have related the rise in blood pressure with age to psychosocial stress.

Eighteen pressure curves have been selected.

Their characteristics permit their juxtaposition in six vertical columns, each column being made up of three examples. From top to bottom, each trio is arrayed in order of rate of rise of blood pressure with age. From left to right, the first two sets involve Americans and Western Europeans, and Russians, Poles, and Czechs, respectively. The next set presents Amerindians, followed by persons of Negro descent, Japanese and Chinese, and, finally, Indians, both in India and outside the country. A brief caption in each diagram epitomizes the origin of that particular survey.

These studies were undertaken by different observers, and obviously no standardization of measurement technique was possible. Some of the differences shown can then be due to observer variation. It seems unlikely, though, that this could account for the marked and regular differences shown in the relationship between age and blood-pressure level. For these differences to be due to observer variation would mean that the observers in the top six studies were systematically underreading pressures, particularly in

Fig. 11-8. — Contrasting rates of change of blood pressure with age can be found in all races. In general, blood pressure is lower where the culture is stable, traditional forms are honored, and the group members are secure in their roles and adapted to them by early experience. (From Henry, J. P., and Cassel, J. C.: Am. J. Epidemiol. 90(No. 3):189, Fig. 9, 1969.)

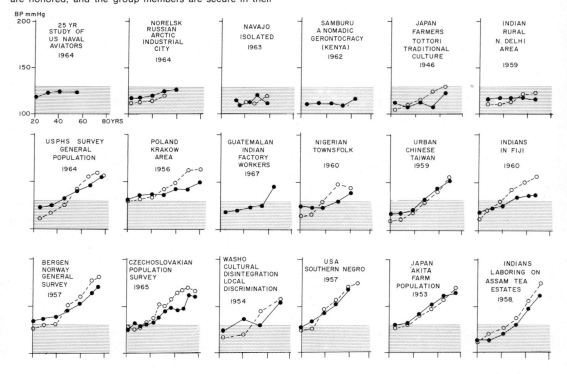

old-age groups, in comparison with observers of the middle or bottom six studies. Such a proposition, while theoretically feasible, appears most unlikely.

All the work is relatively recent; indeed, one half of the observations have been made in the last eight years. The distinction between them does not depend on the presence or absence of a high state of technology and social sophistication; rather it appears to turn on the issue whether the society or group has an established tradition with a social structure that remains unchallenged during the lifetime of the oldest subjects. It is during childhood, adolescence, and early adult life that society inculcates its value systems. Stress develops when the aging individual finds himself or herself in a social milieu to which it is hard to adapt because these values are not supported. Typically, this occurs after a social and cultural revolution or when he is away from his homeland.

Contrasting the top, intermediate, and bottom rows, we find that in general this thesis holds. The U.S. Naval aviators were a select group of 1,000 men who entered flying training during World War II. Careful testing chose only men thoroughly adapted from youth to the demands of a technological society.

We may hazard the guess that the population of Norelsk is also composed of self-selected persons, well adapted by early experience to their life in an arctic industrial environment. The elderly, isolated Navajo were persons who had elected to stay in their ancient homeland and continue their traditional culture. The Samburu have been recently the subject of a detailed and insightful anthropological study. They are a well-integrated and traditional group of pastoral nomads in the northern Kenyan desert country. Related to the Masai, they are ruled by elders and still have a warrior caste; they are living in an isolated ecological niche, relatively undisturbed by the social and technological revolution in the world around them. A low set of pressures with no significant rise with age is seen in the data from a small farming village near the northern coast of Japan. It is believed that these people had retained much of their traditional culture and, at the time of measurement, had not been exposed to the same intensity of change that has swept over the cities and countryside of Japan in the last 20 years. A similar picture is found in recent observations of the blood pressure of a group of villagers in the countryside near New Delhi.

The contrast between the first set of six curves, which remain without a major increase with age; those of the Norwegian city of Bergen, surveyed in 1957; and those for an extensive survey of the general population of Czechoslovakia, made in 1964, is clear-cut. The next in the set with the highest pressures is of data showing the rise in the disintegrating, formerly migratory Washo tribe, evicted by sociocultural events and economic pressures from their homeland in the Lake Tahoe area and living in squatters' shacks outside Carson City. Similarly, the constant blood pressure of the Samburu Kenyan Negroes may be contrasted with a detailed 1957 survey of blood pressures of Negroes in the southern United States. The elevation of pressure among elderly persons living on the increasingly uneconomic farms of the northern Japanese province of Akita can be contrasted with the traditional farming group in nearby Tottori province 20 years before. Finally, there is a sharp rate of rise of pressure of indentured laborers expatriated to Assam from India a generation ago. In their new location, they lost many of their caste affiliations and much of the traditional Hindu culture, as they worked on the rigidly controlled tea plantations in Assam.

Interpolated between the six extremes above and below, comes the general population of the United States, which perhaps today is, at length, adapting to the (for them) 100-year-old technological revolution and developing new traditions to deal with a science-based culture. The next two diagrams, disparate as they seem, i.e., the area around Krakow and a factory in the Guatemalan highland country town of Quezaltenango employing Indians, nevertheless, have in common rural people who, while adapting to cultural change, still have strong traditions from the past. Nigerian townsfolk and the urban Chinese in Taiwan represent people who, while seeking to adjust to great changes within their lifetime, also retain some traditional ties. The final diagram, of the expatriate colony of Indians in Fiji, represents men and women who have a good measure of social satisfaction, yet live in racial conflict with the native Fijians. Born on the island and adapted to their new status as members of this pleasant community, they have, however, lost, for better or for worse, the complex caste structure in which their traditions as socially integrated and religiously oriented orthodox Hindus would have been embedded two generations ago.

Analysis of Groups with Unexpected Blood Pressure Changes with Age

A deleterious social situation in which high blood pressure might appear could be one in which aspirations are blocked, meaningful human intercourse is restricted, and the outcome of important events in the lives of individuals is uncertain. Most social situations inevitably lead to repetitive stimuli. These, if they are symbolically important events, lead to blood pressure responses. Even if a change that occurs in the value system or dogmas of the group of which he is a member is a positive and realistic one, the older or less-favored individual often cannot adapt, and he overresponds to the event. The schema or pattern by which the event has now become an inappropriate autonomic stimulus for him was learned and fixed during his early experience.

For each person, his aspirations and related meaningful events will differ in accordance with the exact circumstances in which he grew up. In a deleterious situation, he will experience repetitive hypothalamic arousals involving the defense-alarm reaction, similar to those of Folkow and Rubinstein's rats. They have shown that their cumulative effects eventually lead to a sustained elevation of blood pressure.

This hypothesis of Folkow and Rubinstein has been used to explain the results of an 11-year prospective study of the role of the interaction of personality and stress in the pathogenesis of essential hypertension. This work is especially important because it arrives at the same conclusions as earlier studies that, however, lacked the advantage of a longitudinal approach. It was found that prehypertensive college women were more likely to experience abrasive, tense, and hostile interactions with other people than a control group with lower pressure. Significantly, they were less attractive, accepted the feminine role less readily, and had more unsatisfactory marriages. Showing less social poise and ease, they are described as having a provocative "chip-on-the-shoulder attitude" and yet tried to hide their emotions, which, when aroused, lasted unduly long. Such personality characteristics might well have been determined by non-nurturant features of their parental and adolescent environments. Individuals of this "temperament" could be expected to adjust less gracefully to progressive change or deficiency in their sociocultural environment than the less "abrasive" controls with their superior social integration.

It may well be a related difference in interaction between personality and environment that determines the markedly different rates of blood pressure increment per annum described for a 30-year prospective study of insurance firm employees. The presumably more adaptable and more favorably socially situated "senior officers" of the firm had a rate of rise of systolic blood pressure of only 0.6 mm Hg/annum, i.e., less than 20 mm Hg in 30 years; whereas that for the firm's clerical workers was 1.9 mm Hg, and that for clerical workers with stomach ulcer was a formidable 2.9 mm Hg/annum or 87 mm Hg in 30 years.

The foregoing throws some light on the puzzling data shown in Figure 11-9.

The first pair of diagrams deals with a study in the 1930's of the blood pressures of convicts and guards at San Quentin maximum security prison in California. There is an apparent paradox here in that the guards have more pressure elevation than the prisoners. However, this study was carried out when the prison administration was moving from a somewhat repressive and authoritarian to a strongly liberal humanitarian bias. Earlier, no doubt, the pressures of the guards and the prisoners might have been reversed. At the point in time of the survey, however, the prisoners had relative security and more hope for the future. The guards, on the other hand, may have experienced frustration at the change in traditions, as well as anxieties generated by the fear that the prisoners' new mood demanded enhanced vigilance.

The contrast between the blood pressures of Trappist monks in Bavarian monasteries a generation ago and those of American contemplative monks today may be related to the fact that the Christian church is currently going through a period of intense self-evaluation, as evidenced by the Second Vatican Council. The fact that the Trappist rule of silence has recently been relaxed would suggest that the older members of this small social group may feel a challenge to the roots of their faith. Certainly, the abbots report opposition from the older monks who resent any departure from tradition.

The next set of curves in Figure 11-9 is for

HIGH BLOOD PRESSURE

two small Pacific islands, both populated by Polynesians living more or less in the traditional style. Puka Puka is a tiny atoll group in a large lagoon, isolated by hundreds of miles of ocean. The few hundred inhabitants are living in their ancient homeland and following a traditional culture that has been relatively undisturbed, despite the upheavals of centuries of Western technological invasion of the Pacific. Niihau is one of the last refuges of traditionalist Hawaiians seeking a place to follow their vanishing cultural patterns. A privately owned and autocratically controlled island, its inhabitants are reported as having difficulty in partaking freely in the life of the nearby, larger Hawaiian islands. The fact that the oldsters' pressures are lower than those of younger men may be a reflection of the characteristics of a cross-sectional survey. Other surveys show such a falling-off of pressure with older members. They were small, traditionally oriented groups in which the younger persons were experiencing conflict between the attractions of the nearby, technologically advanced culture and their loyalty to their parental traditions.

The final diagrams of Figure 11-9 are for two contrasting metropolitan populations, which were both measured approximately 16 years ago. The English data are derived from approximately 1,000 outpatients of a big London hospital who were complaining of minor illnesses and conditions not directly related to the cardiovascular system or blood pressure; i.e., they were chosen at random from cases attending the dental, skin disease, and varicose vein clinics. Coming from the less successful classes, they were living in a depressed urban area with run-down housing in west-central London.

The data from Russia are from a comprehensive study in which over 40,000 healthy working people were measured. They ranged from engineers and administrators to cashiers, bookkeepers, salespeople, and telecommunications workers; the former, in general, had lower pressures than the latter. It has already been indicated that diet or exercise are not likely to be responsible for the sharp difference between the two sets of curves. Pressure elevations in still-healthy persons have been attributed by Russian

Fig. 11-9.—The diets of the populations involved in each of these pairs of curves are approximately the same. The level of psychosocial stimulation might also be interpreted as similar or even as higher in one or more of those in the upper row. These apparent anomalies are discussed in the text. (From Henry, J. P., and Cassel, J. C.: Am. J. Epidemiol. 90(No.3):193, Fig. 10, 1969.)

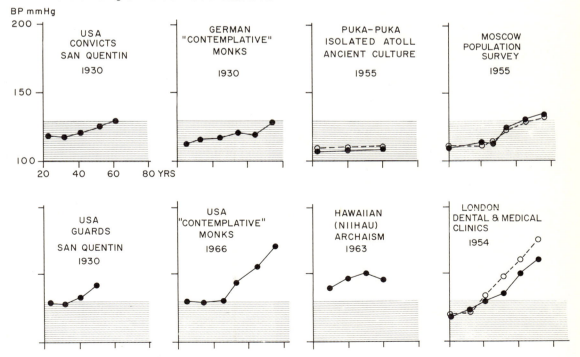

authorities to "difficulties in living, working, and housing conditions and to unfavorable aspects of family life." Evidence accumulated over the years has led these authorities to propose a theory of the "psychoemotional" origins of high blood pressure and to speak of hypertension to some extent as the "atonement" for "civilization." It remains to be seen whether the population in Moscow found adaptation to its social milieu less difficult and demanding than did these particular Londoners.

Certainly, animal experimental evidence shows that, if the defense-alarm reaction is repeatedly alerted, it will cause prolonged sympathetic arousal and sustained high blood pressure. Such may be the case in persons living in a milieu for which their culture and early experience gives them no adequate preparation. Such an environment can, of course, be overwhelming for the best defenses if the stimuli are sufficiently intense. Perhaps the World War II Libyan campaign previously mentioned was such an example, for in warfare the sympathetic system receives a very severe and prolonged stimulation.

Figure 11-10 is an illustration of a situation that appears to support this theory of the etiology of hypertension. A recent World Health Organization-sponsored survey indicates that the mortality from this condition is far higher in some South American cities than in others; the data suggest a relation with the rate at which they are growing. Certainly, a high growth rate can be taken to imply a probability of inadequate housing and a need for facilities such as public transportation, schools, hospitals, and even stores, plus a high influx of immigrants, i.e., those unused to the demands and expectations of city life.

Strong and repeated threatening stimuli may result from such competitive and unfavorably disordered situations. The aged frequently suffer in the competition. A significant percentage of the aged in the "exploding" populations of such cities will fail to achieve the goals they desire in spite of all their striving and effort. The stimulation of the sympathetic system that they will experience may well be sustained and intense and lead to unfavorable responses, as outlined in the beginning of this chapter.

Conclusions

Given vigorous, repeated, and sustained elevation of the blood pressure by mechanisms operating from above down upon the defense-alarm response mechanism, the stage is set for the development of all the complicating and perpetuating disturbances that have been described as the consequence of sustained high blood pressure. Thus the symptoms that bring the patient to the physician with the development of the final kidney, heart, or central nervous system breakdown may be only the last phase in a complex chain of events whose start lies buried in the early experience of the individual and his culturally determined patterns of response to an environment that is becoming increasingly dissonant.

The stimuli that lead to activation of the defense-alarm reaction are not necessarily associated with conscious "fight or flight" responses. Indeed, visceromotor and hormonal responses may take place without emotional disturbance or awareness on the part of the organism. Within any social group, there are systematic differences in the level of stimulation and hence of neuroendocrine arousal depending on their genetically determined responsiveness and their individual positions in the social field of force. Further, group life tends to promote similar responses, with those in subordinate positions tending to

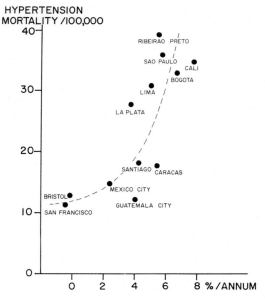

Fig. 11-10.—Preliminary observations suggest that the rate of growth of a city may be related to the incidence of hypertension in the general population. (From Henry, J. P., and Cassel, J. C.: Am. J. Epidemiol. 90(No.3):195, Fig. 11, 1969.)

respond in a more extreme fashion to similar stimuli. Finally, the effect of a given stimulus is determined by the organism's perception, which, in turn, depends on the past history of stimulation and, in particular, upon its early experience. It will be especially the aged, faced with new patterns conflicting with the culture to which they were adjusted in youth, who will find their status ambiguous and fail to adapt, and so meet the criteria first laid down by Scotch for the development of high blood pressure.

REFERENCES

Axelrod, J., Mueller, R. A., Henry, J. P., and Stephens, P.: Psychosocial Stimulation: Changes in Enzymes Involved in the Biosynthesis and Metabolism of Nor-adrenalin and Adrenalin, Nature, London 225:1059–1060, 1970.

Charvat, J., Dell, P., and Folkow, B.: Mental Factors and Cardiovascular Diseases, Cardiologia 44:124–141, 1964.

Folkow, B., and Rubinstein, E. H.: Cardiovascular Effect of Acute and Chronic Stimulations of the Hypothalamic Defense Area in the Rat, Acta Physiol. Scandinav., pp. 28–48, 1966.

Friedberg, C. K.: *Diseases of the Heart,* 3d ed. (Philadelphia: W. B. Saunders Co., 1966), pp. 1474–1517.

Goldblatt, H.: *The Renal Origin of Hypertension* (Springfield, Ill.: Charles C Thomas, Publisher, 1948).

Henry, J. P., Meehan, J. P., and Stephens, P. M.: The Use of Psychosocial Stimuli to Induce Prolonged Hypertension in Mice, Psychosom. Med. 29:408–432, 1967.

Page, I. H., and McCubbin, J. W.: The Physiology of Arterial Hypertension, in Hamilton, W. F. (ed.): *Handbook of Physiology: Circulation* (Washington: American Physiological Society, 1965), Vol. III, chap. 61, pp. 2163–2208.

Page, I. H., and McCubbin, J. W.: *Renal Hypertension* (Chicago: Year Book Medical Publishers, Inc., 1968).

Pickering, W. G.: *High Blood Pressure,* 2d ed. (New York: Grune & Stratton, Inc., 1968), pp. 204–220.

Scotch, N. A., and Geiger, H. J.: Epidemiology of Essential Hypertension: Psychologic and Sociocultural Factors in Etiology, J. Chron. Dis. 16:1183–1213, 1963.

Shapiro, A. P.: Experimental Pyelonephritis and Hypertension, Ann. Int. Med. 59:37–52, 1963.

Smirk, F. H.: The Pathogenesis of Hypertension, in Schlittler, E. (ed.): *Antihypertensive Agents* (New York: Academic Press, Inc., 1967), pp. 2–58.

Stamler, J., Stamler, R., and Pullman, T. N.: *The Epidemiology of Hypertension* (New York: Grune & Stratton, Inc., 1967).

12

Cardiovascular Changes in Certain Adaptive States: A Summary

Reflex Mechanisms and Their Integration

DESCRIPTION OF DIAGRAMS

FOUR BASIC STATES in which there is a sharp deviation from the physiology of the resting organism present an opportunity in this final chapter to delineate the closely coordinated controls of the high- and low-pressure systems. They are exercise, reduced central blood volume, heart failure, and high blood pressure.

Exercise and reduced central blood volume involve the normal interplay of all of the regulatory mechanisms. The former requires increases in cardiovascular performance paced by the increased metabolic needs imposed. By way of contrast, the latter requires conservation of cardiovascular effort, along with the initiation of mechanisms directed toward the expansion of the central blood volume.

Congestive heart failure and hypertension are states in which cardiovascular control mechanisms are operating in a nonphysiologic manner. In congestive failure, the function of the volume-sensing mechanisms of the low-pressure system may be disturbed by changes in the action of the heart, with a maladaptation resulting in the characteristic picture of salt and water retention. Hypertension involves accommodations of the regulatory mechanisms of the high-pressure system. These may be initiated by excessive emotional reaction to environmental stimuli; they are maintained by the continuing need for physiologic levels of peripheral blood flow.

In what follows, the responses that occur will be sketched out by using two series of diagrams (Figs. 12-1 to 8) that seek to portray in a highly symbolized form the feedbacks involved in the regulation of the cardiovascular system. These diagrams are based on the approach presented in the preceding chapters.

Figures 12-1 to 4 are roughly divided into four columns. The first, in passing from left to right, represents the receptors that play upon the central nervous system, bringing information both from the environment and from the organism. Only the eyes and ears are symbolized; however, the sensors for equilibration, touch, smell, and taste are also involved in the information flow. A very important source is the kinesthetic muscle and joint sense. In addition, there are afferents from the lungs and other viscera and from the skin giving temperature information.

All is funneled into the central nervous system, here symbolized by a longitudinal section through the hemispheres, medulla, and spinal cord. The autonomic system is indicated by the chain of sympathetic ganglia.

In the different states, the arrows connecting the sensors with the central nervous system have different values. Thus in a state of high environmental temperature, which is not depicted here, a heavy discharge from the nerve endings in the skin could be anticipated. External objects or events observed or heard that have a strong emotional significance for the organism would be represented by heavy arrows from the eyes and ears. The central nervous system is divided into the cortical analyzer, subcortical regions involved in emotional responses, and the hypothalamus, midbrain, and medulla, with progressively more and more tightly restricted concern with the internal housekeeping of the organism, i.e., with reflex mechanisms involved in maintaining basic equilibria.

The next column—that to the right of the central nervous system proper—is devoted to the effector mechanisms especially responsible for the regulation of the cardiovascular system. From above downward come the arterioles, the heart, and the kidney with its several pathways for regulation of both blood pressure and the salt and water content of the body. The posterior pituitary, which is under control of information from the hypothalamus, is depicted as regulating the level of antidiuretic hormone, which, in turn, regulates water excretion and hence plays a part in determining the body water content. Below this are shown the pre- and post-capillary resistances, which are modulated by information from the autonomic system, and, in turn, determine the flow of fluid between the intra- and extravascular spaces. A final arrow points to the capacitance veins whose tonus eventually increases when the amount of blood available in the thoracic region becomes so deficient that a fall in blood pressure threatens. In man with his erect posture, this can happen in orthostasis when gravity is moving fluid away from this area.

In the various states, differing values will be assigned to the drive emanating from the autonomic nervous system and to the hormones activating the controls of the cardiovascular system. This results in a second set of arrows, all pointing toward the final column that depicts important and readily measurable functions of the cardiovascular system. Arterial pressure is monitored by the sinoaortic receptors, whereas venous blood pressure and blood volume are related to the CUE and end-net receptors of the low-pressure system. The extracellular fluid volume is an integral part of this final column, for the interstitial space has the same distensibility and is functionally so closely related to the blood-volume compartment that they are probably served by the same sets of stretch receptors.

Exercise

The results of a sharp change in muscular activity are expressed by the various weights given to the arrows connecting the symbols that have just been outlined (Fig. 12-1). One most important feature of the vascular adjust-

Fig. 12-1.—Exercise: Illustration of the variety and extent of information arriving at the cardiovascular control centers in the diencephalon. Important components derive from the muscles and joints, and possibly from the regions evaluating the body temperature. The adrenergic system is strongly stimulated and, in turn, passes on direct cardiac sympathetic, arteriolar, and venous responses. Renin and antidiuretic hormonal levels rise, and there is some adjustment of fluid equilibrium across the vascular bed.

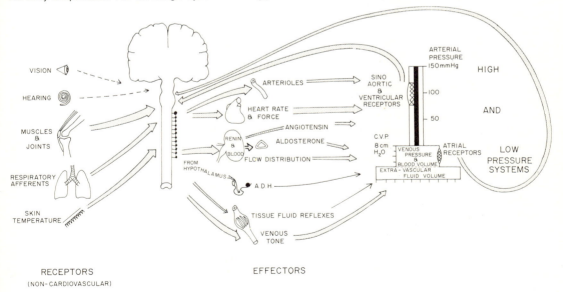

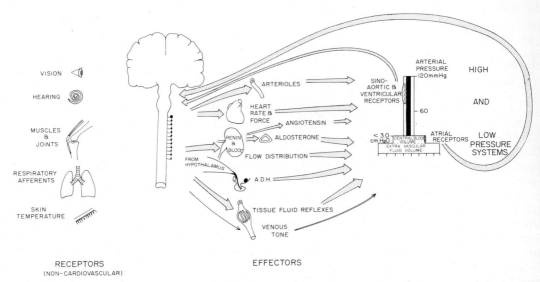

Fig. 12-2.—Reduced central blood volume: When central blood volume is reduced as a result of actual blood loss or footward displacement of blood by the erect posture, there is a sharp response from the low-pressure system in the form of a decreased atrial afferent impulse rate, and, later, from the high-pressure system stretch receptors—as first the pulse pressure and, then, the systolic and mean arterial pressures fall. Intense stimulation of the cardiovascular controls leads to a vigorous adrenergic response that induces positive effects on heart activity, increased arteriolar and venous tone, and renin release. In addition, antidiuretic hormone causes fluid retention; tissue fluid is reabsorbed because of the change in pre- to postcapillary resistance.

Fig. 12-3.—Congestive heart failure: Theoretical schema indicating response patterns in congestive heart failure. Body temperature may relate to heat production and hence to work demands. Brain stem responses activate the sympathetic and adrenal systems inducing an increase in ADH levels and activating the reflexes controlling tissue fluid content. Despite the inotropic effect of the enhanced sympathetic drive, the weakened ventricle cannot perform the needed stroke work. Increased venous tone and ADH and aldosterone levels lead to fluid retention with increased central venous pressure and extravascular fluid volume.

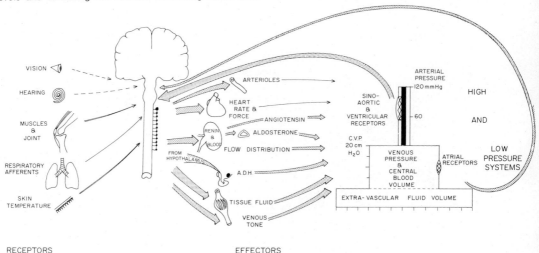

ment to exercise is the local vasodilator effect of accumulated metabolites. However, at higher levels of integration, information resetting the brain stem centers arises from the muscles and joints involved in the exertion. Breathing patterns change, and there is an elevation of central core temperature as the work represented by the action of the muscles results in greater heat production. A major response to this changed information flow is a great enhancement in the sympathetic drive, resulting in increased cardiac frequency and contractility. There is redistribution of blood flow within the kidney and, eventually, a sharp over-all reduction in the blood flow to this and other viscera, whereas the muscle blood flow in those segments involved will greatly increase. Despite the huge alterations in flow distribution, there is usually only a moderate increase in systemic arterial pressure and no significant change in central venous pressure, so that the mechanical receptors in the cardiovascular system are less affected than might be expected.

Reduced Central Blood Volume

A reduction in central blood volume can readily occur as a result of too-strict immobility when warm and when standing erect, i.e., orthostasis. A common condition leading to a similar effect is loss of blood volume, as after a wound. In hemorrhage, there is an absolute decrease of blood and tissue fluid volume. In orthostasis, a displacement occurs so that actually there is an increase in one region while there is a deficiency in the critical area where the sensing mechanisms are located. In the early stages of hemorrhage, which Figure 12-2 illustrates, systemic arterial pressure is not significantly changed (Figs. 7-11 and 7-3) but there is a sharp fall in central venous pressure and in extravascular fluid volume. This fall in venous pressure is associated with a change in afferent impulses from the atrial CUE stretch receptors that, in turn, feed back strongly to the central nervous system, leading to an increase in antidiuretic hormone level. A rise in sympathetic drive results in the usual effects of increased cardiac contractility and stroke work, arteriolar constriction—especially in the viscera—and redistribution of blood flow as, for example, in the kidney. An increased renin level and a sharp fall in sodium output ensue. Antidiuretic hormone levels rise sharply and tissue fluid reflexes act to return fluid into the vascular bed. In the early stages, before more than 20% of the total blood volume has been lost, there is little change in venous tone. As the volume loss progresses and a fall in arterial pressure

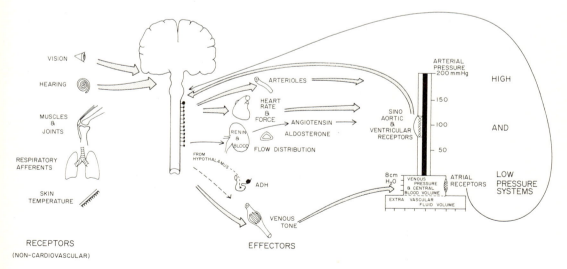

Fig. 12-4.—Essential hypertension: Influences at work in a case of essential hypertension. The early phases are reversible and include cardiac sympathetic effects, constriction of arterioles in the viscera with dilation in the muscle bed, and some increase in venous tone. The result is a sustained elevation of arterial pressure without significant change in extravascular fluid volume and central venous pressure.

threatens, there is a sharp constriction of the veins, helping to sustain central blood volume.

Congestive Heart Failure

In congestive heart failure, there are some moderate changes in the left-hand column symbolizing the state of the afferents (Fig. 12-3). Central venous pressure and the extravascular fluid volume are greatly increased.

The arterial pressure may be somewhat diminished at rest; however, the stroke-work performance of the ventricle falls off as the vigor of contractility flags. This is especially disastrous in exercise and other situations requiring increased cardiac performance. It is probable, though as yet not established, that the performance of the ventricle in systole is sensed by the sinoaortic receptors and by the ventricular end nets, as well as by receptors on the atrioventricular valves.

The venous pressure is increased, and, consequently, both the intravascular and the interstitial fluid volumes are increased. Chronic increases in central venous pressure result in dilation of the atria. When the atria are sufficiently stretched, the signals from the various subendocardial atrial stretch receptors actually diminish due to decreased movement of the atrial wall. The true state of atrial filling is thereby not indicated; for this response indicates the opposite situation, namely that the atria are underfilled. Consequently, the picture in terms of effector drive via the sympathetic system to the heart, kidney, and blood vessels is very similar to that holding for precisely the opposite condition—fluid volume loss.

There is no doubt that the adrenergic system is strongly activated. Indeed, there is an amelioration of the fluid and salt retention when the adrenergic drive is cut off by drugs, when the

Fig. 12-5.—In exercise, the organism is aware of the environmental demands; in addition to direct inflow from peripheral receptors, there is a conscious evaluation of the demands and threats posed by the environment that frequently leads to emotional arousal, which adds its contribution to the over-all adrenergic response.

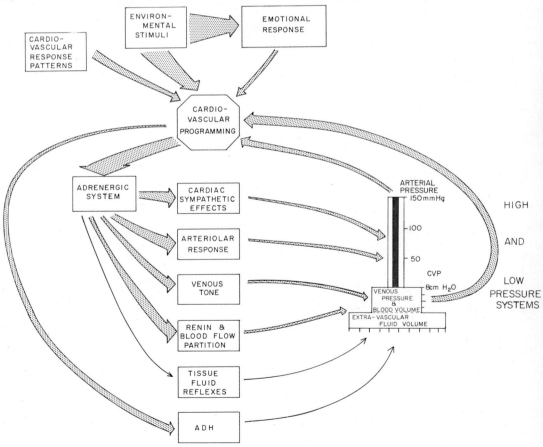

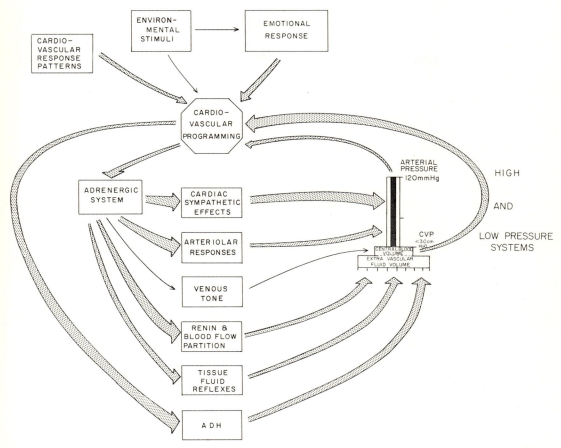

Fig. 12-6.—Conscious awareness of the circumstances of reduced blood volume. Either posture or trauma may contribute to the information flow resulting in adrenergic stimulation.

vascular congestion is relieved by cuffs, when anxiety and discomfort are allayed, and when the appropriate medication improves cardiac function.

Essential Hypertension

The fourth example of an adaptive state with increased adrenergic drive is essential hypertension. Here, extravascular fluid volume and central venous pressure are normal; despite the very high systemic arterial pressure, the drive from the baroreceptors in the great arteries can be shown to have adapted so that it is down to normal levels (Fig. 12-4), possibly as a result of intervention at olivary levels. There is no elevation of antidiuretic hormone level, and the tissue fluid reflexes are not set for the storage of fluid. However, once again, there is evidence of increased drive from the adrenergic system. In the early stages, cardiac output is often increased, perhaps due to excessive contractility. Later, the arterioles create increased peripheral resistance, especially in the visceral circulation. Venous pressure is normal but venous tone is mildly elevated; the blood flow distribution in the kidney is probably on the verge of a juxtamedullary increase, for the handling of sodium by the essential hypertensive shows commencing problems.

Conclusions: Levels of Integration of Cardiovascular Function

In Figures 12-1 to 4, the concept of columns arranged from right to left was used to emphasize the great physiological significance of the sequence receptor-neuropile-effector, i.e., of the reflex element. The diagrams aim to draw attention to the complex of closely interlocking reflex mechanisms that knit the cardiovascular system together.

In Figures 12-5 to 8, the same concepts are presented, but they are redrawn to focus attention on a different facet of these interrelationships. The new series depicts the same information as the other set, but it does so with an emphasis on the hierarchy in the central nervous system, i.e., on the different "levels" that are involved in the over-all regulatory process. No attempt has been made to symbolize the most basic of these modes, autoregulation or the local regulation of blood flow by metabolites that act directly on the small vessels. At the next step, which was the focus of attention in Figures 12-1 to 4, the cardiovascular system is coordinated by means of strategically located stretch receptors. These provide the information for reflexes that meet the housekeeping requirements of the organism. They operate with controls that are for the most part located in the midbrain and hindbrain, extending thence through the autonomic and endocrine systems. Acting in large part below the level of awareness, the responses involve appropriate sympathetic arousal with its complex of accompanying effects upon blood pressure and blood distribution, i.e., upon the heart and blood vessels, and upon the kidney and the regulation of salt-and-water balance.

Figures 12-5 to 8 draw attention to the continuing role of a third set of responses, higher than those of autoregulation and even of volume and pressure regulation, by using boxes placed above the cardiovascular controls. These boxes not only represent the integration of environmental data with respiratory, blood, and body temperature information, but they also involve cardiovascular response patterns that are genetically programmed in the organism. Furthermore, as the legends indicate, the perception

Fig. 12-7.—In congestive heart failure, an awareness of difficulty in meeting environmental demands is fed by afferents from the muscles, joints, and lungs as the individual attempts to do physical work. The normal patterns of response may be available for reference as acquired and inherited schemata stored in the brain.

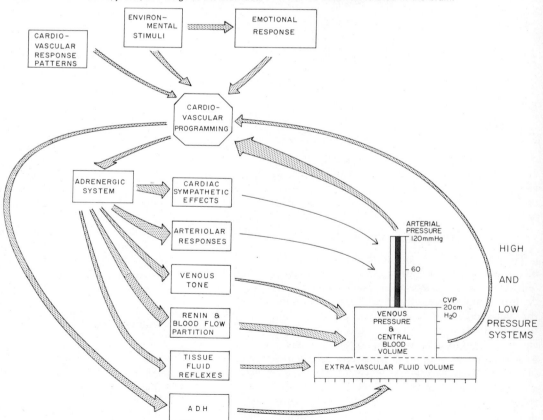

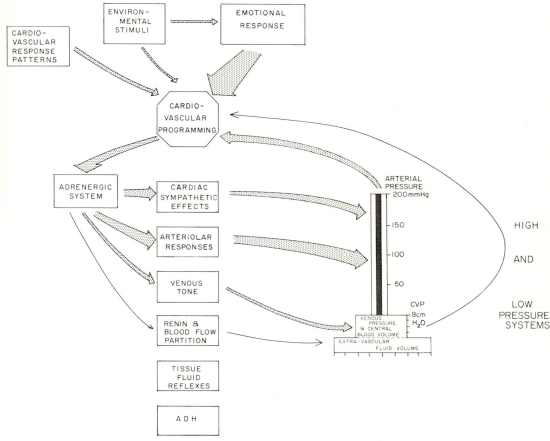

Fig. 12-8.—Essential hypertension indicating the strong role played by environmental stimuli in eliciting emotional responses that interact with the cardiovascular control system to produce sustained adrenergic stimulation.

of events in the environment can be a source of powerful inputs, depending on the significance of that particular perception to that particular individual.

The prior experience of the individual determines the emotional response that any particular stimulus arouses and hence the drive furnished by the stimulus to the diencephalic controls. In addition, the cardiovascular response patterns of certain stereotyped reactions are programmed into the organism. They include fainting, i.e., vasovagal syncope; sexual reactions; and the defense-alarm response. When faced with the requirement to adapt to an environmental stimulus, the organism may assume the flight-or-fight mode or may even collapse in syncope. The exact performance is not readily predictable since it involves learned responses stored in the central nervous system peculiar to each individual. Nevertheless, these adaptations develop on a level independent from those induced by the pressure and volume regulatory system.

In exercise (Fig. 12-5), the organism responds to the awareness that the activity is in progress. The interplay between this awareness and respiratory, kinesthetic, and other senses involves the higher levels of brain organization. Figure 12-6 indicates that, when blood volume is reduced as by hemorrhage, the intensity of the response is in part determined by the awareness that something is not going as it should. In Figure 12-7, not only does information flow from the peripheral receptors into the central transactional component of the nervous system, but the cardiovascular response pattern, the perception of environmental stimuli, and the generation of emotional responses are also involved. In the condition of congestive heart failure, there may be a comparison within the brain between the current disturbed flow of impulses with more normal schemata or cardiovascular response patterns that have already become programmed. Some of these comparisons may involve the higher levels of brain function.

In the early stages of essential hypertension (Fig. 12-8), the condition is predominantly determined by the responses made in the higher levels of the nervous system. Patterns based on earlier responses determine the significance to the organism of the particular environmental information received at any moment. This significance then determines the arousal that occurs. It is postulated that, as a result of unfavorable early experience, the organism becomes sensitized to many events that repeatedly face it later in life. These occurrences do not necessarily evoke consciously experienced emotion, but, nevertheless, they may be strongly arousing to the autonomic system, i.e., they may be "symbolically" significant. Such stimuli can lead to sustained and repeated responses of the cardiovascular control system. A stimulus to which a man has made inadequate defenses will be threatening and evoke a defense-alarm reaction, activating the sympathetic and the pituitary adrenal system. The individual may be unaware of this, but, nevertheless, the response sets into action the cardiovascular patterns appropriate for "fight or flight." This will occur although there is no physical activity to require such adrenergic stimulation. If sufficiently frequent, intense, and long sustained, the effects of successive alarm responses will overlap each other, leading to a continuous hypertensive state. Eventually, if the systemic arterial pressure is sufficiently elevated and is raised for a long enough period, pathological changes set in that render the pressure rise self-sustaining.

The responses demanded from the organism by the social environment are as important as preconditions for normal adaptation as is the internal environment. The purpose of the final set of diagrams is to emphasize that, in addition to the autoregulatory reflexes controlling tissue nutrition and the reflexes controlling blood pressure, volume, and other cardiovascular parameters operating at the first and second levels of integration, there is a third repertoire available to the organism. This is based on responses deriving from the demands to cope with events in the outside world. The intricacies of this hierarchical network are so far only very partially understood.

Index

A

Absorption: capillary, 76
ADH (antidiuretic hormone), 116
  reduction
    blood and, 171
    blood volume reduction and, 124
Adrenergic activity: and congestive heart failure, 165-168
Afferent pathways, 115
Age
  blood and
    flow, cerebral, 133
    pressure changes, 186-190
  influencing pressure-volume curve of aorta, 67
Angiogram: coronary, 130
Angiotensin: infusion, and left-ventricular function curves, 166
Ankle: vein, pressure changes during single step, 106
Antidiuretic hormone (*see* ADH (antidiuretic hormone))
Aorta
  ascending, pressure waves in, 72
  baroreceptors, response to progressive blood loss, 124-126
  elastic reservoir function of, 66-68
  fiber, showing change in burst number with progressive hemorrhage, 115
  pressure
    determination of mean pressure, 73
    —volume curve of, age influencing, 67
    wave transmission and, 68
  regurgitation, 34
  stenosis, 34
Arm
  countercurrent heat exchanger in, 156
  forearm (*see* Forearm)

Arrhythmia: cardiac, 56
Arterioles
  breakdown of, 78
  resistance, regulation of, 119
Artery(ies)
  brachial, and paroxysmal atrial tachycardia, 172
  comparison of pressure and flow pulses in, 70
  coronary, distribution of, 129
  femoral, impedance graph of (in dog), 71
  iliac, mean blood pressure of, determination, 73
  pressure
    systolic (in mice), 180
    Valsalva maneuver and, 146
  pulse (*see* Pulse, arterial)
  tree, branching of, 60
Atrium
  baroreceptors, response to progressive blood loss, 124-126
  fiber, record of membrane potentials of, 49
  firing rate, 113
    atrial pressure and, 169
  pressure
    atrial firing rate and, 169
    changes, and balloon, 122-124
    right-, and blood volume alteration, 94
    tachycardia and, paroxysmal atrial, 172
Attitude hypoxia, 153-154
Auscultation: and heart sounds, areas for, 33

B

Bainbridge reflex, 120-121
Ballistocardiography, 31
Baroreceptors, response to progressive blood loss
  aortic, 124-126
  atrial, 124-126
Beat, heart (*see* Heart, beat)
Bed rest: and blood volume 104-105
Birth: circulation changes at, 145
Blood
  ADH in, reduction, 124, 171
  flow, 17-18
    cerebral (*see* Cerebrum, blood flow in)
    feet and, 80
    liver, measurement of, 138-139
  loss, (*see* Hemorrhage)
  pressure (*see* Pressure)
  return to central reservoir, 92-109
  viscosity of, 19-20
    viscometers and, 20
  volume
    ADH level in blood and, 124
    alteration affecting right-atrial pressure, 94
    bed rest and, 104-105
    central, 95-97
    central nervous system regulating, 121
    central reduced, 196-198
    circulation and, extrathoracic, 97-98
    distribution in different regions, 20-21
    distribution, orthostasis influencing, 99-103
    divisions of, 93-98
    orthostasis and (*see* Orthostasis, blood volume in)
    regulatory responses, 116-118
    relation between interstitial fluid space and, 98
    relationship with mean intrathoracic vascular pressures, 96
    renal vascular redistribution and, 117-118
    renin and, 117-118
    thirst and, 116-117
    weightlessness and, 104-105
Body: weight, and guanethidine, 166

203

INDEX

Bradykinin
  formation in forearm skin during body warming, 137
  vasodilator effects, and skin circulation, 136
Breathing pressure
  negative (NPB), effects on urine flow under chloralose (in dog), 122
  partial pressure suit and, 148
Burst number: aortic fiber showing change with progressive hemorrhage, 115

C

Calf pump: action of, 106-107
Capillary(ies)
  absorption, 76
  "average limb," schematic diagram of, 85
  filtration, 76
  function, 75-81
    general considerations, 75-76
  muscle, diagram of fine structure in, 89
  permeability to lipid soluble molecules, 90-91
  pressure
    functional changes of, 80-81
    hydrostatic, 76-77
  wall
    exchange of substances through, 75-91
    osmotic pressure of proteins and lymphatics, 84-86
Cardiovascular control centers: of diencephalon, information arriving at, illustration, 195
Cardiovascular function
  integration of, central, 110-128
  integration levels of, conclusions, 199-200
  regulation of, local, 110-128
Cardiovascular system
  changes in certain adaptive states, 195-202
  control in, 21-22
    efferent nervous, 22
    hormonal, 22
  efferent pathways in, 116-121
  exercises and, posture, 150-151
  high-pressure system of (see High-pressure system)
  hormones controlling, 116-121
  integration in, 21-22
    information and, exteroceptive and interoceptive, 22
  low-pressure system of (see Low-pressure system)
  receptors in, stretch (see Stretch receptors in cardiovascular system)
  responses of, special, 147-159
  schematic diagram of, 16
Carotid sinus: perfusion experiments, 121-122

Cells: juxtaglomerular, 141
Central nervous system: regulation of blood pressure and volume, 121
Cerebrum
  blood flow in
    age and, 133
    factors affecting, diagrammatic summary of, 134
  circulation, 133-135
    methods of measuring flow, 133-134
Chloralose: effects of negative pressure breathing on urine flow under (in dog), 122
Cholinergic sympathetic vasodilator outflow: and skeletal muscles, 151
Circulation
  cerebral, 133-135
    methods of measuring flow, 133-134
  changes at birth, 145
  compartments of, estimated capacity of, 95
  coronary, 129-133
  defense-alarm response and, 157
  digestion and, 154
  emotion and, 157-159
  exposure and
    cold, 155-157
    heat, 154-155
    underwater, 152-153
  extrathoracic, blood volume of, 97-98
  failure, 160-173
    factors inducing, 161-162
    treatment of, 164
  fetal, 144-145
  general properties of, 15-23
  interstitial fluid, 86-90
  intestines and, 139
  laws and, Poiseuille's, applicability to, 61
  local, characteristics of responses of, 129-145
  placental, 144-145
  portal-liver, 138
  pulmonary
    hypoxia and, 143
    regulation of, 142-143
    vasomotor nerves and, 142-143
  regulation, pressure and volume, diagram of principles of, 127
  renal, 140, 141-142
  reproductive system, 143-145
  resistances of, parallel, 60, 61
  in skin (see Skin, circulation in)
  splanchnic, 138-142
  spleen and, 140
  stomach, 139
  venous, respiration influencing, 99
City: growth rate, and hypertension, 192
Clothing: and metabolic rate, 155
CNS: regulation of blood pressure

and volume, 121
Cold exposure: and circulatory changes, 155-157
Color: skin, and skin circulation, 136-137
Commissurotomy dilutional syndrome: postmitral, 171
Conduction: disturbances, 55-57
Conductive system: heart, 47-58
Congestive heart failure, 164-173, 196, 198-199
  adrenergic activity and, 165-168
  environment and, 200
  exercise and, 165-168
  nor-epinephrine and, 167
  receptors in, 168-170
  symptoms of, 164
  treatment of, 170-171
Constriction: velocity and lateral pressure at, 18
Constrictor response: correlation with stimulation rate, 119
Contractile mechanism: activation of, 37-38
Contractility, heart muscle
  studies of, 41-43
    after-loaded isotonic, 41
    clinical aspects, 46-47
    variations versus effects of preloading, 44-45
Contraction
  muscular, mechanism of, 35-37
  myocardial, ventricular changes during, 24
Coronary
  angiograms, 130
  arteries, distribution of, 129
  circulation, 129-133
  innervation, 132
  phasic flow, 131-132
    diagram of, 131
  vessels
    characteristics of, 129-131
    collaterals of, 130
Coughing, 147
Cranium: and rigidity, 134-135
CUE of Nonidez
  location of, 112
  relationship between pericardium and, 118
Culture: and blood pressure, 188

D

Defense-alarm
  center, diencephalic, in hypothalamus (in mammal), 178
  response, and circulation, 157
Diastole
  flow patterns during, 26
  frequency, and systole, 28
  heart rate and, 28
Dibenzyline and excretion (in dog)
  sodium, 168
  water, 168
Diencephalon
  cardiovascular control centers in,

INDEX

illustration of information arriving at, 195
defense-alarm center, in hypothalamus, 178
Diet: and blood pressure, 191
Diffusion: net, of water, 88
Digestion: and circulation, 154
Dilator: relaxing precapillary sphincter, 78
Disease: and high blood pressure, 184-185
Dissociation curves, hemoglobin
 adult, 145
 fetal, 145

E

Efferent pathways, 116-121
Einthoven: equilateral triangle, and standard limb leads, 51
Elastic(s)
 behavior of, 64
 forces, 30
 reservoir
  action of, demonstration, 66
  function of aorta, 66-68
 -type vessels, behavior of, 62
Elasticity
 coefficient, volume, 65
 vascular bed, 20
Electrical activity: in heart, 48
Electrical axis: of heart, determination of, 52-53
Electrocardiogram, 47-58
 showing time relationships, 51
Electrodes: exploring, 53-54
Emotion
 circulatory changes in, 157-159
 stress, and mental arithmetic, 179
End net: diagrammatic representation of, 112
Environment
 blood pressure and, high, 182-186
 exercise and, 198
 heart failure and, congestive, 200
 skin circulation and, 135-136
 water exchanges in man, 155
Epinephrine: and heart, 49
Equation: Laplace's, 30
Erectile tissues, 143
Excitatory system: heart, 47-50
Exercise(s), 148-152
 blood pressure and
  high, 182-183
  low, 182-183
 cardiovascular changes and, 151-152, 195-197
 environmental demands and, 198
 heart and, 150
  failure, congestive, 165-168
 peripheral vascular bed and, 150
 respiration and, 148-150
Exposure and circulatory changes (see Circulation, exposure and)

F

Fat: and hypertension, 184

Feet
 blood flow through, 80
 venous pressure in, factors regulating, 105-106
Fetus
 circulation in, 144-145
 hemoglobin, dissociation curves for, 145
Filtration
 capillary, 76
 glomerular, protein osmotic pressure for, 83
 in lungs, 77
 rate, forearm, as measured by pressure plethysmography, 87
Firing rate, atrial, 113
 atrium pressure and, 169
Fluid(s)
 exchange network, morphology of, 77-80
 interstitial, 84-90
  circulation of, 86-90
  compartment, pressure in, 84
  proteins and lymphatics, 84-86
  space, and relation between blood volume, 98
 vascular bed, inflow and outflow of, 79
Force-velocity-length relationship: heart muscle, diagrams of, 45-46
Forearm
 filtration rates as measured by pressure plethysmography, 87
 skin, bradykinin formation during body warming, 137
Frank-Starling law of heart, 38-39

G

Gases: respiratory, capillary permeability to, 90-91
Glomerular filtration: significance of protein osmotic pressure for, 83
Guanethidine
 body weight and, 166
 heart rate and, 166
 sodium balance and, 166
 venous pressure and, 166

H

Hand: vessels, pressure-volume diagram of, 63
Heart
 (See also Cardiovascular)
 arrhythmias, 56
 beat
  role of sympathetic system in regulating force of, 119-120
  vagal regulation of rate of, 120
 chambers
  as muscular pumps, 24-26
  as reservoir of low-pressure system, 28-29
 conductive system of, 47-50
 cycle, sequence of events in, 26-28
 efficiency, 30
 electrical activity in, 48
 electrical axis of, determination, 52-53
 epinephrine and, 49
 excitatory system of, 47-50
 exercise and, 150
 failure
  chronic (see Congestive heart failure)
  congestive (see Congestive heart failure)
  straining and, 147-148
 fibers, cathodal stimuli applied to, 49
 filling, pericardial assistance to, 25
 function, intrinsic and extrinsic, determinants of, 35-47
 innervation, influence of, 57-58
 ions and, 56-57
 law of
  exceptions to, 39-41
  Frank-Starling, 38-39
 -lung preparation, effect of increasing arterial resistance on pressures in, 39
 medullary cardiac afferent locations, 115
 murmurs, 33
 muscles
  arrangement of, 24-25
  contractility of (see Contractility, heart muscle)
  differences between skeletal muscle and, 47
  force-velocity-length relationship diagrams, 45-46
  method of study of after-loaded isotonic contraction of, 41
  work versus power, 46
 output, 30
  factors, determining, 28-31
  heart rate and, 29
 performance, posture influencing, 103
 as pump, 24-34
 rate
  cardiac output and, 29
  control of, 29
  duration of systole and diastole in relation to, 28
  guanethidine and, 166
  sympathetic stimulation and, 120
 as reservoir, 24-34
 rhythm, abnormalities of, 54-55
 sounds, 31-34
  audible, 31
  auscultation of, areas for, 33
  causes of, 32-33
  jugular vein pulse and, 108
  timing of, 32

INDEX

Heart (cont.)
  as specialized muscle, 35-58
  syncope, 161
  transplantation, 170
  valves
    function of, 25-26
    ring, movement of, 25
  work of, 30-31
Heat
  countercurrent heat exchanger in arm, 156
  exposure, and circulation, 154-155
Hemoglobin dissociation curves
  adult, 145
  fetal, 145
Hemorrhage
  nonhypotensive, mechanism for compensatory responses during, 162-163
  progressive
    aortic fiber showing change in burst number with, 115
    responses of atrial and aortic baroreceptors to, 124-126
    spleen size and, 125
    venous pressure change in, 93
Hepatic (see Liver)
Heredity: and high blood pressure, 186
High-pressure system, 15-17, 59-74
  components of, illustration, 95
  receptors in, stretch, 21-22, 111-114
HIP (hydrostatic indifference point), 99-103
Hormones
  antidiuretic (see ADH (antidiuretic hormone)
  cardiovascular system and, 22, 116-121
Hydrodynamic flow: of water, 88
Hydrostatic
  indifference point (HIP), 99-103
  pressure, 17
    capillary, 76-77
Hypertension, 174-193
  disease and, 184-185
  environmental factors and, 182-186
  essential, 199
    influences at work in, illustration, 197
  exercise and, 182-183
  experimental observations demonstrating role of subhypothalamic mechanisms in development of, 175-177
  fat and, 184
  heredity and, 186
  hypothalamus and, 174-175, 177-182
  malnutrition and, 184
  obesity and, 185-186
  protein and, 184
  rate of growth of cities and, 192

salt and, 183
smoking and, 186
Hypotension: orthostatic, 160-161
Hypothalamus
  diencephalic defense-alarm center in (in mammal), 178
  hypertension and, 174-175, 177-182
Hypovolemia, 158
Hypoxia
  attitude, 153-154
  circulation and, pulmonary, 143

I

Iliac artery: mean blood pressure of, 73
Impedance
  graphs, femoral artery (in dog), 71
  vascular, and arterial pulse, 70-72
Infusion
  angiotensin, and left-ventricular function curves, 166
  venous pressure change in, 93
Innervation (see Nerves)
Interstitial fluids (see Fluid(s), interstitial)
Intestines: circulation in, 139
Intramural tension, 19
Ions: and heart, 56-57
Irreversible shock, 163

J

Jugular vein: pulse in, relationship to heart sounds, 108
Juxtaglomerular cells, 141

K

Kidney
  circulation in, 140, 141-142
  tachycardia and, paroxysmal atrial, 172
  vascular redistribution, and blood volume, 117-118

L

Laplace
  equation of, 30
  relation, practical aspects of, 63-64
Law(s)
  of heart
    exceptions to, 39-41
    Frank-Starling, 38-39
  Poiseuille's, applicability to circulation, 61
  van't Hoff's, physiological significance of deviations from, 83
Leads, precordial
  unipolar, location of, 55
  Wilson's central terminal, connections for, 54
Liver

blood supply, measurement, 138-139
portal-, circulation, 138
Low-pressure system, 15-17, 92-109
  components of, illustration, 95
  heart chambers as reservoir of, 28-29
  receptors in, stretch, 21-22, 111-114
  ventricle in, left, position of, 97
Lung(s)
  circulation in (see Circulation, pulmonary)
  filtration in, 77
  heart-lung preparation, effect of increasing arterial resistance on pressures in, 39
Lymphatics
  function, and proteins in interstitial fluid, 84-86
  role of, 75-91

M

Malnutrition: and high blood pressure, 184
Mean blood pressure
  determination
    aorta, 73
    iliac artery, 73
  estimation of, 73
Menstruation, 143
Metabolism: rate, and clothing, 155
Mitral
  postcommissurotomy dilutional syndrome, 171
  regurgitation, 34
  stenosis, 34
Molecules: lipid soluble, capillary permeability to, 90-91
Murmurs: heart, 33
Muscle(s)
  capillary, diagram of fine structure in, 89
  contraction
    heart, after-loaded isotonic, study of, 41
    mechanism of, 35-37
  heart (see Heart, muscle)
  pump
    orthostasis and, 105-107
    properties of, 106
  skeletal
    comparison with heart muscle, 47
    intercerebral course of cholinergic sympathetic vasodilator outflow to, 151
    stretching of, effects, 38
  specialized, heart as, 35-58
  ventricular, stretching of, 38
  vessels, behavior of tissues in wall of, 65
Myocardium: contraction, changes in ventricles during, 24

N

Negative pressure breathing (NPB): effects on urine flow under chloralose (in dog), 122
Nephrons: and blood flow distribution, 140
Nerve(s)
  coronary, 132
  heart, influence of, 57-58
  skin circulation and, 136
  vagus, regulation and rate of heart beat, 120
  vasomotor, and pulmonary circulation, 142-143
Nets: end, diagrammatic representation of, 112
Nonidez, CUE of (*see* CUE of Nonidez)
Nor-epinephrine: and congestive heart failure, 167
NPB (negative pressure breathing): effects on urine flow under chloralose (in dog), 122

O

Obesity: and hypertension, 185-186
Orthostasis, 92-109
  blood volume in
    changes of, 102-103
    distribution of, 99-103
    redistribution of, 102-103
  hypotension and, 160-161
  muscle pump and, 105-107
  water immersion as antagonist of, 101
Osmometer: Basic principles of, 81
Osmotic pressure (*see* Protein(s), osmotic-pressure)
Oxygen: uptake, and ventilation, 149

P

Patent ductus arteriosus, 34
Pathways
  afferent, and central representation, 115
  efferent, 116-121
Perfusion: carotid sinus, experiments, 121-122
Pericardium
  pouch, distension of
    sodium excretion and, 117
    urine flow and, 117
    relationship with CUE of Nonidez, 118
Phonocardiograms, 33
Placenta
  circulation in, 144-145
  diagram of, 144
Plethysmograph, 62
  pressure
    filtration rate in forearm measured by, 87
    volume diagram of legs at various temperatures of, 102

Poiseuille's law: and circulation, 61
Postmitral commissurotomy dilutional syndrome, 171
Posture
  erect, effects on cardiovascular system, 150-151
  heart performance and, 103
  supine, effects on cardiovascular system, 150-151
Precordial leads (*see* Leads)
Pressure
  age and, 186-190
  arterial (*see* Artery(ies), pressure)
  atrial (*see* Atrium, pressure)
  capillary (*see* Capillary(ies), pressure)
  causes of variations in, 72-73
  central nervous system regulating, 121
  culture and, 188
  curve, arterial pulse, 69
  diet and, 191
  elevation (in mice), 181
  flow relationships in vascular bed, 17-21
  high (*see* Hypertension)
  increase, and psychosocial stimuli, 187-192
  low, and exercise, 182-183
  mean (*see* Mean blood pressure)
  pulse and, 59-61
  race and, 188
  regulatory responses, 118-121
  responses of Gemini 4 command pilot, 105
  systems (*see* High-pressure system, Low-pressure system)
  systolic, 187
  vascular (*see* Vessel(s), pressure)
  venous (*see* Vein(s), pressure)
  -volume curve, aorta, age influencing, 67
  -volume diagrams, vessels, 64-68
    hand, 63
  -wave transmission, aorta, 68
Protein(s)
  blood pressure and, high, 184
  osmotic-pressure
    concentration curve, 82
    glomerular filtration and, 83
    in interstitial fluid, and lymphatics, 84-86
    plasma, 82-83
Psychosocial stimuli: and blood pressure increase, 187-192
Pulse
  arterial, 68-72
    comparison of pressure and flow, 70
    contour, 68-70
    pressure curve of, 69
    vascular impedance, 70-72
    wave reflection, 70-72
    wave velocity, 68
  blood pressure and, 59-61
  jugular vein, relationship to heart sounds, 108

transmission, mechanism of, 61
Pump(s)
  calf, action of, 106-107
  heart as, 24-34
  muscle
    cardiac chambers as, 24-26
    orthostasis and, 105-107
    properties of, 106
  thigh, action of, 106-107

R

Race: and blood pressure, 188
Radius: and intramural tension, 19
Ratio (*see* Resistance ratio)
Receptors
  heart failure and, congestive, 168-170
  stretch (*see* Stretch receptors)
Reflex
  Bainbridge, 120-121
  mechanisms, 194-199
  spinal vasomotor, 115
Regurgitation
  aortic, 34
  mitral, 34
Renal (*see* Kidney)
Renin: and blood volume, 117-118
Reproductive system
  circulation in, 143-145
  erectile tissues in, 143
Reservoir
  central, blood return to, 92-109
  elastic
    action of, demonstration, 66
    function of aorta, 66-68
  heart as, 24-34
  heart chambers as, and low-pressure system, 28-29
Resistance ratio, control of
  post-capillary, 116
  pre-capillary, 116
Respiration
  circulation and, venous, 99
  exercise and, 148-150
  gases, capillary permeability to, 90-91
Rhythm: heart, abnormalities of, 54-55

S

Salt: and hypertension, 183
Shock, 160-173
  irreversible, 163
Skeletal muscles (*see* Muscle(s), skeletal)
Skin
  bradykinin and, 136, 137
  circulation in, 135-137
    diagrammatic representation of, 135
    environmental factors, 135-136
    nervous control and, 136
    skin color and, 136-137
    triple response in, 137
    white reaction of skin and, 137

INDEX

Skin *(cont.)*
  color, and skin circulation, 136-137
  white reaction, and skin circulation, 137
Smoking: and hypertension, 186
Sodium
  balance, and guanethidine, 166
  excretion
    dibenzyline and (in dog), 168
    distension of pericardial pouch and, 117
    relationship between urine flow and inflation of balloon in left atrium, 123
Sounds *(see* Heart, sounds)
Spine: vasomotor reflexes, 115
Splanchnic circulation, 138-142
Spleen
  circulation in, 140
  hemorrhage and, 125
Starling law, 38-39
Stenosis
  aortic, 34
  mitral, 34
Stimulation
  rate, and correlation with constrictor response, 119
  sympathetic, and heart rate, 120
Stimuli: psychosocial, and blood pressure increase, 187-192
Stomach: and circulation, 139
Straining, 146-152
  heart failure and, 147-148
  intrathoracic pressure elevation and, 146-147
Stress: emotional, 179
Stretch receptors in cardiovascular system, 21-22
  high-pressure system of, 21-22, 111-114
  low-pressure system of, 21-22, 111-114
Sympathetic system: role in regulating force of heart beat, 119-120
Sympathetic vasodilator pathways: courses of, 152
Syncope, 160-173
  cardiac, 161
  vasodepressor, 158-159
Systole
  arterial (in mice), 180
  flow patterns during, 26
  heart rate and, 28
  influencing of frequency on the ratio of diastole to, 28
  ventricular, 26-28

T

Tachycardia, paroxysmal atrial, 173
  atrial pressure and, 172
  brachial arterial pressure and, 172
  renal response to, 172
Tension: intramural, 19
Thigh pump: action of, 106-107
Thirst: and blood volume, 116-117

Tilt-table: responses of Gemini 4 command pilot, 105
Transplantation: heart, 170

U

Underwater exposure: circulatory changes during, 152-153
Urine flow
  negative pressure breathing and, under chloralose (in dog), 122
  pericardial pouch distension and, 117
  sodium excretion and atrium, 123

V

Vagal regulation: rate of heart beat, 120
Valsalva maneuver, 146-148
  arterial pressure and, 146
Valves, cardiac
  function of, 25-26
  mitral *(see* Mitral)
  ring, movement of, 25
van't Hoff's law: physiological significance of deviations from, 83
Vasodepressor: syncope, 158-159
Vasodilator
  effects of bradykinin and skin circulation, 136
  outflow, cholinergic sympathetic, and skeletal muscles, 151
  sympathetic pathways, courses of, 152
Vasomotor
  nerves, and pulmonary circulation, 142-143
  reflexes, spine, 115
Vectorcardiography, 53
Vein(s)
  circulation, respiration influencing, 99
  jugular, pulse in, relationship to heart sounds, 108
  pressure
    changes during single step in ankle, 106
    foot, factors regulating, 105-106
    gradient, 98-99
    guanethidine and, 166
    hemorrhage and, 93
    infusion and, 93
    measurements, 107-108
    renal, redistribution, and blood volume, 117-118
    tone, 103-104
    control of, 116
    sympathetic outflow of, 116
Velocity
  at constriction, 18
  critical, change in type of fluid flow at, 18
  pulse wave, 68
Ventilation: and oxygen uptake, 149

Ventricle(s)
  changes during myocardial contraction, 24
  force-velocity-volume relationship diagram for, 44
  function curve, 40
  ranges, and angiotensin infusion, 116
  left, position in low-pressure system, 97
  muscle, stretching effects of, 38
  systole, 26-28
Vessel(s)
  (See also Cardiovascular)
  bed
    elasticity of, 20
    exercise and, 150
    inflow and outflow of fluid from, 79
    pressure flow relationships in, 17-21
  coronary *(see* Coronary, vessels)
  cylindrical, diagram of forces operating in equilibrium of wall of, 19
  hand, pressure-volume diagrams of, 63
  muscular, behavior of tissues in wall of, 65
  pressure
    intrathoracic, relationship with volume changes, 96
    volume diagram of, 64-68
  wall of
    elastic-type, behavior of, 62
    elements in, 61-63
Viscoelastics: behavior of, 64
Viscometers: and blood viscosity, 20
Viscosity, 19-20, 30
  viscometers and, 20
Viscous material: behavior of, 64

W

Water
  exchanges in man, and environment, 155
  excretion, and dibenzyline (in dog), 168
  hydrodynamic flow of, 88
  immersion as antagonist of orthostasis, 101
  net diffusion of, 88
  underwater exposure, circulatory changes during, 152-153
Wave
  pressure, and ascending aorta, 72
  reflection, arterial pulse, 70-72
Weight: body, and guanethidine, 166
Weightlessness: and blood volume, 104-105
White reaction: skin, and skin circulation, 137
Wilson's central terminal precordial leads: connections for, 54